Emerging Updates of Radiation Oncology for Surgeons

Editor

ADAM RABEN

SURGICAL ONCOLOGY CLINICS OF NORTH AMERICA

www.surgonc.theclinics.com

Consulting Editor
NICHOLAS J. PETRELLI

July 2017 • Volume 26 • Number 3

ELSEVIER

1600 John F. Kennedy Boulevard • Suite 1800 • Philadelphia, Pennsylvania, 19103-2899

http://www.theclinics.com

SURGICAL ONCOLOGY CLINICS OF NORTH AMERICA Volume 26, Number 3
July 2017 ISSN 1055-3207, ISBN-13: 978-0-323-53156-6

Editor: John Vassallo (j.vassallo@elsevier.com)
Developmental Editor: Meredith Madeira

Surgical Oncology Clinics of North America (ISSN 1055-3207) is published quarterly by Elsevier Inc., 360 Park Avenue South, New York, NY 10010-1710. Months of publication are January, April, July, and October. Business and Editorial Offices: 1600 John F. Kennedy Blvd., Ste. 1800, Philadelphia, PA 19103-2899. Customer Service Office: 3251 Riverport Lane, Maryland Heights, MO 63043. Periodicals postage paid at New York, NY and additional mailing offices. Subscription prices are $296.00 per year (US individuals), $490.00 (US institutions) $100.00 (US student/resident), $337.00 (Canadian individuals), $620.00 (Canadian institutions), $205.00 (Canadian student/resident), $418.00 (foreign individuals), $620.00 (foreign institutions), and $205.00 (foreign student/resident). Foreign air speed delivery is included in all *Clinics* subscription prices. All prices are subject to change without notice. **POSTMASTER**: Send address changes to *Surgical Oncology Clinics of North America,* Elsevier Health Science Division, Subscription Customer Service, 3251 Riverport Lane, Maryland Heights, MO 63043. **Customer Service: 1-800-654-2452 (US and Canada). 314-447-8871 (outside US and Canada). Fax: 314-447-8029. E-mail: journalscustomerservice-usa@elsevier.com (for print support); journalsonline support-usa@elsevier.com (for online support).**

Reprints. For copies of 100 or more, of articles in this publication, please contact the Commercial Reprints Department, Elsevier Inc., 360 Park Avenue South, New York, New York 10010-1710. Tel. 212-633-3874; Fax: 212-633-3820; E-mail: reprints@elsevier.com.

Surgical Oncology Clinics of North America is covered in *MEDLINE/PubMed (Index Medicus) and EMBASE/ Excerpta Medica, Current Contents/Clinical Medicine, and ISI/BIOMED.*

Contributors

CONSULTING EDITOR

NICHOLAS J. PETRELLI, MD, FACS
Helen F. Graham Cancer Center & Research Institute, Christiana Care Health Systems, Newark, Delaware

EDITOR

ADAM RABEN, MD
Chairman, Department of Radiation Oncology, Helen F. Graham Cancer Center, Christiana Care Health System, Newark, Delaware

AUTHORS

KAMRAN A. AHMED, MD
Resident, Department of Radiation Oncology, H. Lee Moffitt Cancer Center and Research Institute, Tampa, Florida

SHAHED N. BADIYAN, MD
Department of Radiation Oncology, University of Maryland School of Medicine, Baltimore, Maryland

SERGUEI A. CASTANEDA, MD
Department of Radiation Oncology, Helen F. Graham Cancer Center & Research Institute, Christiana Care Health System, Newark, Delaware; Department of Radiation Oncology, Drexel University College of Medicine, Philadelphia, Pennsylvania

RICHARD CHOO, MD
Professor, Department of Radiation Oncology, Mayo Clinic, Rochester, Minnesota

MICHAEL D. CHUONG, MD
Department of Radiation Oncology, Miami Cancer Institute, Baptist Health South Florida, Miami, Florida

TU DAN, MD
Department of Radiation Oncology, University of Texas Southwestern, Dallas, Texas

BRIAN J. DAVIS, MD, PhD
Professor, Department of Radiation Oncology, Mayo Clinic, Rochester, Minnesota

LANA DE SOUZA LAWRENCE, MD
Radiation Oncology Physician, Department of Radiation Oncology, Christiana Care Health Services, Newark, Delaware

CHRISTOPHER L. DEUFEL, PhD
Assistant Professor, Department of Radiation Oncology, Mayo Clinic, Rochester, Minnesota

PATRICK K. HA, MD
Professor, Division of Head and Neck Surgical Oncology, Department of Otolaryngology-Head and Neck Surgery, University of California-San Francisco, San Francisco, California

LOUIS B. HARRISON, MD
Senior Member and Chair, Department of Radiation Oncology, H. Lee Moffitt Cancer Center and Research Institute, Tampa, Florida

ERIC M. HORWITZ, MD
Professor and Chairman, Department of Radiation Oncology, Fox Chase Cancer Center, Philadelphia, Pennsylvania

LISA A. KACHNIC, MD
Professor and Chair, Department of Radiation Oncology, Vanderbilt University Medical Center, Nashville, Tennessee

ADEEL KAISER, MD
Department of Radiation Oncology, University of Maryland School of Medicine, Baltimore, Maryland

ERIC KEMMERER, MD, MS
Department of Radiation Oncology, Drexel University College of Medicine, Philadelphia, Pennsylvania

SUNGJUNE KIM, MD, PhD
Assistant Member, Department of Radiation Oncology, H. Lee Moffitt Cancer Center and Research Institute, Tampa, Florida

JON MALLEN-ST. CLAIR, MD, PhD
Clinical Fellow, Division of Head and Neck Surgical Oncology, Department of Otolaryngology-Head and Neck Surgery, University of California-San Francisco, San Francisco, California

JOSHUA E. MEYER, MD
Associate Professor, Department of Radiation Oncology, Fox Chase Cancer Center, Philadelphia, Pennsylvania

JASON K. MOLITORIS, MD, PhD
Department of Radiation Oncology, University of Maryland Medical Center, Baltimore, Maryland

LANCE A. MYNDERSE, MD
Assistant Professor, Department of Urology, Mayo Clinic, Rochester, Minnesota

ARTI PAREKH, MD
Department of Radiation Oncology and Molecular Radiation Sciences, Johns Hopkins University, Baltimore, Maryland

WILLIAM F. REGINE, MD
Department of Radiation Oncology, University of Maryland School of Medicine, Baltimore, Maryland

LINDSAY B. ROMAK, MD
Department of Radiation Oncology, Helen F. Graham Cancer Center & Research Institute, Christiana Care Health System, Newark, Delaware

SUNJAY SHAH, MD
Department of Radiation Oncology, Christiana Care, Newark, Delaware

TALHA SHAIKH, MD
Resident Physician, Department of Radiation Oncology, Fox Chase Cancer Center, Philadelphia, Pennsylvania

CLAYTON A. SMITH, MD, PhD
Assistant Professor, Division of Radiation Oncology, University of South Alabama Mitchell Cancer Institute, Mobile, Alabama

BRADLEY J. STISH, MD
Assistant Professor, Department of Radiation Oncology, Mayo Clinic, Rochester, Minnesota

JON STRASSER, MD
Department of Radiation Oncology, Helen F. Graham Cancer Center & Research Institute, Christiana Care Health System, Newark, Delaware

NOELLE L. WILLIAMS, MD
Department of Radiation Oncology, Thomas Jefferson University, Philadelphia, Pennsylvania

JEAN L. WRIGHT, MD
Associate Professor, Department of Radiation Oncology and Molecular Radiation Sciences, Johns Hopkins University, Baltimore, Maryland

SUE S. YOM, MD, PhD, MAS
Associate Professor, Departments of Radiation Oncology and Otolaryngology-Head and Neck Surgery, University of California-San Francisco, San Francisco, California

Contents

Foreword **xiii**

Nicholas J. Petrelli

Preface: Update of Practical Radiation Oncology Management Trends for Surgeons **xv**

Adam Raben

Update on Radiotherapy for Central Nervous System Malignancies **347**

Eric Kemmerer and Sunjay Shah

Malignancies arising from the central nervous system are rare. Brain metastases, in contrast, are perhaps the most common neurologic complication of cancer. Radiotherapy, as part of combined modality therapy, continues to evolve with the advancement of stereotactic radiosurgery indications, the addition of new technologies, such as alternating electric field therapy, and mounting advances in the complex biology of these entities. The explosion of new clinical trials combined with newly discovered molecular markers suggest the beginning of a paradigm shift in the management of these challenging malignancies that will allow for future risk-stratification strategies.

Controversies in Postoperative Irradiation of Oropharyngeal Cancer After Transoral Surgery **357**

Sue S. Yom, Jon Mallen-St. Clair, and Patrick K. Ha

Transoral surgery (TOS) is a novel technology whose adoption is expanding in the United States and other countries. TOS offers the possibility of a minimally invasive surgical approach to head and neck cancers. Its most frequent application has been in oropharyngeal cancers (OPC), of which most are associated with human papillomavirus (HPV). For HPV-associated OPC, where high response and survival rates are expected, deintensification of standard therapy is a major area of clinical research. In HPV-OPC, traditional pathologic risk factors indicating a need for adjuvant radiation or chemoradiation may not apply as strongly.

Updates in the Treatment of Breast Cancer with Radiotherapy **371**

Serguei A. Castaneda and Jon Strasser

Breast-conserving therapy is one of the most remarkable achievements of modern cancer care. The authors review the evidence supporting the role of adjuvant radiotherapy as the standard of care for breast cancer after breast-conserving surgery, consensus guidelines for margins in invasive cancer disease and ductal carcinoma in situ, the role of partial-breast irradiation and hypofractionated whole-breast irradiation, and the evolving indications for postmastectomy radiation therapy and extent of nodal coverage. Areas of research include specific methods of partial-breast irradiation, interactions between neoadjuvant chemotherapy and radiotherapy, and integration of molecular profiles with the selection of the best treatment modality and timing.

Updates in Postmastectomy Radiation **383**

Jean L. Wright and Arti Parekh

Although the use of postmastectomy radiation therapy (PMRT) is widely accepted in certain clinical situations, areas of controversy persist for some clinical scenarios. In addition, with significant shifts in the management of breast cancer, including omission of axillary nodal dissection in select sentinel node–positive patients and increased use of neoadjuvant chemotherapy, new clinical challenges have arisen regarding the role of PMRT. This article reviews the data to support current recommendations for postmastectomy radiation and explores areas of controversy and the studies that guide clinicians in these scenarios.

Management of Stage I Lung Cancer with Stereotactic Ablative Radiation Therapy **393**

Tu Dan and Noelle L. Williams

Early stage non–small cell lung cancer is a growing clinical entity with evolving standards of care. With the adoption of lung screening guidelines, the incidence of early stage disease is expected to increase. Surgical resection for early stage disease has been considered standard of care; however, there is evidence that stereotactic ablative radiation therapy (SABR) may be a viable alternate to surgery. In the last decade, advances in image guidance, treatment planning systems, and improved spatial accuracy of treatment delivery have converged to result in the effective use of SABR in the treatment of early stage lung cancer.

Optimal Use of Combined Modality Therapy in the Treatment of Esophageal Cancer **405**

Talha Shaikh, Joshua E. Meyer, and Eric M. Horwitz

Esophageal cancer is associated with a poor prognosis with 5-year survival rates of approximately 15% to 20%. Although patients with early stage disease may adequately be treated with a single modality, combined therapy typically consisting of neoadjuvant chemoradiation followed by esophagectomy is being adopted increasingly in patients with locally advanced disease. In patients who are not surgical candidates, definitive chemoradiation is the preferred treatment approach. All patients with newly diagnosed esophageal cancer should be evaluated in the multidisciplinary setting by a surgeon, radiation oncologist, and medical oncologist owing to the importance of each specialty in the management of these patients.

The Role of Radiation Therapy for Pancreatic Cancer in the Adjuvant and Neoadjuvant Settings **431**

Shahed N. Badiyan, Jason K. Molitoris, Michael D. Chuong, William F. Regine, and Adeel Kaiser

Pancreatic cancer is the third leading cause of cancer-related death in the United States. Although surgery remains the only curative treatment, chemotherapy and radiation therapy are frequently used. In the adjuvant setting, radiation is usually delivered with chemotherapy to eradicate residual microscopic or macroscopic disease in the resection bed. Neoadjuvant radiation therapy has become more frequently utilized. This article reviews the historical and modern literature regarding radiation therapy in the neoadjuvant and adjuvant settings, focusing on the evolution of radiation therapy techniques and clinical trials in an attempt to identify patients best suited to receiving radiation therapy.

Evolving Role of Radiotherapy in the Management of Rectal Carcinoma **455**

Clayton A. Smith and Lisa A. Kachnic

Management of locally advanced rectal cancer has evolved over time from surgical resection alone to multimodality therapy with preoperative radiation, chemotherapy, and total mesorectal excision resulting in excellent local control rates. Refinements in neoadjuvant therapies and their sequencing have improved pathologic complete response rates such that consideration of selective radiation and nonoperative management are now active clinical trial questions. Advances in radiation treatment planning and delivery techniques may allow for further reduction in acute treatment-related toxicity in select patient populations. Collectively, therapeutic strategies remain focused on improving outcomes for patients with higher-risk disease and reducing the morbidity of treatment.

Radiotherapy for Anal Cancer: Intensity-Modulated Radiotherapy and Future Directions **467**

Serguei A. Castaneda and Lindsay B. Romak

The treatment of anal cancer has evolved remarkably in the past 30 years. Definitive chemoradiotherapy is the standard of care, allowing organ preservation and maintenance of continence for most patients. This article reviews recent advances in radiotherapy planning and delivery that have resulted in improvements in treatment-related toxicity. Most notably, the advent and wide adoption of intensity-modulated radiotherapy provides a superior toxicity profile compared with older techniques, while maintaining similar oncologic outcomes. Current areas of active research include optimizing and individualizing treatment intensity and possible integration of biologic agents and immunotherapies in the treatment of anal cancer.

Radiation Oncology Management of Stage I–III Cervix Cancer **477**

Lana de Souza Lawrence

Radiotherapy plays a critical role in the management of cervix carcinoma, in the adjuvant setting for patients with high-risk pathologic features and in the definitive setting for locoregionally advanced disease. External beam radiotherapy fields encompass potential areas of microscopic disease spread in addition to known areas of gross disease. In the presence of gross disease, however, escalation of dose is required that is best accomplished using a brachytherapy boost to spare surrounding normal organs from toxicity. This article addresses indications for radiotherapy in the management of nonmetastatic cervix cancer and reviews various radiotherapy techniques, with a heavy focus on brachytherapy.

Brachytherapy in the Management of Prostate Cancer 491

Bradley J. Stish, Brian J. Davis, Lance A. Mynderse, Christopher L. Deufel, and Richard Choo

Brachytherapy is performed by directly inserting radioactive sources into the prostate gland and is an important treatment option for appropriately selected men with prostate adenocarcinoma. Brachytherapy provides highly conformal radiotherapy and delivers tumoricidal doses that exceed those administered with external beam radiation therapy. There is a significant body of literature supporting the excellent long-term oncologic and safety outcomes achieved when brachytherapy is used for men in all risk categories of nonmetastatic prostate cancer. This article highlights some important considerations and published outcomes that relate to brachytherapy and its role in the treatment of prostate cancer.

Novel Opportunities to Use Radiation Therapy with Immune Checkpoint Inhibitors for Melanoma Management 515

Kamran A. Ahmed, Sungjune Kim, and Louis B. Harrison

Immunotherapy has revolutionized the systemic management of numerous malignancies. Nowhere has the proven benefit of these agents in clinical practice been more evident than in the management of advanced melanoma. Numerous preclinical studies have revealed the potential benefit of immune-priming radiotherapy in stimulating tumor-specific immune responses. This signal for immune activation may lead to clinically relevant synergy with immune checkpoint inhibitors against malignant cells. In this review, the authors summarize the current data outlining the role radiation therapy may play in the management of advanced melanoma alongside immune checkpoint inhibitors.

SURGICAL ONCOLOGY CLINICS OF NORTH AMERICA

FORTHCOMING ISSUES

October 2017
Clinical Trials in Surgical Oncology
Elin R. Sigurdson, *Editor*

January 2018
Changing Paradigms in Breast Cancer Diagnosis and Treatment
Kelly K. Hunt, *Editor*

April 2018
Colon Cancer
Mark W. Arnold, *Editor*

RECENT ISSUES

April 2017
Advances in Esophageal and Gastric Cancer
David H. Ilson, *Editor*

January 2017
Anal Canal Cancers
Cathy Eng, *Editor*

October 2016
Contemporary Management and Controversies of Sarcoma
Chandrajit P. Raut, *Editor*

RELATED INTEREST

Surgical Clinics of North America, April 2017 (Vol. 97, Issue 2)
Multidisciplinary Management of Gastric Neoplasms
Kelly L. Olino and Douglas S. Tyler, *Editors*
http://www.surgical.theclinics.com/

Foreword

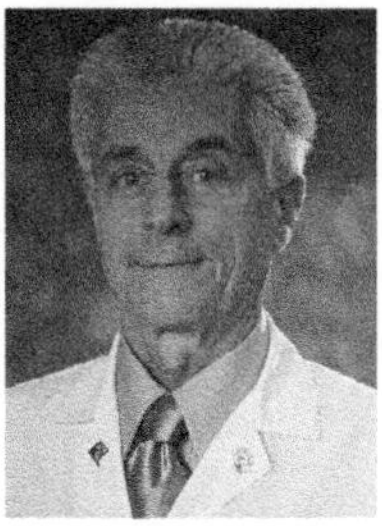

Nicholas J. Petrelli, MD, FACS
Consulting Editor

This issue of the *Surgical Oncology Clinics of North America* is devoted to radiation oncology. The guest editor is Adam Raben, MD. Dr. Raben is Chair of the Department of Radiation Oncology at the Helen F. Graham Cancer Center and Research Institute at Christiana Care Health System in Newark, Delaware. Dr Raben received his undergraduate degree from Duke University followed by his medical degree from Wake Forest University. He completed his residency in radiation oncology at Memorial Sloan Kettering Cancer Center in New York. Dr Raben's department has received the Research Excellence and Top Radiation Oncology Accrual Award from the Radiation Therapy Oncology Group over a 4-year period from 2005 to 2013.

Dr Raben has assembled an outstanding group of clinicians and investigators in this issue of the *Surgical Oncology Clinics of North America*. This issue was long overdue because the last topic on radiation oncology was in July of 2013.

The variety of topics organized by Dr Raben is excellent. As an example, the article on "Updates in Post Mastectomy Radiation," by Drs Wright and Parekh includes a discussion of postmastectomy radiation in a subgroup of patients with node-negative disease who have high-risk features. Another example is the article by Drs Dan and Williams entitled, "Management of Stage I Lung Cancer with Stereotactic Ablative Radiation Therapy." The last example is the article by Drs Yom, St Clair and Ha entitled, "Controversies in Post Operative Irradiation of Oropharyngeal Cancer after Transoral Surgery." One of the areas emphasized by this article is transoral surgery, which is expanding in the United States and other countries.

I would like to take this opportunity to thank Dr Adam Raben for an outstanding and comprehensive issue in the *Surgical Oncology Clinics of North America*. I encourage

Surg Oncol Clin N Am 26 (2017) xiii–xiv
http://dx.doi.org/10.1016/j.soc.2017.02.001
1055-3207/17/© 2017 Published by Elsevier Inc.

our readers to share this information with all of their trainees, and I appreciate the time and effort put into this issue by all contributors.

Nicholas J. Petrelli, MD, FACS
Helen F. Graham Cancer Center & Research Institute
Christiana Care Health Systems
4701 Ogletown-Stanton Road, Suite 1233
Newark, DE 19713, USA

E-mail address:
npetrelli@christianacare.org

Preface

Update of Practical Radiation Oncology Management Trends for Surgeons

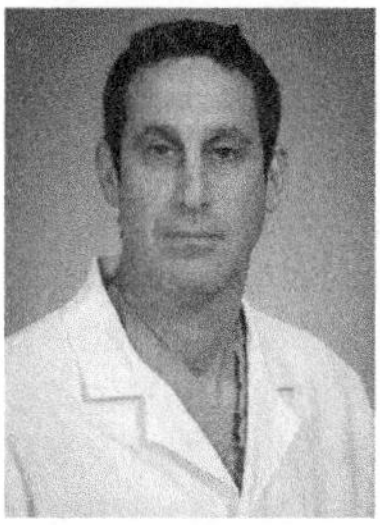

Adam Raben, MD
Editor

In this latest issue of *Surgical Oncology Clinics of North America*, updated and emerging trends in the management of selected malignancies with radiation therapy, relevant to surgeons in the modern era of multidisciplinary care, are presented in 12 selected articles. The authors were chosen to reflect a diversity of training experiences and expertise from respected university- and community-based programs in the country. In addition, several of the authors have led investigators of important national clinical trials, or have participated in the design and discussion of clinical and translational trials at the cooperative group level with their surgical colleagues that have shaped current standards. Many of the articles highlight important trials that have closed or are ongoing that are practice changing. The importance of a prospective multidisciplinary approach to cancer has never been more important, with the rapid changes in technology, surgical techniques, genomics, targeted agents, immunotherapy, and imaging, and the rapid expansion of short-course, extremely precise radiotherapy that may have implications for local control and systemic cure.

Recent advances that have dramatically changed the landscape in the management of adult central nervous system (CNS) malignancies are reviewed by Drs Kemmerer and Shah. This includes emerging data challenging the need for comprehensive CNS radiotherapy after surgery for oligo-brain metastases in favorable selected cases, in which stereotactic body radiation therapy can be effectively utilized after surgery or as an alternative to spare patients from late cognitive and memory deficits, without compromising survival. Exciting new survival data with PCV chemotherapy redefine the standard of care for low- and intermediate-risk gliomas after gross total or subtotal resection. Finally, important genomic characterization of CNS primary tumors is

Surg Oncol Clin N Am 26 (2017) xv–xvii
http://dx.doi.org/10.1016/j.soc.2017.04.001
1055-3207/17/© 2017 Published by Elsevier Inc.

exploding and is being incorporated into clinical trials for HG gliomas to improve outcomes after surgery and radiotherapy.

The recognition of HPV+16 cancers of the oropharynx as a distinct biologic disease, with a favorable prognosis, is discussed by Drs Yom, Mallen-St Clair, and Ha, where they review new deescalation strategies that combine advanced surgical robotic technology (transoral robotic surgery, TORS) with reduced dose and site radiotherapy, and alternatives to chemotherapy. Trials to determine if TORS can reduce late toxicity compared with a full course of radiotherapy in a younger population are underway and will be critical in defining new standards of care.

Several articles reflect emerging and novel use of advanced technology in the field of Radiation Oncology that have resulted in an improved therapeutic ratio of cancers, such as lung and anus, and in the case of breast, shorter treatment courses that improve patient convenience and compliance. Maturing data presented in this issue now demonstrate meaningful opportunities to provide value-based care (reduced cost with improved or equipoise outcomes compared with protracted treatment courses) without compromising cancer-specific survival. Landmark trials reported in the last 5 years have demonstrated that prolonged courses of radiotherapy as part of breast conservation are not necessary for many patients, resulting in reduced cost, equivalent cosmesis and local control, and improved convenience. The article by Drs Castaneda and Strasser provides evidence of the rapid evolution of accelerated whole and partial breast radiotherapy techniques, with mature data for ductal carcinoma in situ and invasive disease that are changing the landscape of breast conservation management. The controversies regarding the value and efficacy of postmastectomy radiotherapy for locally advanced breast cancer are discussed by Drs Wright and Parekh, highlighted by review of landmark trials to give guidance to the surgical community.

This issue also updates the global adoption and effectiveness of stereotactic ablative radiotherapy (SABR) for non–small cell lung cancer. Advancements in image guidance, treatment planning systems, and improved spatial accuracy of treatment delivery have all converged to result in the effective use of SABR in the treatment of early-stage lung cancer. This paradigm-shifting approach allows significant reduction of treatment volumes, facilitating the use of high-dose radiation and increased biologic effective doses delivered to tumors. Drs Dan and Williams present compelling data demonstrating clinical equipoise between SABR and surgery for medically inoperable patients as well as a number of multi-institutional trials underway, investigating the direct comparison of SABR as an alternative to surgical resection.

For locally advanced esophageal cancer, trimodality treatment is now the new standard. Radiation with chemotherapy for locally advanced disease is suboptimal when surgery is omitted. Drs Shaikh, Meyer, and Horwitz reveal the results of the landmark CROSS trial, a contemporary well-designed phase 3 trial with modern staging, systemic chemotherapy, and radiotherapy resulting in a doubling of survival compared with surgery alone. Important biomarkers are expressed in esophageal cancer that may hold promise in improving survival. They reveal that nearly 20% of esophageal cancers have overexpression of HER2, a transmembrane tyrosine kinase receptor. Recent trials have shown improved survival with the addition of Trastuzumab, while new studies are underway to evaluate other mutations.

The changing landscape of management of pancreatic cancer over the last 4 years is presented by Dr Badiyan and colleagues. Current trials attempting to redefine the role of radiotherapy with systemic chemotherapy before or after surgery as well as its role in the unresectable setting and the controversy of its impact on survival are presented. In particular, the technological advance of SABT and image guidance to deliver equivalent local control in a shorter period of time without significant toxicity is practice changing.

Drs Castaneda and Romak update recent cooperative trials in anal cancer demonstrating the favorable role of intensity-modulated radiation therapy versus standard three-dimensional conformal radiotherapy in reducing significant acute and late-toxicity, risk adaptive-deescalation strategies combining local excision and lower radiotherapy stratified by margins in less advanced disease, and describe current areas of active research investigating the integration of biologic and immunotherapies in the treatment of ASCC.

Dr Stish and colleagues contribute an excellent summary of the long-term results of published brachytherapy experiences in the modern screening era for prostate cancer in both the favorable, intermediate, and high-risk setting that demonstrate improved risk group assessment, value-based care, and favorable outcomes in the high-risk setting when brachytherapy is added to external beam, based on exciting new data from a large phase 3 randomized trial that establishes a new standard of care.

Prospective multidisciplinary management of esophageal cancer, cervical cancer, and rectal/anal cancers has ushered in a greater cooperation and partnership between Radiation Oncologists, Surgeons, and Medical Oncologists.

Finally, Drs Ahmed, Kim, and Harrison articulate the emerging role and research of immunotherapies with radiation in the treatment of melanoma (that are now being applied to other malignancies), and why novel local delivery of radiation may be essential for systemic cancer cure.

I would like to thank Dr Nicholas Petrelli for the opportunity to participate as guest editor of this issue. I also would like to extend my sincere appreciation to the contributing authors, and the time and effort they gave into presenting such well-written and comprehensive articles, that I hope will be meaningful to our surgical colleagues.

Adam Raben, MD
Department of Radiation Oncology
Helen F. Graham Cancer Center
Christiana Care Health System
Suite 1109, HFGCC-CCHS
4701 Ogletown-Stanton Road
Newark, DE 19713, USA

E-mail address:
araben@christianacare.org

Update on Radiotherapy for Central Nervous System Malignancies

Eric Kemmerer, MD, MS[a,*], Sunjay Shah, MD[b]

KEYWORDS

- Brain tumors • Glioblastoma • Brain metastases

KEY POINTS

- Although whole-brain radiotherapy (WBRT) remains an important tool for the treatment of brain metastases, strategies for avoidance of the hippocampal neural stem cell compartment and the use of memantine can minimize the cognitive effects of WBRT. Stereotactic radiosurgery (SRS) without WBRT is appropriate in selected patients.
- Adjuvant treatment with alternating cranial electric fields after standard radiotherapy, a new treatment modality, can extend progression-free survival in patients with glioblastoma multiforme.
- Adjuvant procarbazine, CCNU, and vincristine in the treatment of low-grade glioma demonstrates a marked survival benefit.
- In 2016, the World Health Organization (WHO) classification of brain tumors was updated with the addition of various molecular markers prognostic for outcome.

INTRODUCTION

Malignancies arising from the central nervous system (CNS) are rare, representing 1.4% of cancer cases, with approximately 24,000 new cases estimated in 2016 leading to approximately 16,000 attributable deaths.[1] Brain metastases, in contrast, are perhaps the most common neurologic complication of cancer,[2] with an estimated incidence rate of up to 200,000 per year in the United States.[3] Radiotherapy, as part of combined modality therapy, continues to evolve with the advancement of stereotactic radiosurgery (SRS) indications; addition of new technologies, such as alternating electric field therapy; and mounting advances in the complex biology of these entities.

The authors have nothing to disclose.

[a] Department of Radiation Oncology, Drexel University College of Medicine, 245 North 15 Street, Philadelphia, PA 19102, USA; [b] Department of Radiation Oncology, Christiana Care, 4701 Ogletown-Stanton Rd, Newark, DE 19713, USA

* Corresponding author.

E-mail address: Eric.Kemmerer@drexelmed.edu

Surg Oncol Clin N Am 26 (2017) 347–355

http://dx.doi.org/10.1016/j.soc.2017.01.003 surgonc.theclinics.com

BRAIN METASTASES

Decision-making with respect to the treatment of brain metastases is a function of many factors, including patient age, performance status, comorbid conditions, symptoms, extracranial disease extent, and histopathology of the primary tumor. Treatment options include resection, whole-brain radiotherapy (WBRT), SRS, or some combination of these modalities. Work has been done to stratify patients into various prognostic groups, identifying cut-points of three factors prognostic for overall survival: (1) Karnofsky performance status (KPS), (2) age, and (3) presence of extracranial metastases.[4] More recently, a diagnosis-specific graded prognostic assessment (GPA)[5] has been developed, reflective of the strong role of primary tumor histopathology. Algorithms have been proposed using the functional status, systemic disease status, and number of metastases, such that patients with the worst prognosis are identified and recommended WBRT only, in contrast to patients with more favorable factors who may be recommended surgery or SRS, possibly followed by WBRT.[6]

WBRT is a well-established and widely used treatment of brain metastases. In a landmark trial comparing the effect of surgical resection in addition to WBRT, Patchell and colleagues[7] randomized a total of 48 patients with a single brain metastasis to either surgical resection or a biopsy only (in patients with supratentorial disease) followed by WBRT. The radiation was delivered to a total dose of 36 Gy through two parallel-opposed lateral portals, with the treatment field including the entire brain and meninges to the level of foramen magnum. Patients receiving surgery and WBRT had a significantly longer survival than those not receiving surgery, with a median survival of 40 weeks versus 15 weeks, respectively ($P<.01$). On multivariate analysis, only surgical treatment of brain metastasis was associated with a better functional status and quality of life on multivariate analysis.[7] Patchell and colleagues later performed a multicenter randomized trial of treatment of a single brain metastasis with surgical resection followed by radiotherapy versus surgical resection alone.[7] A total of 49 patients were randomized to postoperative WBRT and 46 patients to resection alone, with WBRT given to a total dose of 50.4 Gy via parallel-opposed lateral fields. They demonstrated a significantly decreased rate of recurrence at the operative bed and remainder of the brain with receipt of WBRT. Moreover, patients who received postoperative WBRT were significantly less likely to die of neurologic causes, although no difference in overall survival was shown.

WBRT, however, is associated with long-term permanent neurocognitive effects and adverse effects on quality of life. DeAngelis and coworkers[8] described WBRT-induced dementia causing severe disability in 1.9% to 5.1% of patients receiving a total dose ranging from 25 Gy to 39 Gy, attributing this to large fractions of radiation (3–6 Gy per day) delivered. More recently, Chang and colleagues[9] examined neurocognitive outcomes as assessed by a formal tool, the Hopkins Verbal Learning Test-Revised, in patients with one to three brain metastases randomized to SRS alone versus SRS with the addition of WBRT. Although 73% of patients who received SRS followed by WBRT were free from CNS recurrence at 1 year, compared with 27% who received SRS alone, the trial met early stopping rules because of a significant predicted decline in learning and memory function.

To ameliorate the neurocognitive effects of WBRT, the use of memantine, an *N*-methyl-D-aspartate-receptor antagonist, has been explored in the setting of a randomized, double-blinded, placebo-controlled trial.[10] This randomized patients receiving WBRT to memantine (20 mg/d) versus placebo, for a total of 24 weeks, with the observation of significantly longer time to cognitive decline in patients receiving memantine and a strong trend toward less decline in delayed recall in the memantine arm at

24 weeks (P = .059). The probability of cognitive function failure at 24 weeks was 53.8% in the memantine arm and 64.9% in the placebo arm. Better results were seen in the memantine arm for executive function, processing speed, and delayed recognition at 24 weeks. Memantine was well tolerated and had a toxicity profile similar to placebo.

Other efforts directed toward the preservation of neurocognitive function include the use of conformal radiotherapy, specifically through the use of intensity modulated radiation therapy to spare the hippocampal neural stem-cell compartment, for which radiation-induced damage has been implicated in causing cognitive decline.[11] This hypothesis was examined in Radiation Therapy Oncology Group (RTOG) 0933, a single-arm, phase 2 multi-institutional trial that enrolled recursive partitioning analysis (RPA) class I-II patients with no brain metastases within a 5-mm margin around either hippocampus and examined the primary end point of Hopkins Verbal Learning Test-Revised delayed recall.[12] Use of hippocampal-avoiding intensity modulated radiation therapy was associated with a 7% mean relative decline in this metric from baseline, significantly lower compared with the historical control, and additionally, without reported decline in patient-reported quality-of-life scores. Given these encouraging positive results, and observed benefit with the use of memantine, NRG-CC001, a randomized phase 3 trial of memantine and WBRT with or without hippocampal avoidance, launched in July of 2015 and is presently accruing.

SRS, the administration of highly conformal high dose external beam radiotherapy typically in one to five total fractions, is another frequently used modality for the treatment of brain metastases. Common treatment platforms include gamma knife, cyber knife, and linear accelerator based SRS. SRS alone, WBRT alone, and both SRS and WBRT have all been noted to have level 1 evidence to support their use in patients with multiple brain metastases less than 3 to 4 cm in size with a life expectancy of greater than 3 months.[13]

European Organisation for Research and Treatment of Cancer trials 22952–26001 examined patients with one to three metastases who underwent surgical resection or SRS, and were then randomized to WBRT versus observation.[14] No difference in median time to loss of functional independence (World Health Organization [WHO] performance status >2) was noted. Although intracranial progression caused death in 44% of patients in the observation arm and in 28% of patients in the WBRT arm, no difference was observed in overall survival between groups. Conversely, the addition of an SRS boost to WBRT was examined in RTOG 9508, in which patients with one to three brain metastases were randomized to receive WBRT with or without SRS.[15] Patients in the SRS boost group were more likely to have a stable or improved KPS score at 6-month follow-up than were patients allocated WBRT alone (43% vs 27%, respectively; P = .03). In addition, the authors noted a survival benefit in the SRS group in recursive partitioning analysis class I patients. This suggests that the local control afforded by WBRT alone is suboptimal, at least in a subgroup of patients.

The results of these two trials, together with other data, including the aforementioned work by Chang and colleagues[9] highlighting the adverse neurocognitive effects of WBRT, has led to ongoing interest in the avoidance of WBRT in favor of SRS alone in favorable subsets of patients. A recent individual patient meta-analysis pooling multiple phase 3 trials examining the addition of WBRT to SRS has generated considerable interest in this regard. Identifying a total of 364 patients, the authors demonstrated that the use of SRS alone was associated with improved survival in patients age 50 or younger, and that avoidance of WBRT in this population did not result in increased failure elsewhere in the brain.[16]

The cost-effectiveness of WBRT has recently been investigated in the QUARTZ study, which examined patients with metastatic non–small cell lung cancer with brain metastases unsuitable for either surgical resection or SRS who were randomly assigned to WBRT and dexamethasone versus best supportive care.[17] The authors noted a benefit in terms of mean quality-adjusted life-year of only 4.7 days with WBRT. Thus, hospice care should be strongly considered in unfavorable patient subsets, for which WBRT seems to offer minimal benefit.

PRIMARY BRAIN MALIGNANCIES

Traditionally, characterization of brain tumors has relied on histopathologic features, such as morphology, immunohistochemistry, and other testing to describe tumor histogenesis and degree of differentiation. With recent advances in the molecular characterization of various primary CNS malignancies, the WHO classification of brain tumors has undergone a major restructuring.[18] Although a full description of the various changes being instituted is beyond the scope of this article, highlights include restructuring of diffuse gliomas, such as glioblastoma multiforme (GBM), to include genetic prognostic factors of isocitrate dehydrogenase (IDH) mutation wild-type versus IDH-mutant and H3 K27M–mutant diffuse midline glioma. Ependymoma is further characterized by the presence of RELA gene fusion and medulloblastoma is further characterized by molecular subtype as WNT-activated versus SHH-activated. Embryonal tumors with multilayered rosettes are characterized by upregulation of the oncogenic miRNA cluster C19MC.[19] These exciting changes herald an era when perhaps molecular characteristics may supercede traditional clinicopathologic characteristics in terms of prognostic and therapeutic significance.

HIGH-GRADE GLIOMA

GBM is the most common primary malignant brain malignancy of adulthood, and the most devastating, with a median survival of 15 months, occurring with an average incidence rate of approximately 3 per 100,000 people, and with a median age at diagnosis of 64.[20] The exploration of the use of radiotherapy to treat GBM in the 1970s with radiotherapy demonstrated a more than doubling of median survival in comparison with best supportive care.[21] The standard of care treatment of WHO grade 4 GBM remains maximal safe resection followed by chemoradiation with concurrent and adjuvant temozolomide delivered to the resection cavity and residual tumor. This treatment regimen was established by the seminal trial of Stupp and colleagues,[22] which randomized 573 patients with histologically proven debulked GBM to receive focal brain radiation of 60 Gy in 30 fractions over 6 weeks, versus the same radiation with concurrent daily temozolomide followed by adjuvant temozolomide for six 28-day cycles. With a median follow-up of 28 months, the median survival was 14.6 months with radiotherapy plus temozolomide and 12.1 months with radiotherapy alone. Perhaps even more striking was a reported 2-year overall survival rate of 26.5% with radiotherapy plus temozolomide and 10.4% with radiotherapy alone, which on longer follow-up, demonstrated a 5-year overall survival of 9.8% with combined treatment versus 1.9% with radiotherapy alone.[23] Thus, the addition of concurrent temozolomide and adjuvant temozolomide to radiotherapy led to an approximate five-fold increase in 5-year overall survival, a historic advance in the treatment of GBM.

One of the seminal findings in the Stupp and colleagues[22] trial was the prognostic importance of methylation of the O6-methylguanine–DNA methyltransferase (MGMT) DNA repair enzyme. Epigenetic silencing via promoter methylation of MGMT, whose gene product is an enzyme that catalyzes the removal of alkyl groups from the O6 position of guanine, impairs the ability of tumor cells to repair DNA damage.[24] Patients with MGMT promoter methylation who received radiotherapy and temozolomide had a 2-year overall survival of 46%, whereas only 23% of patients with the MGMT promoter methylation who were assigned to radiotherapy alone were alive at 2 years. However, patients without MGMT promoter methylation had 2-year overall survival of 14% receiving radiotherapy and temozolomide versus less than 2% in those receiving radiotherapy only.

Treatment of GBM in the elderly, who have a bleak prognosis, has also been examined. A 2007 trial randomized good performance status patients 70 or older to 50 Gy of focal radiotherapy versus supportive care only and demonstrated a marked survival benefit. The hazard ratio of death in the radiotherapy group was 0.42 with a *P* value of 0.002.[25] Roa and colleagues[26] randomized 100 patients age 60 or older to receive surgical resection and standard radiotherapy (60 Gy in 30 fractions for 6 weeks) versus a shortened course of radiotherapy (40 Gy in 15 fractions for 2 weeks) without temozolomide. No difference in median survival from diagnosis was noted (5.9 months and 6.1 months in the standard and shortened course, respectively). Additionally, no difference was seen between the two groups in KPS scores tracked over time. More recently, Roa and colleagues[26] examined a further radiotherapy dose reduction in elderly and/or frail patients, comparing their previously examined 15 fraction treatment with a schedule of 25 Gy in five daily fractions for 1 week. In terms of overall survival, progression-free survival, and quality of life measures, the five-fraction regimen was noninferior. Thus, elderly patients with GBM can be reasonably afforded a 1-week course of radiotherapy without the burden of an extended course of treatment. Finally, in the elderly patient population, consideration can be given to temozolomide only. The NOA-08 study group of the German Cancer Society examined temozolomide versus radiotherapy in patients older than 65 and with a KPS of at least 60 with anaplastic astrocytoma or GBM.[27] This demonstrated a median survival of 8.6 months in the temozolomide group and 9.6 months in the radiotherapy group, within their 25% margin of noninferiority. Examining tumor MGMT methylation status, patients with methylation who received temozolomide had a superior event-free survival compared with patients who underwent radiotherapy. Thus, temozolomide alone in this patient population is yet another option, with the selection of patients informed by MGMT status.

An exciting recent development in the treatment of GBM has been the advent of alternating electric fields technology. Specifically, the use of low-intensity, intermediate frequency (100–300 kHz) has been investigated and shown to induce growth inhibitory effects in proliferating cells and cell death in neoplastic cells by disrupting the polymerization and depolymerization of microtubules in mitosis.[28] Stupp and colleagues[29] examined the addition of tumor-treating fields to conventional chemoradiation in the initial treatment of GBM. This EF-14 trial randomized a total of 466 patients in a 2:1 fashion who had undergone resection and radiotherapy with temozolomide, stratified by extent of resection and MGMT status, to receiving adjuvant temozolomide and 200-kHz treatment field therapy delivered via transducer arrays applied to the shaved scalp. Examining a primary end point of progression-free survival, the trial met a prespecified stopping rule for experimental treatment success, with a median progression-free survival in the intent-to-treat population of 7.1 months in the alternating electric fields plus temozolomide group (n = 196) versus 4.0 months in the temozolomide alone group (n = 84), with an estimated hazard ratio of 0.62 for progression (*P* = .001). Even more striking was a benefit in median overall survival, with a median survival of 20.5 months in the alternating electric fields plus temozolomide group and 15.6 months in the temozolomide alone group, with an estimated hazard ratio of

0.64 for death ($P = .004$). Moreover, alternating electric field was well tolerated, with a chief toxicity of grade 1 to 2 skin reaction characterized by localized dermatitis underneath the area of the transducer leads from the alternating electric field device in 43% of patients and more severe skin reaction (grade 3) in 2% of patients.

Despite some logistical challenges, these results represent a paradigm shift in the locoregional treatment of GBM, and perhaps herald the addition of this exciting new technology to the therapeutic armamentarium in other malignancies. For instance, the PANOVA trial is currently ongoing, which seeks to examine the safety and preliminary efficacy of the use of tumor-treating fields with chemotherapy in the setting of unresectable pancreatic cancer.

A major advance in immuno-oncology has been the development of checkpoint inhibitors, specifically the development of targeted agents directed at programmed death cell 1 (PD-1) protein and its ligand (PD-1L), an inhibitory cell surface receptor involved in inhibiting T-cell effector function and maintaining normal tissue tolerance.[30] The use of radiotherapy, particularly SRS, in conjunction with immune checkpoint blockade is an evolving therapeutic strategy. Preclinical data suggest concurrent PD-1 blockade potentiates not only the local effect of radiotherapy, but also possibly a secondary downstream systemic or abscopal effect in melanoma and renal cell carcinoma models.[31] Zeng and colleagues[32] examined the combination of anti-PD-1 immunotherapy with SRS in a mouse orthotopic GBM model where mice underwent treatment with anti-PD-1 immunotherapy only, SRS only, or SRS with anti-PD-1 immunotherapy, with a control group undergoing no treatment. The median survival in the control group of mice was 25 days, compared with 27 days in the anti-PD-1 antibody arm, 28 days in the radiation arm, and 53 days in the radiation plus anti-PD-1 ($P<.05$). Perhaps even more striking was the observation that only mice in the combined modality treatment had long-term survival beyond 180 days. MEDI473 is a phase 2 trial currently recruiting patients with newly diagnosed unmethylated MGMT GBM investigating an anti-PD-L1 monoclonal antibody with standard chemoradiation.

LOW-GRADE GLIOMA

Low-grade gliomas are rare tumors, accounting for about 15% of all brain tumors, although predominately occurring in a younger population (35–44 years of age) in comparison with high-grade glioma.[33] The presenting symptom in approximately 80% of patients diagnosed with low-grade glioma is seizures. Low-grade gliomas consist of a group of WHO grade 1-2 tumors (ie, astrocytomas, oligodendrogliomas, mixed oligoastrocytomas), for which the optimal management has been somewhat controversial.[34] In addition to surgical resection, radiotherapy has played an important role in the management of low-grade gliomas in the adjuvant setting.[35]

European Organisation for Research and Treatment of Cancer trials have identified clinicopathologic high-risk features in patients with low-grade glioma. Specifically, age 40 or older, astrocytoma histology, tumor diameter 6 cm or larger, tumor crossing the midline, and presence of neurologic deficit before surgery were identified as unfavorable prognostic factors for survival.[36] Daniels and colleagues[37] subsequently quantified survival with a low-risk group of low-grade glioma (0–2 unfavorable prognostic factors) and a high-risk group (>2 unfavorable prognostic factors) with median survival of 10.8 years versus 3.9 years, respectively. Furthermore, the cytogenetic abnormality of codeletion of 1p19q correlates favorably with survival, with median survival of 12.6 years versus 7.2 years in patients with codeletion versus noncodeletion, respectively.

Recently there has been a significant paradigm shift with the addition of procarbazine, lomustine (CCNU) and vincristine, demonstrating a clinically significant survival benefit. Buckner and colleagues[38] examined a total of 258 patients from 1998 to 2002 with grade 2 astrocytoma, oligoastrocytoma, or oligodendroglioma. Specifically, subtotally resected patients younger than 40 years and patients 40 years or older were randomized to radiotherapy alone versus radiotherapy with six cycles of adjuvant procarbazine, CCNU, and vincristine (PCV). At a median follow-up of 11.9 years, the median overall survival was significantly improved in patients receiving radiotherapy and adjuvant PCV compared with radiation therapy alone (13.3 vs 7.8 years, $P = .003$, respectively). The use of temozolomide instead of PCV in low-grade glioma is of considerable interest, because temozolomide is an easily administered oral agent and bears a more favorable toxicity profile.[31] The addition of temozolomide to radiotherapy in progressive or symptomatic low-grade glioma is currently being investigated in Eastern Cooperative Oncology Group E3F05/RTOG 1072, a phase 3 randomized trial.

Molecular subtyping through genomic analysis is allowing for improved risk stratification and may lead to better tailoring of therapy for patients with low-grade glioma.

Results of a comprehensive genomic analysis of diffuse low-grade gliomas by the Cancer Genome Atlas Research Network[39] demonstrated that patients with an IDH (*IDH1* or *IDH2* gene) have a much better prognosis than do wild-type tumors. Codeletion of chromosome 1p/19q has also been identified as a positive prognostic factor. The median survival was 1.7 years in patients with *IDH* wild-type tumors, 6.3 years in *IDH* mutant patients without 1p/19q codeletion, and 8.0 years in patients with both mutant *IDH* and 1p/19q codeletion.

SUMMARY

Recent advances have dramatically changed the landscape in the management of adult CNS malignancies. The hope is that genomic characterization will allow use of more targeted and less toxic therapies. For example, missense mutations of the B-raf proto-oncogene (*BRAF*), specifically the V600E mutation, have been identified in 66% of WHO grade 2 pleomorphic xanthoastrocytomas.[40] In a small series of four patients with recurrent pleomorphic xantroastrocytoma with BRAF V600E mutations, vemurafenib (Food and Drug Administration–approved for the treatment of metastatic or unresectable melanoma with the BRAF V600E mutation) demonstrated activity with a median progression-free survival of 5 months.[41] The explosion of new clinical trials combined with newly discovered molecular markers suggest the beginning of a paradigm shift in the management of these challenging malignancies that will allow for future risk-stratification strategies.

REFERENCES

1. Surveillance, Epidemiology, and End Results Program. Fast Stats. Available at: http://seer.cancer.gov/faststats/. Accessed September 10, 2016.
2. Nayak L, Lee EQ, Wen PY. Epidemiology of brain metastases. Curr Oncol Rep 2011;14(1):48–54.
3. Gavrilovic IT, Posner JB. Brain metastases: epidemiology and pathophysiology. J Neurooncol 2005;75(1):5–14.
4. Gaspar L, Scott C, Rotman M, et al. Recursive partitioning analysis (RPA) of prognostic factors in three Radiation Therapy Oncology Group (RTOG) brain metastases trials. Int J Radiat Oncol Biol Phys 1997;37(4):745–51.
5. Sperduto P, Chao S, Sneed P, et al. Diagnosis-specific prognostic factors, indices, and treatment outcomes for patients with newly-diagnosed brain

metastases: a multi-institutional analysis of over 5000 patients. Int J Radiat Oncol Biol Phys 2009;75(3):S225.
6. Eichler AF, Loeffler JS. Multidisciplinary management of brain metastases. Oncologist 2007;12(7):884–98.
7. Patchell RA, Tibbs PA, Walsh JW, et al. A randomized trial of surgery in the treatment of single metastases to the brain. N Engl J Med 1990;322(8):494–500.
8. DeAngelis LM, Delattre J-Y, Posner JB. Radiation-induced dementia in patients cured of brain metastases. Neurology 1989;39(6):789–96.
9. Chang EL, Wefel JS, Hess KR, et al. Neurocognition in patients with brain metastases treated with radiosurgery or radiosurgery plus whole-brain irradiation: a randomised controlled trial. Lancet Oncol 2009;10(11):1037–44.
10. Brown PD, Pugh S, Laack NN, et al. Memantine for the prevention of cognitive dysfunction in patients receiving whole-brain radiotherapy: a randomized, double-blind, placebo-controlled trial. Neuro Oncol 2013;15(10):1429–37.
11. Monje ML, Mizumatsu S, Fike JR, et al. Irradiation induces neural precursor-cell dysfunction. Nat Med 2002;8(9):955–62.
12. Gondi V, Pugh SL, Tome WA, et al. Preservation of memory with conformal avoidance of the hippocampal neural stem-cell compartment during whole-brain radiotherapy for brain metastases (RTOG 0933): a phase II multi-institutional trial. J Clin Oncol 2014;32(34):3810–6.
13. Tsao MN, Rades D, Wirth A, et al. Radiotherapeutic and surgical management for newly diagnosed brain metastasis(es): an American society for radiation oncology evidence-based guideline. Pract Radiat Oncol 2012;2(3):210–25.
14. Kocher M, Soffietti R, Abacioglu U, et al. Adjuvant whole-brain radiotherapy versus observation after radiosurgery or surgical resection of one to three cerebral metastases: results of the EORTC 22952-26001 study. J Clin Oncol 2011; 29(2):134–41.
15. Andrews DW, Scott CB, Sperduto PW, et al. Whole brain radiation therapy with or without stereotactic radiosurgery boost for patients with one to three brain metastases: phase III results of the RTOG 9508 randomised trial. Lancet 2004; 363(9422):1665–72.
16. Sahgal A, Aoyama H, Kocher M, et al. Phase 3 trials of stereotactic radiosurgery with or without whole-brain radiation therapy for 1 to 4 brain metastases: individual patient data meta-analysis. Int J Radiat Oncol Biol Phys 2015;91(4):710–7.
17. Mulvenna P, Nankivell M, Barton R, et al. Dexamethasone and supportive care with or without whole brain radiotherapy in treating patients with non-small cell lung cancer with brain metastases unsuitable for resection or stereotactic radiotherapy (QUARTZ): results from a phase 3, non-inferiority, randomised trial. Lancet 2016;388(10055):2004–14.
18. Louis DN, Perry A, Reifenberger G, et al. The 2016 World Health Organization classification of tumors of the central nervous system: a summary. Acta Neuropathol 2016;131(6):803–20.
19. Ceccom J, Bourdeaut F, Loukh N, et al. Embryonal tumor with multilayered rosettes: diagnostic tools update and review of the literature. Clin Neuropathol 2014;33(01):15–22.
20. Thakkar JP, Dolecek TA, Horbinski C, et al. Epidemiologic and molecular prognostic review of glioblastoma. Cancer Epidemiol Biomarkers Prev 2014;23(10): 1985–96.
21. Walker MD, Alexander E, Hunt WE, et al. Evaluation of BCNU and/or radiotherapy in the treatment of anaplastic gliomas. J Neurosurg 1978;49(3):333–43.

22. Stupp R, Mason WP, Bent MJVD, et al. Radiotherapy plus concomitant and adjuvant temozolomide for glioblastoma. N Engl J Med 2005;352(10):987–96.
23. Stupp R, Hegi ME, Mason WP, et al. Effects of radiotherapy with concomitant and adjuvant temozolomide versus radiotherapy alone on survival in glioblastoma in a randomised phase III study: 5-year analysis of the EORTC-NCIC trial. Lancet Oncol 2009;10(5):459–66.
24. Hegi ME, Diserens A-C, Gorlia T, et al. MGMT gene silencing and benefit from temozolomide in glioblastoma. N Engl J Med 2005;352(10):997–1003.
25. Keime-Guibert F, Chinot O, Taillandier L, et al. Radiotherapy for glioblastoma in the elderly. N Engl J Med 2007;356(15):1527–35.
26. Roa W, Brasher P, Bauman G, et al. Abbreviated course of radiation therapy in older patients with glioblastoma multiforme: a prospective randomized clinical trial. J Clin Oncol 2004;22(9):1583–8.
27. Wick W, Platten M, Meisner C, et al. Temozolomide chemotherapy alone versus radiotherapy alone for malignant astrocytoma in the elderly: the NOA-08 randomised, phase 3 trial. Lancet Oncol 2012;13(7):707–15.
28. Kirson ED. Disruption of cancer cell replication by alternating electric fields. Cancer Res 2004;64(9):3288–95.
29. Stupp R, Taillibert S, Kanner AA, et al. Maintenance therapy with tumor-treating fields plus temozolomide vs temozolomide alone for glioblastoma. JAMA 2015;314(23):2535.
30. Keir ME, Butte MJ, Freeman GJ, et al. PD-1 and its ligands in tolerance and immunity. Annu Rev Immunol 2008;26(1):677–704.
31. Park SS, Dong H, Liu X, et al. PD-1 restrains radiotherapy-induced abscopal effect. Cancer Immunol Res 2015;3(6):610–9.
32. Zeng J, See AP, Phallen J, et al. Anti-PD-1 blockade and stereotactic radiation produce long-term survival in mice with intracranial gliomas. Int J Radiat Oncol Biol Phys 2013;86(2):343–9.
33. Central Brain Tumor Registry of the United States. Statistical report: primary brain tumors in the United States, 2000–2004. Available at: http://www.cbtrus.org/reports/2007-2008/2007report.pdf. Accessed September 2, 2016.
34. Pouratian N, Schiff D. Management of low-grade glioma. Curr Neurol Neurosci Rep 2010;10(3):224–31.
35. Chang EF, Potts MB, Keles GE, et al. Seizure characteristics and control following resection in 332 patients with low-grade gliomas. J Neurosurg 2008;108(2):227–35.
36. Pignatti F. Prognostic factors for survival in adult patients with cerebral low-grade glioma. J Clin Oncol 2002;20(8):2076–84.
37. Daniels TB, Brown PD, Felten SJ, et al. Validation of EORTC prognostic factors for adults with low-grade glioma: a report using Intergroup 86-72-51. Int J Radiat Oncol Biol Phys 2011;81(1):218–24.
38. Buckner JC, Shaw EG, Pugh SL, et al. Radiation plus procarbazine, CCNU, and vincristine in low-grade glioma. N Engl J Med 2016;374(14):1344–55.
39. Comprehensive, integrative genomic analysis of diffuse lower-grade gliomas. N Engl J Med 2015;372(26):2481–98.
40. Schindler G, Capper D, Meyer J, et al. Analysis of BRAF V600E mutation in 1,320 nervous system tumors reveals high mutation frequencies in pleomorphic xanthoastrocytoma, ganglioglioma and extra-cerebellar pilocytic astrocytoma. Acta Neuropathol 2011;121(3):397–405.
41. Chamberlain MC. Salvage therapy with BRAF inhibitors for recurrent pleomorphic xanthoastrocytoma: a retrospective case series. J Neurooncol 2013;114(2):237–40.

Controversies in Postoperative Irradiation of Oropharyngeal Cancer After Transoral Surgery

Sue S. Yom, MD, PhD, MAS[a,b,*], Jon Mallen-St. Clair, MD, PhD[b], Patrick K. Ha, MD[b]

KEYWORDS

- Transoral robotic surgery • Transoral laser microscopy • Oropharyngeal cancer
- Human papillomavirus • Chemotherapy • Radiation

KEY POINTS

- Transoral surgery (TOS) is a minimally invasive approach to the management of early- and intermediate-stage head and neck squamous cell carcinomas, whose adoption is expanding in the United States and other countries.
- Human papillomavirus (HPV)-associated oropharyngeal cancer is increasing in incidence, coincident with development of the technology and expertise necessary for TOS.
- Pathologic features traditionally considered to be indications for postoperative radiation or postoperative chemoradiation for other head and neck cancers may apply to HPV-associated oropharyngeal cancer to a lesser extent.
- Clinical trials of TOS are focused on defining the contribution of surgery in potentially de-intensifying treatment of HPV-associated patients with oropharyngeal cancer, in comparison to traditional upfront radiation or chemoradiation.

TRANSORAL SURGERY IN OROPHARYNGEAL CANCER TREATMENT

Transoral endoscopic surgery (TOS) encompasses 2 different techniques, transoral laser microsurgery (TLM) and transoral robotic surgery (TORS), both of which provide a minimally invasive surgical approach to the pharynx.[1] TOS offers superior

Disclosure Statement: The authors have nothing to disclose.

[a] Department of Radiation Oncology, University of California-San Francisco, 1600 Divisadero Street, H1031, San Francisco, CA 94143-1708, USA; [b] Division of Head and Neck Surgical Oncology, Department of Otolaryngology-Head and Neck Surgery, University of California-San Francisco, 550 16th Street, Box 3213, San Francisco, CA 94158, USA
* Corresponding author. Department of Radiation Oncology, University of California-San Francisco, 1600 Divisadero Street, H1031, San Francisco, CA 94143-1708.
E-mail address: yoms@radonc.ucsf.edu

Surg Oncol Clin N Am 26 (2017) 357–370
http://dx.doi.org/10.1016/j.soc.2017.01.006 surgonc.theclinics.com

oncologic and functional outcomes compared with the traditional open surgical approach.[2,3] TLM, originally developed in the 1970s for the ablation of laryngeal papillomas, has expanded into the oropharynx and oral cavity, but its application has been limited by the requirements of line-of-sight visualization and occupation of one hand to operate the laser. Meanwhile, TORS, approved by the US Food and Drug Administration in 2009 for removal of benign and malignant early-stage pharyngeal tumors, has experienced rapid adoption. Advantages of TORS over TLM include improved wide-field visualization, especially useful at the base of tongue, and greater stability and subtlety of movement in a virtual, magnified, 3-dimensional surgical environment. The surgeon is seated at a console remote from a patient-side cart equipped with robotic arms that deliver the surgical instruments and endoscope. TORS allows for bimanual manipulation and en bloc excision of tumors. In the United States, TORS has increasingly been used as part of a curative-intent treatment plan for oropharyngeal squamous cell carcinomas (OPSCC),[4] and its use is increasing in Europe and other parts of the world.[5]

The emergence of transoral surgery as an upfront management strategy has coincided with the recognition of human papillomavirus (HPV) as an etiologic and prognostic factor in OPSCC, leading to several interrelated uncertainties pertinent to postoperative management. At present, single-modality treatment (using either radiation therapy or TOS) is clearly appropriate for early- and intermediate-stage (T1-2, N0-1) OPSCC, but it has proven more complex to identify indications for TOS in the management of advanced-stage cancers, which have been traditionally managed with chemoradiation (CRT) over the past 2 decades.[6] In locally or regionally advanced oropharyngeal cancers, complete extirpation may be more challenging, and by current standards of care, postoperative radiation or CRT is required in most cases.[7] Thus, investigators are rigorously examining the indications for adjuvant therapy following initial surgical management for advanced OPSCC. The hypothesis is that histopathologic information from upfront surgery will result in an improved precision of adjuvant therapy decisions, thereby improving function and quality-of-life outcomes over upfront radiation-based treatment in patients who are pathologically downstaged and receive deintensified adjuvant therapy.

IMPACT OF HUMAN PAPILLOMAVIRUS ON PROGNOSIS AND STAGING OF OROPHARYNGEAL CANCER

HPV was confirmed in 2000 by DNA polymerase chain reaction detection to be an etiologic agent of OPSCC.[8] It is now known that greater than 60% of OPSCC are exclusively associated with HPV-16 (which accounts for 86.7% of HPV detected in OPSCC) or HPV-18, although other "high-risk" strains that are detected at a low frequency include HPV-31, -33, -35, -39, -45, and -52, for an overall proportion of greater than 70% of OPSCC that is HPV related.[9,10] These findings are reinforced by a distinct clinical profile of patients with HPV-associated OPSCC that differs dramatically from patients with conventional head and neck cancer. Patients with HPV-OPSCC have been found more likely to be younger, nonsmokers, and with higher rates of marijuana and sexual exposure than other patients with head and neck cancer.[11] They tend to have a higher socioeconomic status and level of education.[12] HPV-OPSCC has a distinctive molecular profile as well, demonstrating a lack of p53 mutations and overexpression of p16 caused by inhibition of retinoblastoma protein pRB by HPV E7 protein.[13,14] Unlike the stability or declines seen in the incidence of other head and neck cancers in Western countries consequent to decreases in the rate of cigarette smoking, the incidence of HPV-OPSCC is countering the trend with a rising incidence.[15,16]

An important recursive partitioning analysis of Radiation Therapy Oncology Group (RTOG) 0129, a CRT-based cooperative group clinical trial, showed that compared with other OPSCC patients, patients with HPV-OPSCC were at “low risk” for death, due to the responsiveness of their cancers to CRT and their lower risk for development of distant metastases.[17] The 3-year overall survival (OS) rates were 82.4% for HPV-OPSCC patients versus 57.1% for patients with HPV-negative tumors, with HPV positivity conferring a 58% reduction in the risk of death and risk of death increasing for each additional pack-year of tobacco smoking. In the low-risk group, defined by HPV positivity and either $\leq$10 pack-years of smoking or greater than 10 pack-year history with stage N0-N2a, the 3-year OS was 93%. Given the exceptional response of HPV-OPSCC to standard therapy and the lengthy survivorship seen in this patient population with a higher relative risk of long-term morbidity from potential overtreatment, recently conceived clinical trials for this population have focused on “deintensification” of therapies (**Table 1**). The clinical trial landscape for this category of patients is very active, with a large number of competing proposed interventions and no new singular standard of care that has clearly emerged.

One major change that is universally accepted is that p16 status is now considered a basic mandatory stratification factor in clinical trials for oropharyngeal cancer. Diffuse nuclear and cytoplasmic p16 protein staining set at a cutoff of greater than 70% of tumor cells has approximately 90% correlation with HPV status as determined by in situ hybridization and quantitative and consensus polymerase chain reaction.[18] Because p16 immunohistochemistry is less costly and reliably standardizes across laboratories, p16 graded by H-score, rather than HPV DNA status, has been used for stratification in most clinical trials.[19] A complicating issue is that although p16 remains the most commonly accepted biomarker for HPV status, it is itself a tumor suppressor protein. Therefore, p16 positivity may be reflective of a biological process independent of HPV status. One large study of aggregated clinical trial data showed a prognostic value of p16 in oral, laryngeal, and hypopharyngeal squamous cell carcinomas, but the prognosis of these cancers was not as dramatically improved by p16 positivity as was OPSCC, and p16 positivity in these nonoropharyngeal cancers showed less correlation with HPV DNA status.[20] Therefore, no proposals for changes to standard treatment have been made for nonoropharyngeal head and neck cancers on the basis of either p16 or HPV status. p16 has also been identified in other cancers, which can metastasize to the lymph nodes of the head and neck, such as skin cancer, wherein p16 positivity does not affect prognosis and is not associated with HPV in these cancers.[21]

Parallel to the evolution in clinical trials is a change in the American Joint Committee on Cancer (AJCC) staging system for OPSCC. In the AJCC 8th edition, which will take effect in the national cancer registries on January 1, 2018, HPV-OPSCC has its own unique staging system separate from other OPSCC. HPV-OPSCC patients who would formerly have been considered to have stage IVA oropharyngeal cancer will mostly be reclassified to have stage I or stage II, reflecting that they are at a low risk for death when appropriately treated. Because the staging system is an international system that must be used worldwide, the definition of HPV-OPSCC for staging purposes will rely on p16 immunohistochemistry. It is also important to note that OPSCC staging, whether HPV-associated or not, remains distinct from staging for cancers of the oral cavity.

Table 1
Completed and accruing clinical trials testing deintensified regimens for patients with HPV-associated oropharyngeal cancer

Trial	Phase	Inclusion Criteria	Study Arms	Primary Outcome
Surgically based				
SiRS (NCT02072148)	2	T1-2N0-N2b, with level 2 adenopathy, ECE-, <20 pack-years with >10 y tobacco-free	Low risk: observation; intermediate risk: 50 Gy; high risk: 56 Gy with weekly cisplatin	3- and 5-y DFS and LRC
ECOG 3311 (NCT01898494)	2	Stage III-IVB	Low risk: observation; intermediate risk: randomized to 50 vs 60 Gy; high risk: 66 Gy with weekly cisplatin	2-y PFS
PATHOS (NCT02215265)	2	T1-T3N0-2b, current smokers with N2b disease ineligible	Low risk: observation; intermediate risk: randomized to 50 Gy vs 60 Gy; high risk: randomized to 60 Gy with or without weekly cisplatin	1-y MDADI score; planned expansion to phase 3 for OS
ADEPT (NCT01687413)	3	T1-4aN+, ECE+	Randomized to 60 Gy RT with or without weekly cisplatin	2-y DFS and LRC
ORATOR (NCT01590355)	2	T1-2N0-N2, ECE−	Randomized to 70 Gy ± cisplatin vs TORS-ND ± IMRT	1-y QOL
Radiotherapy-based				
NRG-HN002 (NCT02254278)	2	T1-2N1-2b or T3N0-2b, <10 pack-years	Randomized to 60 Gy with or without weekly cisplatin	2-y PFS
UNC-UFL (NCT01530997)	2	T1-3N0-2c, <10 pack-years or >5 y tobacco-free	60 Gy with weekly cisplatin, followed by biopsies and ND	Pathologic CR

ECOG 1308 (NCT01084083)	2	Stage IIIA-IVB	Induction cisplatin-paclitaxel-cetuximab + RT (54 Gy for CR, 69.6 Gy for partial/no response) with cetuximab	2-y PFS in CR patients
The Quarterback Trial (NCT01706939)	3	Stage III-IVB, unknown primary or nasopharyngeal cancer eligible, active smokers or >20 pack-years ineligible	Induction TPF, then responders randomized 2:1 to carboplatin with 56 Gy vs 70 Gy	3-y PFS
RTOG 1016 (NCT01302834)	3	T1-2N2a-3 or T3-4	Randomized to 70 Gy with cetuximab vs cisplatin	5-y OS
De-ESCALaTE (NCT01874171)	3	T3N0-T4N0 or T1N1-T4N3, >10 pack-years with N2b-N3 ineligible	Randomized to 70 Gy with cetuximab vs cisplatin	2-y grade 3 toxicity
TROG 12.01 (NCT01855451)	3	Stage III (excluding T1-2N1) or IV (excluding T4, N3, M1), if >10 pack-years nodal disease must be N0-N2a	Randomized to 70 Gy with cetuximab vs cisplatin	MDASI-HN symptom severity through wk 20

Abbreviations: CR, complete response; DFS, disease-free survival; LRC, locoregional control; MDADI, MD Anderson Dysphagia Inventory; MDASI-HN, MD Anderson Symptom Inventory–Head and Neck Module; ND, neck dissection; PFS, progression-free survival; QOL, quality of life; TORS-ND, transoral robotic surgery-neck dissection; RT, radiation therapy; TPF, taxane-platinum-fluorouracil.

SAFETY AND ONCOLOGIC OUTCOMES OF TRANSORAL ROBOTIC SURGERY FOR OROPHARYNGEAL CANCER

TORS represents an interesting case study in the assessment of quality in head and neck cancer care. TORS emerged in a time of close monitoring of outcome measures by health care systems and regulatory agencies. An initial study of TORS using measures from the American College of Surgeons' National Surgical Quality Improvement Program (NSQIP) revealed a low rate of postoperative complications of 7.9%.[22] However, the NSQIP measures were not ideal to assess TORS, because common complications were not specifically measured. Postoperative bleeding was measured through the surrogate of transfusion requirement, and other metrics of quality, such as need for reoperation, were difficult to assess because of the often-staged nature of TORS operations. Furthermore, metrics of quality specific to head and neck cancer such as speech and swallowing outcomes were not included. This study highlighted the need for specialty-specific NSQIP measures to allow more relevant analyses of quality for TORS.

For TORS, as for many surgical techniques, increased volume has been associated with a lower rate of complications and improved quality outcomes. Multiple case series describe a decreased risk of complications after TORS with increasing experience,[23,24] and increased TORS experience correlates with decreased operative time, length of intubation, and hospital stay.[25] The risk of complications appears to be lower in surgeons who have performed more than 50 TORS procedures.[26] As a result, there has been considerable effort by the American Academy of Otolaryngology-Head and Neck Surgery and the American Head and Neck Society to set up an independent credentialing committee to standardize training.[27] Previous credentialing methods were institution-dependent and highly reliant on industry.[28] Establishment of national standards will enable follow-up analyses of adherence to guidelines and impact on quality.

At present, TORS has been evaluated most thoroughly in single- and multi-institutional studies conducted by major academic centers. Although the available data suggest very favorable oncologic outcomes,[29–32] no randomized controlled studies have been completed comparing the outcomes of upfront TOS and upfront CRT or radiation. This direct comparison is the goal of the ORATOR (NCT01590355) randomized phase 2 clinical trial, which is based on a head-to-head randomization of surgery versus radiation-based treatment. One large, influential, multi-institutional series found 2-year locoregional control and OS rates of TOS-treated patients to be 91.8% and 91%, respectively.[32] A systematic review of 11 studies could not clearly report long-term local control due to variable follow-up but identified 9 studies reporting gastrostomy tube dependence for an aggregate 12-month rate of only 5%.[31] On head-and-neck–specific quality-of-life surveys, outcomes of upfront TOS followed by adaptive adjuvant therapy appear to be roughly equivalent to, and in cases when no adjuvant therapy or adjuvant radiation alone can be given, superior to, concurrent CRT.[33–36] However, attempts at direct comparison may be affected by selection bias given resectability and better performance status of surgically eligible patients.

Complicating the issue of comparative evaluation further is the fact that most patients with OPSCC, even those with locoregionally advanced cancers who receive CRT, tend to experience quite favorable long-term survival outcomes with low rates of severe toxic effects.[37–39] The differences separating patients treated with variably sequenced forms of multimodal therapy may be subtle and difficult to distinguish.[40] An additional complicating factor is that the standard of CRT is evolving, with large institutional experiences indicating that T1-T2 node-positive HPV-OPSCC patients achieve high 5-year survival rates (90%) when treated with radiation alone, potentially making comparisons of TOS to radiation alone or other "deintensified" radiation-based treatments currently under study more valid in the future than comparisons to standard CRT.

To address these questions, clinical trials such SiRS (NCT02072148), ECOG 3311 (NCT01898494), and PATHOS (NCT02215265), all studies of upfront TOS followed by histopathologically directed adjuvant therapy, are investigating the role of upfront TOS for the purpose of decreasing adjuvant radiation dosage. Other trials such as ADEPT (NCT01687413) are examining the feasibility of decreasing or eliminating adjuvant chemotherapy intensity in surgically staged HPV-OPSCC patients. These clinical trials will record outcomes prospectively in HPV-OPSCC patients treated with TOS, providing a higher-quality evidence base for meaningfully crediting the contribution of surgery in well-controlled clinical scenarios.

CONTROVERSIES IN ADJUVANT THERAPY FOLLOWING TRANSORAL SURGERY FOR OROPHARYNGEAL CANCER

The coincident identification of HPV-OPSCC in the context of increasing management of OPSCC by TOS has resulted in several complex intersecting questions about the relevance of traditional postoperative therapy for this patient population. Major areas of uncertainty in postoperative management include determination of the necessary indications for the addition of concurrent chemotherapy and radiation therapy dose and field size in relation to surgical extent.

In the National Comprehensive Cancer Network (NCCN) guidelines, indications for postoperative radiation therapy include pathologic T3-4 or N2-N3 stage, nodal disease in levels IV or V, perineural invasion, or lymphovascular invasion.[41] Concurrent CRT is recommended for extracapsular extension (ECE), and for positive resection margins in T2 cancers, either re-resection or CRT is to be considered, whereas for positive margins in stage T3-T4, it is recommended. The recommendations for CRT are derived from a combined analysis of 2 phase 3 trials, RTOG 9501 and European Organisation for Research and Treatment of Cancer 22931, which established the survival benefit of adding concurrent cisplatin to postoperative radiation therapy in patients with these pathologic findings.[42] These 2 clinical trials included oral cavity, oropharynx, hypopharynx, and larynx cancers, did not test patients for HPV status at entry, and were completed in an era predating minimally invasive TOS.[43,44]

Small studies in the modern era have not reliably identified a survival benefit to concurrent CRT among HPV-OPSCC patients meeting the entry criteria of these trials, leading to controversy about whether these phase 3 data truly apply to the HPV-OPSCC population.[44,45] Clarification of the indications for adjuvant radiation versus CRT is important because it is clear that intensity of adjuvant therapy delivered after TOS affects functional and patient-reported outcomes.[46–48]

Although it may be premature at this point to endorse the removal of chemotherapy from adjuvant treatment for margin-positive or ECE-positive patients, it is probable that there are some HPV-OPSCC patients currently falling into these categories for whom adjuvant CRT may be of less benefit. Awareness of these issues has led to a re-examination of both of these classifications, which may benefit from more specificity and gradation in their clinical application.

MARGIN STATUS IN THE DETERMINATION OF ADJUVANT THERAPY AFTER TRANSORAL SURGERY

The definition of a "clear" surgical margin for head and neck cancers was traditionally considered to be greater than 5 mm measured at the mucosal and deep aspects of the tumor on a formalin-fixed specimen, as specified by the original reporting standards from the Royal College of Pathologists (RCP) in 1998, which was updated in 2005.[49] In the classic RCP definition, 1 to 5 mm is defined as "close" and less than 1 mm is called "involved." In practice, these cutoffs have been loosely translated into categories of "intermediate" or "high" risk for which adjuvant radiation or CRT would be indicated, respectively. However, substantial differences of interpretation exist around these definitions, as demonstrated in a survey of the American Head and Neck Society membership,[50] which confirmed that the most common definition of a clear margin was indeed greater than 5 mm but with variability and qualifications of the responses. Among major centers of head and neck TOS, definitions of a clear margin vary and are in many cases specific to anatomic site.

This lack of consensus is reflected in reviews of the medical literature[51,52] and the NCCN guidelines, where the RCP "clear" and "close" definitions are reiterated, but a "positive" margin is defined as carcinoma in situ or invasive carcinoma at the margin, and 1- to 2-mm margins are defined as adequate for glottic cancers. For TLM, it is stated that 1.5 to 2.0 mm "may be achieved with the goal of complete tumor resection," although "with this approach, adequacy of resection may be uncertain" and "such margins would be considered 'close.'"[41] Of note, the NCCN guidelines do not link margin status to any recommendation for postoperative therapy.

Clinical trials designed for the postoperative population have also not reached a consensus on the definition of margins. RTOG 0920 (NCT00956007), a phase 3 study testing the benefit of cetuximab added to postoperative radiation in "intermediate-risk" cases with concerning features that fall short of positive margins or ECE, defines a close margin according to the classical definition of less than 5 mm, which allows patients with p16-positive OPSCC entry into the study. RTOG 1216 (NCT01810913), a phase 2/3 postoperative study of intensified chemotherapy concurrent with postoperative radiation for "high-risk" cases, restricts entry to "tumor on ink," and excludes patients with p16-positive OPSCC. ECOG 3311 defines a clear margin as greater than 3 mm. A positive margin is defined as "carcinoma at the cut-specimen edge" and "extensive" ECE as tumor extension more than 1 mm beyond the lymph node capsule; either of these pathologic findings results in postoperative assignment to concurrent weekly cisplatin and an escalated radiation dose of 66 Gy. In ECOG 3311, if a margin is less than 3 mm but not positive, it is called close and radiation is required, although the patient is entered into the intermediate-risk arm randomizing between 60 Gy and 50 Gy of radiation alone. On the other hand, SiRS and ORATOR require postoperative radiation for a less than 1 mm or less than 2 mm margin, respectively.

Another factor relevant to oropharyngeal resections is that tissue under tension contracts after surgical resection and mucosal margins will shrink on the order of 20% to 25%, with another 10% contraction resulting from formalin fixation and paraffin embedding.[52] Thus, final margins on permanent sections may differ from intraoperative margins or gross specimen margins. These factors and the complex anatomic structure of the tonsillar fossa frequently result in narrow but clear margins for these resections. In ECOG 3311, the superior constrictor is defined as the deep margin for tonsillar fossa cancers and should be resected en bloc with the tumor and be "histologically negative," because it is recognized that this is a natural anatomic boundary to cancer spread.

The status of tonsillar margins is especially important due to the consequences of implementing intensified adjuvant therapy to areas of margin considered close or positive. After oropharyngeal resection, soft tissue necrosis is a particular risk that has been found to affect 23.5% to 28% of patients undergoing TORS and adjuvant radiation, with higher risk related to factors such tonsillar primary site, the depth of the resection, and if the radiation was given at a rate of greater than 2 Gy per day. In these series, more than 60% of the patients had received concurrent chemotherapy with radiation.[53,54]

EXTRACAPSULAR EXTENSION AS A RISK FACTOR AFTER TRANSORAL SURGERY

ECE, also known as extracapsular spread or extranodal extension (ENE), is a well-established high-risk feature in head and neck cancer, and the recommendation for adjuvant CRT is based on a significant OS benefit in the aforementioned phase III randomized trials.[42] Thus, clinically evident ECE is not infrequently considered a disincentive to upfront surgical management, because these patients will likely receive a CRT treatment in the adjuvant setting that is similar to definitive therapy.[55] However, the more common situation occurs in patients who undergo TOS and are discovered to have ECE on pathologic review.

There are single-institution series indicating that ECE may have less prognostic value in HPV-OPSCC and questioning the value of adjuvant CRT in these patients.[56–58] Given that older series may have included a greater proportion of patients with clinically evident ECE and that these patients may have had less radioresponsive, non-HPV-associated oropharyngeal tumors, intensification of adjuvant therapy may be of less benefit in HPV-OPSCC patients with only pathologically identified ECE.

In ECOG 3311, patients with less than 1 mm of ECE are allowed to receive radiation therapy alone, and in fact, enter into the randomized arm of the study where they may receive an experimentally lower postoperative dose of 50 Gy of radiation alone. The ADEPT randomized phase 3 study is explicitly studying the question of CRT, testing for the additional value of concurrent cisplatin added to postoperative radiation in HPV-OPSCC patients found to have ECE. For confirmed ECE, the ADEPT radiation dose is 60 Gy, whereas the ECOG 3311 dose in the "high-risk" arm is 66 Gy, reflecting the lack of consensus about the appropriate intensity of treatment of ECE in HPV-OPSCC patients.

In the AJCC 8th edition staging system, the nodal staging for head and neck cancers has been revised such that ECE is a factor that generally raises a patient's N-stage. However, uniquely for HPV-OPSCC, ECE will not be counted in this way, in keeping with the ongoing investigatory nature about the prognostic value of ECE in these patients.

DOSE AND EXTENT OF RADIATION FIELDS AFTER TRANSORAL SURGERY

There is in vitro evidence that HPV-OPSCC has greater intrinsic radiosensitivity,[59,60] and this has led to translational investigations such as the cooperative group trials of reduced-dose CRT, ECOG 1308 (NCT01084083)[61] and NRG-HN002 (NCT02254278).[62,63] Likewise, it may be feasible to deintensify the postoperative dose of radiation therapy for HPV-OPSCC patients who have undergone TOS. ECOG 3311 and the PATHOS trial are both powered for a randomization of "intermediate-risk" patients to receive either 50 Gy (experimental arm) versus 60 Gy (standard arm) of radiation therapy, and the SiRS trial is also studying dose reductions to 50 Gy of radiation alone or 56 Gy with cisplatin in a single-arm, histopathologically directed manner. In these studies, patient-reported outcomes will be needed to quantify the functional and quality-of-life impact of a lower postoperative radiation dose enabled by TOS.

Most recently, the delineation of the postoperative irradiation fields in relation to the extent of surgery has come under investigation. Postoperative radiation fields are usually larger in size than definitive-intent radiation fields, due to the necessity of covering the entire region of the operative bed. Furthermore, postoperative radiation has traditionally been delivered comprehensively to all anatomic compartments involved in surgery to address potential lymphovascular disruption and microscopic seeding of tumor into hypoxic regions. Investigators at the University of Pennsylvania have initiated a single-arm phase 2 trial (NCT02159703) testing the safety of neck-only radiation, omitting radiation to the primary site in patients with T1-T2 tumors who achieve 2-mm margins with no other negative features. The assumption is that omission of radiation to the pharyngeal area will improve functional outcomes, as was suggested in one retrospective TLM series that showed a reduction in gastrostomy tube rates and a local failure rate of 3% versus 17% among early versus advanced T-stage patients who had omitted primary site radiation.[64]

The success of this approach will likely depend to a great degree on the exact specifics of the definition of the radiation fields. One small dosimetric study did not find that sparing the primary site adequately reduced the radiation dose to the pharyngeal constrictor muscles to a degree that would be likely to result in improved swallowing, although the dose to the oral cavity was substantially reduced.[65] However, even if functional outcomes were not positively affected in a quantifiable manner, adverse events such as severe mucositis or soft tissue necrosis could be lessened with a reduction of dose to an area rendered delicate by recent surgical manipulation. The benefit of this approach remains to be confirmed.

SUMMARY

Transoral surgery, as a remarkable innovation in the management of early-stage oropharyngeal cancers, may fundamentally redefine many traditional precepts that have governed postoperative management. Its development coincident with the rising incidence of HPV-OPSCC has led to a complex intersection of the 2 phenomena, with the initiation of multiple clinical trials aimed at deintensification of current therapies in this unique patient population. As TORS is a nascent technology, the major experience thus far has mostly been limited to select institutions, although dissemination of the equipment and operational expertise is rapidly increasing. Ongoing efforts in standardization, quality assessment, and clinical trial development will be critical in maximizing the potential of this new area of surgical inquiry.

REFERENCES

1. Li RJ, Richmon JD. Transoral endoscopic surgery: new surgical techniques for oropharyngeal cancer. Otolaryngol Clin North Am 2012;45(4):823–44.
2. Ford SE, Brandwein-Gensler M, Carroll WR, et al. Transoral robotic versus open surgical approaches to oropharyngeal squamous cell carcinoma by human papillomavirus status. Otolaryngol Head Neck Surg 2014;151(4):606–11.
3. Lee SY, Park YM, Byeon HK, et al. Comparison of oncologic and functional outcomes after transoral robotic lateral oropharyngectomy versus conventional surgery for T1 to T3 tonsillar cancer. Head Neck 2014;36(8):1138–45.
4. Chen MM, Roman SA, Kraus DH, et al. Transoral robotic surgery: a population-level analysis. Otolaryngol Head Neck Surg 2014;150(6):968–75.
5. Lorincz BB, Laban S, Knecht R. The development of TORS in Europe. HNO 2013;61(4):294–9 [in German].
6. Gourin CG, Frick KD. National trends in oropharyngeal cancer surgery and the effect of surgeon and hospital volume on short-term outcomes and cost of care. Laryngoscope 2012;122(3):543–51.

7. Duek I, Billan S, Amit M, et al. Transoral robotic surgery in the HPV era. Rambam Maimonides Med J 2014;5(2):e0010.
8. Gillison ML, Koch WM, Capone RB, et al. Evidence for a causal association between human papillomavirus and a subset of head and neck cancers. J Natl Cancer Inst 2000;92(9):709–20.
9. Kreimer AR, Clifford GM, Boyle P, et al. Human papillomavirus types in head and neck squamous cell carcinomas worldwide: a systematic review. Cancer Epidemiol Biomarkers Prev 2005;14(2):467–75.
10. Steinau M, Saraiya M, Goodman MT, et al. Human papillomavirus prevalence in oropharyngeal cancer before vaccine introduction, United States. Emerg Infect Dis 2014;20(5):822–8.
11. Fakhry C, Gillison ML. Clinical implications of human papillomavirus in head and neck cancers. J Clin Oncol 2006;24(17):2606–11.
12. Dahlstrom KR, Bell D, Hanby D, et al. Socioeconomic characteristics of patients with oropharyngeal carcinoma according to tumor HPV status, patient smoking status, and sexual behavior. Oral Oncol 2015;51(9):832–8.
13. Westra WH, Taube JM, Poeta ML, et al. Inverse relationship between human papillomavirus-16 infection and disruptive p53 gene mutations in squamous cell carcinoma of the head and neck. Clin Cancer Res 2008;14(2):366–9.
14. Rayess H, Wang MB, Srivatsan ES. Cellular senescence and tumor suppressor gene p16. Int J Cancer 2012;130(8):1715–25.
15. Shiboski CH, Schmidt BL, Jordan RC. Tongue and tonsil carcinoma: increasing trends in the U.S. population ages 20-44 years. Cancer 2005;103(9):1843–9.
16. Chaturvedi AK, Engels EA, Pfeiffer RM, et al. Human papillomavirus and rising oropharyngeal cancer incidence in the United States. J Clin Oncol 2011; 29(32):4294–301.
17. Ang KK, Harris J, Wheeler R, et al. Human papillomavirus and survival of patients with oropharyngeal cancer. N Engl J Med 2010;363(1):24–35.
18. Gronhoj Larsen C, Gyldenlove M, Jensen DH, et al. Correlation between human papillomavirus and p16 overexpression in oropharyngeal tumours: a systematic review. Br J Cancer 2014;110(6):1587–94.
19. Jordan RC, Lingen MW, Perez-Ordonez B, et al. Validation of methods for oropharyngeal cancer HPV status determination in US cooperative group trials. Am J Surg Pathol 2012;36(7):945–54.
20. Chung CH, Zhang Q, Kong CS, et al. p16 protein expression and human papillomavirus status as prognostic biomarkers of nonoropharyngeal head and neck squamous cell carcinoma. J Clin Oncol 2014;32(35):3930–8.
21. McDowell LJ, Young RJ, Johnston ML, et al. p16-positive lymph node metastases from cutaneous head and neck squamous cell carcinoma: no association with high-risk human papillomavirus or prognosis and implications for the workup of the unknown primary. Cancer 2016;122(8):1201–8.
22. Su HK, Ozbek U, Likhterov I, et al. Safety of transoral surgery for oropharyngeal malignancies: an analysis of the ACS NSQIP. Laryngoscope 2016;126(11): 2484–91.
23. Genden EM, Desai S, Sung CK. Transoral robotic surgery for the management of head and neck cancer: a preliminary experience. Head Neck 2009;31(3):283–9.
24. Lawson G, Matar N, Remacle M, et al. Transoral robotic surgery for the management of head and neck tumors: learning curve. Eur Arch Otorhinolaryngol 2011; 268(12):1795–801.

25. White HN, Frederick J, Zimmerman T, et al. Learning curve for transoral robotic surgery: a 4-year analysis. JAMA Otolaryngol Head Neck Surg 2013;139(6):564–7.
26. Chia SH, Gross ND, Richmon JD. Surgeon experience and complications with Transoral Robotic Surgery (TORS). Otolaryngol Head Neck Surg 2013;149(6):885–92.
27. Gross ND, Holsinger FC, Magnuson JS, et al. Robotics in otolaryngology and head and neck surgery: recommendations for training and credentialing: a report of the 2015 AHNS education committee, AAO-HNS robotic task force and AAO-HNS sleep disorders committee. Head Neck 2016;38(Suppl 1):E151–8.
28. Zhang N, Sumer BD. Transoral robotic surgery: simulation-based standardized training. JAMA Otolaryngol Head Neck Surg 2013;139(11):1111–7.
29. Weinstein GS, Quon H, Newman HJ, et al. Transoral robotic surgery alone for oropharyngeal cancer: an analysis of local control. Arch Otolaryngol Head Neck Surg 2012;138(7):628–34.
30. Moore EJ, Olsen SM, Laborde RR, et al. Long-term functional and oncologic results of transoral robotic surgery for oropharyngeal squamous cell carcinoma. Mayo Clin Proc 2012;87(3):219–25.
31. Kelly K, Johnson-Obaseki S, Lumingu J, et al. Oncologic, functional and surgical outcomes of primary Transoral Robotic Surgery for early squamous cell cancer of the oropharynx: a systematic review. Oral Oncol 2014;50(8):696–703.
32. de Almeida JR, Li R, Magnuson JS, et al. Oncologic outcomes after transoral robotic surgery: a multi-institutional study. JAMA Otolaryngol Head Neck Surg 2015;141(12):1043–51.
33. Choby GW, Kim J, Ling DC, et al. Transoral robotic surgery alone for oropharyngeal cancer: quality-of-life outcomes. JAMA Otolaryngol Head Neck Surg 2015;141(6):499–504.
34. Dziegielewski PT, Teknos TN, Durmus K, et al. Transoral robotic surgery for oropharyngeal cancer: long-term quality of life and functional outcomes. JAMA Otolaryngol Head Neck Surg 2013;139(11):1099–108.
35. Maxwell JH, Mehta V, Wang H, et al. Quality of life in head and neck cancer patients: impact of HPV and primary treatment modality. Laryngoscope 2014;124(7):1592–7.
36. Chen AM, Daly ME, Luu Q, et al. Comparison of functional outcomes and quality of life between transoral surgery and definitive chemoradiotherapy for oropharyngeal cancer. Head Neck 2015;37(3):381–5.
37. Ward MC, Ross RB, Koyfman SA, et al. Modern image-guided intensity-modulated radiotherapy for oropharynx cancer and severe late toxic effects: implications for clinical trial design. JAMA Otolaryngol Head Neck Surg 2016;142(12):1164–70.
38. Garden AS, Kies MS, Morrison WH, et al. Outcomes and patterns of care of patients with locally advanced oropharyngeal carcinoma treated in the early 21st century. Radiat Oncol 2013;8:21.
39. Setton J, Lee NY, Riaz N, et al. A multi-institution pooled analysis of gastrostomy tube dependence in patients with oropharyngeal cancer treated with definitive intensity-modulated radiotherapy. Cancer 2015;121(2):294–301.
40. de Almeida JR, Byrd JK, Wu R, et al. A systematic review of transoral robotic surgery and radiotherapy for early oropharynx cancer: a systematic review. Laryngoscope 2014;124(9):2096–102.

41. NCCN Clinical Practice Guidelines in Oncology: Head and Neck Cancers: NCCN.org; [Version 1.2017]. Available at: https://www.nccn.org/professionals/physician_gls/PDF/head-and-neck.pdf. Accessed February 16, 2017.
42. Bernier J, Cooper JS, Pajak TF, et al. Defining risk levels in locally advanced head and neck cancers: a comparative analysis of concurrent postoperative radiation plus chemotherapy trials of the EORTC (#22931) and RTOG (# 9501). Head Neck 2005;27(10):843–50.
43. Bernier J, Domenge C, Ozsahin M, et al. Postoperative irradiation with or without concomitant chemotherapy for locally advanced head and neck cancer. N Engl J Med 2004;350(19):1945–52.
44. Cooper JS, Fortpied C, Gregoire V, et al. The role of postoperative chemoradiation for oropharynx carcinoma: a critical appraisal revisited. Cancer 2017;123(1): 12–6.
45. Sinha P, Haughey BH, Kallogjeri D, et al. The role of postoperative chemoradiation for oropharyngeal carcinoma: a critical appraisal revisited. Cancer 2016. [Epub ahead of print].
46. Hutcheson KA, Holsinger FC, Kupferman ME, et al. Functional outcomes after TORS for oropharyngeal cancer: a systematic review. Eur Arch Otorhinolaryngol 2015;272(2):463–71.
47. Leonhardt FD, Quon H, Abrahao M, et al. Transoral robotic surgery for oropharyngeal carcinoma and its impact on patient-reported quality of life and function. Head Neck 2012;34(2):146–54.
48. Ling DC, Chapman BV, Kim J, et al. Oncologic outcomes and patient-reported quality of life in patients with oropharyngeal squamous cell carcinoma treated with definitive transoral robotic surgery versus definitive chemoradiation. Oral Oncol 2016;61:41–6.
49. Standards and Datasets for Reporting Cancers. Datasets for histopathology reports on head and neck carcinomas and salivary neoplasms. London: The Royal College of Pathologists; 2005. Available at: http://www.spitalmures.ro/_files/protocoale_terapeutice/laborator/headneckdatasetjun05.pdf.
50. Meier JD, Oliver DA, Varvares MA. Surgical margin determination in head and neck oncology: current clinical practice. The results of an International American Head and Neck Society Member Survey. Head Neck 2005;27(11):952–8.
51. Alicandri-Ciufelli M, Bonali M, Piccinini A, et al. Surgical margins in head and neck squamous cell carcinoma: what is 'close'? Eur Arch Otorhinolaryngol 2013;270(10):2603–9.
52. Hinni ML, Ferlito A, Brandwein-Gensler MS, et al. Surgical margins in head and neck cancer: a contemporary review. Head Neck 2013;35(9):1362–70.
53. Lukens JN, Lin A, Gamerman V, et al. Late consequential surgical bed soft tissue necrosis in advanced oropharyngeal squamous cell carcinomas treated with transoral robotic surgery and postoperative radiation therapy. Int J Radiat Oncol Biol Phys 2014;89(5):981–8.
54. Lee YH, Kim YS, Chung MJ, et al. Soft tissue necrosis in head and neck cancer patients after transoral robotic surgery or wide excision with primary closure followed by radiation therapy. Medicine (Baltimore) 2016;95(9):e2852.
55. Evans M, Jones TM. Transoral surgery or radiotherapy for oropharyngeal carcinoma—is it either or…? Clin Oncol (R Coll Radiol 2016;28(7):413–20.
56. Yokota T, Onitsuka T, Kusafuka K, et al. Is postoperative adjuvant chemoradiotherapy necessary for high-risk oropharyngeal squamous cell carcinoma? Int J Clin Oncol 2014;19(1):38–44.

57. Maxwell JH, Ferris RL, Gooding W, et al. Extracapsular spread in head and neck carcinoma: impact of site and human papillomavirus status. Cancer 2013; 119(18):3302–8.
58. Sinha P, Lewis JS Jr, Piccirillo JF, et al. Extracapsular spread and adjuvant therapy in human papillomavirus-related, p16-positive oropharyngeal carcinoma. Cancer 2012;118(14):3519–30.
59. Kimple RJ, Smith MA, Blitzer GC, et al. Enhanced radiation sensitivity in HPV-positive head and neck cancer. Cancer Res 2013;73(15):4791–800.
60. Rieckmann T, Tribius S, Grob TJ, et al. HNSCC cell lines positive for HPV and p16 possess higher cellular radiosensitivity due to an impaired DSB repair capacity. Radiother Oncol 2013;107(2):242–6.
61. Marur S, Li S, Cmelak AJ, et al. E1308: phase II trial of induction chemotherapy followed by reduced-dose radiation and weekly cetuximab in patients with HPV-associated resectable squamous cell carcinoma of the oropharynx- ECOG-ACRIN Cancer Research Group. J Clin Oncol 2016 [Epub ahead of print]. JCO2016683300.
62. Mirghani H, Amen F, Tao Y, et al. Increased radiosensitivity of HPV-positive head and neck cancers: molecular basis and therapeutic perspectives. Cancer Treat Rev 2015;41(10):844–52.
63. Cleary C, Leeman JE, Higginson DS, et al. Biological features of human papillomavirus-related head and neck cancers contributing to improved response. Clin Oncol (R Coll Radiol) 2016;28(7):467–74.
64. Sinha P, Patrik P, Thorstad WL, et al. Does elimination of planned postoperative radiation to the primary bed in p16-positive, transorally-resected oropharyngeal carcinoma associate with poorer outcomes? Oral Oncol 2016;61:127–34.
65. Fried D, Lehman-Davis M, Willson A, et al. Dosimetric feasibility of sparing the primary site for oropharyngeal squamous cell carcinoma after transoral laser microsurgery in patients with unilateral positive neck nodes. Pract Radiat Oncol 2013; 3(4):282–6.

Updates in the Treatment of Breast Cancer with Radiotherapy

Serguei A. Castaneda, MD[a,b], Jon Strasser, MD[a,b,*]

KEYWORDS

- Breast cancer • Breast neoplasms • Radiotherapy
- Accelerated partial-breast irradiation • Hypofractionated whole-breast irradiation
- Intensity-modulated radiotherapy • Toxicity

KEY POINTS

- In early stage breast cancer and ductal carcinoma in situ, breast-conserving therapy with breast-conserving surgery and adjuvant radiotherapy is one of the most significant evidence-based advancements of modern cancer care.
- Accelerated partial breast irradiation and hypofractionated whole-breast radiation therapy provide shorter treatments with lower costs, while maintaining oncologic outcomes and cosmetic results.
- Multidisciplinary recommendations for acceptable margin status in invasive and noninvasive disease have been established; similar guidelines have been recently established in the postmastectomy setting.

INTRODUCTION

Breast-conserving surgery followed by radiation therapy is a widely accepted standard approach that allows for organ preservation in most early stage breast cancers.[1–3] Postmastectomy radiation therapy remains a widely accepted standard of care in the management of advanced breast cancer for appropriate indications.[4–6] Over the last several years, multidisciplinary guidelines have been updated to standardize prior controversies in breast cancer management with respect to margin status, use of postmastectomy radiation therapy, and use of advanced therapies, including accelerated partial breast radiation therapy.[7–10] In addition, new advances in the use of hypofractionated treatment are also gaining wide popularity because

[a] Department of Radiation Oncology, Helen F. Graham Cancer Center & Research Institute, Christiana Care Health System, 4701 Ogletown-Stanton Road, S-1110, Newark, DE 19713, USA; [b] Department of Radiation Oncology, Drexel University College of Medicine, 245 North 15th Street, MS #200, Philadelphia, PA 19102, USA
* Corresponding author.
E-mail address: jstrasser@christianacare.org

Surg Oncol Clin N Am 26 (2017) 371–382
http://dx.doi.org/10.1016/j.soc.2017.01.013
surgonc.theclinics.com

of their comparable toxicity profiles and ability to treat patients with a shorter course of therapy, thus adding value and cost savings to the management of breast cancer.[11] This article serves to update the reader with what's new in radiation therapy management of breast cancer with an emphasis on breast-conserving approaches. Please see Jean L. Wright and Arti Parekh's article, "Updates in Postmastectomy Radiation," in this issue, for more information on the topic.

HISTORICAL CONTEXT

Breast-conserving therapy with breast-conserving surgery and adjuvant radiotherapy for early stage breast cancer and ductal carcinoma in situ (DCIS) is one of the most remarkable achievements of evidenced-based modern cancer care. Moving away from the Halsteadian approach to breast cancer with radical mastectomy, Dr Fisher and his collaborators[1] completely changed the approach to management of early stage disease. Standard whole-breast radiotherapy (WBRT) has become the most widely accepted standard of care for most women diagnosed with early stage invasive breast cancer and DCIS who choose a breast-conserving approach. Radiation has been shown to reduce the risk of local recurrence in invasive cancer and noninvasive disease by 60% to 70% and 50% to 60%, respectively, as established by a myriad of trials conducted by the National Surgical Adjuvant Breast and Bowel Project (NSABP), European Organisation for Research and Treatment of Cancer (EORTC), and United Kingdom Coordinating Committee on Cancer Research.[1–3,12,13] The Early Breast Cancer Trialists' Collaborative Group (EBCTCG) meta-analyses have reported 15-year durable results, along with a breast cancer survival advantage in invasive disease.[14] Furthermore, significant evidence has been building on safe strategies to decrease the duration, length, dose, and cost of radiotherapy, while maintaining oncologic and cosmetic outcomes.

In advanced-stage breast cancer, there are more substantial challenges with the use of postmastectomy radiation to eliminate long-term potential complications; however, the evidence continues to support a wide indication for adjuvant radiotherapy with a local control benefit of 60% to 70% relative reduction in recurrence and a 10% improvement in absolute survival.[4–6] Significant technical advances allow delivery of radiation to target regions, including the internal mammary lymph node basin (IMNs), while reducing dose and toxicities to normal structures including the heart. The most recent consensus statement on postmastectomy radiation therapy from the Society of Surgical Oncology (SSO), American Society of Clinical Oncology (ASCO), and the American Society of Radiation Oncology (ASTRO) has potentially expanded the use of postmastectomy radiotherapy.[10]

CONSENSUS GUIDELINES ON MARGINS

Over the last 2 years, there have been significant agreements between several oncologic societies on margin assessment. In an era of multidisciplinary collaboration, the use of no ink on tumor as the standard for an adequate margin in invasive cancer has been endorsed by SSO, ASCO, and ASTRO.[7] This widely accepted consensus guideline aims to lower re-excision rates, improve cosmetic outcomes, and decrease health care costs, while maintaining low rates of ipsilateral breast tumor recurrences.[7] More recently, SSO, ASCO, and ASTRO developed a consensus guideline on margins in DCIS.[8] The standard adequate margin in DCIS treated with breast-conserving surgery and WBRT has been defined as a 2-mm margin from the DCIS edge.[8] This wider margin, compared with invasive disease, is based on the accepted notion that DCIS can have skip lesions and higher rates of recurrence with closer margins. The use of a 2-mm margin is designed to allow for adequate local control, while preserving breast anatomy with the smallest acceptable margins. The major area of continued uncertainty remains in tumors with mixed invasive and DCIS histologies, given the differences between the 2 competing guidelines. The ongoing approaches tend to reflect the predominant disease in the histology, with wider margins (2 mm) for invasive tumors with a large component of DCIS. For invasive tumors with small components of DCIS, no ink on tumor is a reasonable margin, as long as it is focal or involving only one margin. Re-excision would be recommended in patients with multiple close margins with DCIS or with broad fronts of DCIS at the margin edge. In addition, post-lumpectomy mammogram may be useful to identify the presence of residual calcifications, which could signify residual disease necessitating re-excision. The authors' preferred approach with all patients is to use the guidelines in a multidisciplinary approach with careful attention to pathologic details.

SHORT-COURSE BREAST RADIOTHERAPY

Accelerated Partial-Breast Irradiation

Accelerated partial breast irradiation (APBI) encompasses several effective approaches available for radiotherapy after breast-conserving surgery in selected patients with early stage breast cancer. These approaches include brachytherapy approaches with commercial balloon-based devices (MammoSite and Contura; Hologic [Marlborough, MA, USA]), commercial interstitial devices (strut adjusted volume implant [SAVI]; Cianna Medical [Aliso Viejo, CA, USA]), other interstitial catheter approaches, and 3-dimensional conformal external beam delivery approaches. ASTRO recently released a consensus statement based on the evidence-based support for APBI, which is an update to the consensus statement published in 2009, and proposed 3 patient groups: suitable, cautionary, and unsuitable.[9]

- Suitable: patients aged ≥50, negative margins by ≥2 mm, T stage of Tis or T1 (≤2 cm), and DCIS that meets all criteria (screen detected, low to intermediate nuclear grade, size ≤2.5 cm, and negative margins at ≥3 mm).
- Cautionary: patients aged 40 to 49 if all other criteria for "suitable" are met as well as patients aged ≥50 if they have at least 1 of the following criteria (size 2.1–3.0 cm, T stage T2, close margins at less than 2 mm, limited/focal lymphovascular space invasion, estrogen receptor negative, clinically unifocal with total size 2.1–3.0 cm, invasive lobular histology, pure DCIS ≤3 cm if criteria for "suitable" not fully met, and extensive intraductal component ≤3 cm).
- Unsuitable: patients aged ≤40, as well as patients aged 40 to 49 with no "cautionary" criteria, positive margins, and DCIS with size greater than 3 cm.

For the use of ABPI outside of a clinical trial, the Update Task Force proposed that it is acceptable for patients in the suitable group, that caution and concern should be applied when considering in the cautionary group, and it is not generally considered warranted in the unsuitable group. The American Brachytherapy Society consensus statement for APBI is less strict with respect to overall tumor parameters and defines appropriate patient selection through consideration of the following factors: age ≥50 year old, tumor size ≤3 cm, all invasive subtypes and DCIS, negative surgical margins, no lymphovascular space invasion, and negative nodal status.[15] The RTOG 0413/NSABP B39 trial allowed women with invasive or noninvasive disease less than 3 cm with 1 to 3 positive lymph nodes to be randomized to whole breast or APBI. The results of the RTOG 0413/NSABP B39 trial will give definitive results of the safety and efficacy of APBI in a diverse group of early stage patients compared with WBRT. In the authors' institution, they offer APBI for patients with early stage invasive cancer or DCIS, age greater than 50, who are lymph node negative, estrogen receptor positive, Her2/neu negative, with less than 3 cm of disease, and negative margins. The authors do use caution in those who have high-grade DCIS due to the lack of available data in these patients.

Brachytherapy for breast cancer was first developed using multicatheter interstitial implants, which are inserted using a free-hand technique often under image guidance. Significant limitations in terms of complexity, user dependence, logistics, conformality (accurate shape and scale), and reproducibility among patients prompted the development of device-based interstitial brachytherapy. Two of the more widely embraced single-entry catheter devices are multilumen balloon based and SAVI with 6 to 9 catheters. In the authors' experience, multichannel SAVI-based implants markedly reduces the maximum skin and chest wall doses, simultaneously achieving dose coverage to the target volume compared with balloon techniques. Also, differential-source dwell-loading allows modulation in the distribution of the radiation dose that leads to improved dosimetric conformality.[16] SAVI is safe and increases eligibility for APBI over balloon brachytherapy because the device can be safely placed closer to the skin (up to 3 mm) or chest wall with the ability to dose shape precisely.[17] It also has more consistency in the quality of the implant compared with a free-hand technique. Brachytherapy approaches typically deliver less radiation doses to the uninvolved ipsilateral breast, heart, and lung compared with external-beam radiation techniques.[18]

Multiple series have documented excellent clinical outcomes with interstitial APBI and balloon-based brachytherapy. Five-year outcomes demonstrate a 3.8% risk of local recurrence in more than 1400 patients with invasive cancer treated with MammoSite brachytherapy, and in 2.6% at 4 years in 300 patients treated with SAVI brachytherapy.[19,20] The NRG have reported on their experience of multicatheter brachytherapy with a 5.2% risk of local recurrence at 10 years in 100 patients.[21] A similar low risk of recurrence of 2.6% at 5 years was seen in 300 patients with DCIS treated with MammoSite brachytherapy.[22] It is important to note that these series typically reflect very favorable risk patients; however, there have so far been no safety signals from the RTOG/NSABP trial, suggesting this treatment may even become more widely available if the efficacy continues to be favorable.

Intraoperative radiotherapy is typically a single dose of radiation limited to the tumor bed at the time of breast-conserving surgery. Intraoperative radiotherapy can play a role in the decision of some patients of undergoing breast-conserving therapy over mastectomy, especially when factors such as long travel distances to the hospital, advanced age, or socioeconomic status have a significant influence. However, there are concerns about the efficacy of this modality based on the results of the TARGIT A and ELIOT trials that show a higher local recurrence at short follow-up compared with traditional treatment.[23,24] In the TARGIT A trial, local recurrence was 3.3% for intraoperative radiotherapy versus 1.3% for whole-breast radiotherapy, with an equivalent breast cancer mortality.[23] In the ELIOT trial, the local recurrence was within the prespecified margin but higher than with whole-breast radiotherapy, 4.4% versus 0.4%, with no difference in overall survival.[24] One of the principal issues with single fraction radiation is the lack of assessment of margin status at the time of treatment. In addition, there are concerns about dose accuracy, given the lack of imaging to assess that the applicator is intimately opposed to the breast tissues. Recent analyses of these trials reported that intraoperative radiotherapy had a significantly higher risk of ipsilateral breast tumor recurrence compared with WBRT but no significantly higher overall mortality.[25,26] Nonetheless, this treatment has established a foothold globally and in the United States and will likely continue to be used more regularly in selected low-risk patients, albeit with higher potential recurrence rates. However, there is further investigation ongoing to identify the subset of patients who may safely benefit from intraoperative radiotherapy. The previously described consensus guidelines for APBI highlight the importance of the prudent selection of suitable patients with low risk of local recurrence.[9]

External-beam radiotherapy for APBI has been studied with several types of radiation (ie, photons, electrons, and protons) as well as with various types of planning and delivery techniques, that is, 3 dimensional conformal radiotherapy (3D-CRT), intensity-modulated radiotherapy (IMRT), and TomoTherapy. In general, external-beam radiotherapy offers excellent target coverage and dose homogeneity but inferior conformality, when compared with brachytherapy, leading to increased doses to the uninvolved ipsilateral breast, skin, heart, and lung. Proton therapy may decrease the dose to the uninvolved ipsilateral breast, heart, and lung at the expense of a modest decrease in target coverage and an increased risk of skin toxicity.[27] Some of the early reports from the randomized NSABP B-39/RTOG 0413 protocol have demonstrated that 3D-CRT for ABPI resulted in a high rate of moderate to severe late normal tissue effects (10%), despite the relatively brief median follow-up period (15 months).[28] Finally, there is also interest in stereotactic body radiotherapy via CyberKnife as a means of APBI. CyberKnife radiosurgery for breast cancer is considered experimental today; however, early data demonstrate good feasibility and safety in brief median follow-up period (18 months).[29]

Hypofractionated Whole-Breast Irradiation

Prospective, randomized, phase 3 clinical trials evaluating hypofractionated whole-breast irradiation therapy (HWBI) conducted in Canada and the United Kingdom have matured and reported long-term 10-year or greater results.[11,30,31] These studies have established the role of HWBI in early stage breast cancer as an option endorsed by ASTRO in their Choosing Wisely Campaign. Local control has been equal, and cosmetic results and complications have been equal or better with accelerated hypofractionation compared with conventional fractionation with 10-year follow-up.[11,30,31] There are many potential benefits, including patient convenience, less cutaneous toxicity, and reduced cost of care. For these reasons, HWBI is now a standard option as an alternative to conventional fractionation for most women.

However, there has been some limitation in the extension of the overall positive results of HWBI to specific subgroups that were underrepresented in these phase 3 trials, including younger women. Based on the available data, HWBI may be safely offered to most women with DCIS or early stage invasive breast cancer treated by conventional whole-breast irradiation. However, there is still controversy about the use of HWBI in women aged less than 50 years, high-grade cancers, or tumors requiring a sequential tumor bed boost or chemotherapy before or after radiation. Large breast size or chest wall separation (distance from the midline to midaxillary line) is also a relative contraindication because of the heterogeneity of dose distribution in the breast—with larger breast size or separation leading to inhomogeneities of greater than 7%. Based on the Canadian experience, most radiation oncologists use a maximum of 7% inhomogeneity for consideration of HWBI.[11] However, improvements in radiation therapy equipment and planning techniques since the conduct of earlier HWBI studies may allow for previously ineligible patients to be considered for HWBI. Finally, HWBI studies have not included coverage of regional nodes, which increases the radiation volumes substantially, and potentially toxicity. Conventional fractionation remains the standard for women who have dose inhomogeneity greater than 7%, require chemotherapy, or need regional node irradiation.

REGIONAL NODAL MANAGEMENT

Management of the axilla in early stage disease has become more standardized after publication of the results of the ACOSOG Z11 trial.[32] This study randomized 891 women with clinically node negative disease who ultimately had a positive sentinel node biopsy (SNB) (2 or less lymph nodes) to axillary lymph node dissection versus no further surgery. All patients underwent lumpectomy and tangential whole-breast irradiation but they were not supposed to receive axillary-specific radiation. With a median follow-up of 6.3 years, there was no difference in disease-free survival or overall survival, but there were less axillary seromas, wound infections, axillary paresthesias, and lymphedema.[33] Almost immediately, SNB became standard in those with 2 or fewer lymph nodes involved with no clinically apparent axillary disease. Axillary dissection has been reserved for those with 3 or more positive lymph nodes. However, the remaining controversy from the Z11 trial is whether lymph nodes basins were radiated. Although not all radiation records were evaluable, of those that were evaluable, half had high tangents that would have covered some of the low nodal basin and 15% of overall patients had coverage of the supraclavicular region.[34]

High tangential photons increase the superior border of a traditional breast field by about 2 cm to the humeral head and can allow reasonable radiation dose coverage to the level 1 and 2 lymph nodes, without any significant increase in toxicity, particularly lymphedema. Based on this, the authors' institution will often use high tangential photon fields in the setting of 2 or fewer involved sentinel nodes to cover potential subclinical microscopic disease in adjacent lymph nodes. In patients wherein SNB has more than 2 positive lymph nodes, completion axillary lymph node dissection should be performed, and the radiation therapy volumes should be determined by the finding in the breast and regional nodal dissection. In the absence of a completion dissection, the authors recommend more comprehensive nodal irradiation.

When regional lymph nodes are positive, there is also evidence that full regional nodal radiation therapy may be of benefit. The MA.20 trial randomized 1832 women receiving breast-conserving surgery with node positive or high-risk node negative breast cancer (tumor >5 cm or >2 cm with <10 axillary nodes removed) to whole-breast irradiation with or without regional nodal irradiation (inclusive of the axillary nodes, supraclavicular nodes, and IMNs) after surgical resection and axillary dissection with systemic chemotherapy.[35] At 10 years, the addition of regional nodal irradiation increased relative disease-free survival by 24% (absolute 5% improvement) with reductions in both isolated locoregional and distant recurrences. There was no survival difference in the published data, but lymphedema rates in the presence of an axillary dissection and regional nodal radiation were nearly doubled.[35]

The EORTC has also recently published results on regional nodal radiation therapy, inclusive of the IMN and medial supraclavicular nodal basins.[36] This study randomized 4004 patients with medial/central lesions (stage I, II, or III) or those with lateral lesions with axillary involvement to cover regional nodes, including the IMN chain versus no regional nodal irradiation, while still receiving breast or chest wall radiation. With 10 years of follow-up, those receiving IMN radiation had significantly improved disease-free survival of 72.1% versus 69.1%. Distant disease-free survival and breast cancer mortality were also improved at 10 years in the regional nodal irradiation arm, 78% versus 75% and 12.5% versus 14.4%, respectively. Overall survival had a borderline trend significant benefit, 82.3% in the irradiation arm versus 80.7% with a *P* value of 0.06.[36]

The extent of regional nodal radiation remains somewhat controversial. Most major studies that have demonstrated the benefits of regional nodal radiation included the lower and upper axillary lymphatic basins (level 1–3 and supraclavicular lymph nodes) as well as the IMN chain. The Danish Breast Cancer Cooperative Group evaluated node-positive patients in a prospective manner with standard breast/chest wall radiotherapy in the nonresected axilla setting.[37] Although not randomized, patients with right-sided cancer had treatment of the IMNs, while left-sided patients did not have IMN irradiation. The IMN irradiated group demonstrated a statistically improved overall survival at 8 years of 3.7% (72.2% vs 75.9%) and a significant decrease in breast cancer mortality (23.4% vs 20.9%). The benefit appeared to be most significant in the subgroup of high-risk patients with medial/central disease and extensive involvement of axillary nodes. Those with lateral lesions and 1 to 3 lymph nodes appeared to have no benefit.

A similar trial conducted in France evaluated the role of IMN coverage in 1334 patients with positive axillary lymph nodes or central tumors without positive axillary lymph nodes after mastectomy.[38] With a median follow-up of 11.3 years, overall survival was nonsignificant at 62.6% versus 59.3%. The investigators in this study did look at different risk criteria (medial/central and node negative, node positive, and use of chemotherapy). There was no overall survival benefit in any of these subgroups.

IMN irradiation typically increases the volume of tissues radiated fairly significantly. Although there are several techniques for IMN coverage, most techniques increase both lung and heart doses (for left-sided cancers) and potentially increase the complexity of setup. Cardiac toxicity, although overall rare in long-term survivors, is a significant potential toxicity. Darby and colleagues[39] conducted a population-based case-control study in Sweden and Denmark, which evaluated the association between external beam radiation and cardiac dose/events. They identified 963 patients with major coronary events with 44% occurring within 10 years of treatment, 33% occurring at 10 to 19 years, and 23% occurring more than 20 years after treatment. Mean heart doses were as high as 6.6 Gy in women treated with left-sided breast cancer. The rate of major coronary events increased by 7.4% for each increase in mean heart dose of 1 Gy. This study, however, was conducted with patients treated as far back as the 1950s, when computed tomographic–based radiotherapy plans were not available. The authors estimated the actual cardiac doses based on assumptions of little variation in cardiac anatomy in patients. In addition, in modern medicine, there is more control of modifiable risk factors including dyslipidemias treated with statin, hypertension treated with antihypertensives, and smoking with decreased tobacco exposure. Modern series of radiation between right and left breast radiation show no increase in cardiac toxicity.[40] Nonetheless, most radiation oncologists strive to keep heart dose as low as reasonably achievable and a mean dose less than 4 Gy.[39]

In early September 2016, SSO, ASCO, and ASTRO released an updated multidisciplinary consensus statement on the role of postmastectomy radiation therapy.[10] This statement was an update to previous SSO, ASCO, and ASTRO guidelines released in 2001 and reviewed published literature from 2001 to 2015 and the EBCTGC Meta Analysis from 2014.[41] Although this update is focused on postmastectomy patients, there is some relevance to extrapolation to node-positive patients in the breast conservation arena. This update attempted to focus on 4 areas of controversy: 1 to 3 positive lymph nodes, T1/T2 lesions with positive SNB, neoadjuvant chemotherapy, and extent of regional nodal irradiation. For more information on this topic, please see Jean L. Wright and Arti Parekh's article, "Updates in Postmastectomy Radiation," in this issue.

Two current trials are attempting to clarify how to handle patients who convert to nodal negativity or remain node positive and are relevant to both the postmastectomy and breast conservation populations. For patients who are biopsy-proven node positive, the Alliance A011202 trial randomizes women with residual nodal positivity by SNB after neoadjuvant chemotherapy to completion axillary lymph node dissection versus radiation therapy encompassing the regional nodes. In those women who experience a pathologic complete response on SNB to neoadjuvant chemotherapy, they are offered randomization on the NRG 9353 study to regional nodal radiotherapy versus no regional nodal radiotherapy. These trials should help to identify the role of radiation therapy to the axilla based on response of SNB to neoadjuvant chemotherapy.

Finally, the consensus panel attempted to give some guidance on the extent of regional nodal radiation therapy. As previously cited in this article, regional nodal basins include the axillary lymphatics (inclusive of level 1, 2, and 3), the supraclavicular basin, and the internal mammary nodal chain.[35–37] Although there is clear agreement on treating some variation of axillary and supraclavicular nodal basins, based on the finding of axillary sentinel node procedure or dissection, the treatment of the internal mammary nodal basin has been less clear. In the EBCTCG meta-analysis, 20 of 22 trials included the IMN basin, and hence, weighed heavily on the panel's recommendations.[10,42] The data suggest a small benefit (1%–5%) to local recurrence and breast cancer mortality with more extensive regional nodal radiation therapy, albeit with the potential for more toxicity to adjacent organs.[35,36,42] The panel recommended treatment to generally include the supraclavicular and axillary apical nodes as well as the IMNs for patients with positive nodes but acknowledged there may be subgroups with limited benefit.[10] However, given limited evidence, they were unable to define subgroups with limited benefit to inclusion of IMN irradiation. The general consensus in the radiation oncology community is that IMN radiation should be at least strongly considered in women with large medial tumors or with lateral tumors with axillary node involvement.

At the authors' institution, they use a multidisciplinary conference to evaluate the extent of axillary involvement to define the extent of the volumes related to axillary nodal radiation (full axilla vs coverage of just the level 3 and supraclavicular basin). They evaluate factors such as percent of positive involved lymph nodes, presence of lymphatic vascular invasion, and the presence of extracapsular extension. In general, after a complete axillary dissection with more than 10 lymph nodes removed, the authors recommend no coverage of the low basin of axillary lymphatics (levels 1 and 2), as recurrence is generally rare after axillary lymph node dissection and the risks for lymphedema are markedly increased.[43] However, if there is extensive positive lymph node involvement (either clinically or pathologically) or a less than adequate dissection is performed, they would cover the entire axillary nodal basin. After neoadjuvant chemotherapy, they base the extent of axillary coverage on the extent of dissection and cover undissected basins and consider dissected regions if there are residual high-risk features (including extensively involved nodes or extracapsular extension). The authors will consider IMN coverage based on tumor location and presence of axillary involvement as previously mentioned, but also evaluate the potential risks and benefits to adjacent tissues, including heart and lung. Finally, they always consider patients for any open clinical trials that may help to further advance cancer treatment strategies.

SUMMARY

In early stage breast cancer and DCIS, breast-conserving therapy with breast-conserving surgery and adjuvant radiotherapy is one of the most significant evidence-based advancements of modern cancer care. Breast-conserving therapy allows organ preservation while maintaining excellent outcomes for the vast majority of patients. APBI and HWBI provide shorter treatments with lower costs, while maintaining oncologic outcomes and cosmetic results. Multidisciplinary recommendations for acceptable margin status in invasive and noninvasive disease have been established. Similar guidelines have recently also been established in the postmastectomy setting.

The authors have further defined the indications, efficacy, and toxicity of regional nodes irradiation in the breast-conserving surgery setting. Recent advances in radiation oncology treatment planning and delivery have resulted in clinically meaningful reduction in toxicity, in many cases also improving cosmetic results. Most notably, forward-calculation algorithms with field-in-field techniques allow more CRT planning, leading to a decrease in toxicity. Improvement in cardiac dosing with use of IMRT and volumetric-modulated arc therapy is achievable in select patients for the treatment of left-sided breast cancers and chest wall irradiation. IMRT may allow for acceptable coverage of larger volumes of regional nodes.

Ongoing studies aim to further establish the role of specific methods of APBI as well as interactions between radiotherapy and neoadjuvant chemotherapy with the need for coverage of regional lymph nodes based on pathologic response. The future will integrate molecular profiles of specific tumor subtypes with the selection of the best modality and timing of treatments.

REFERENCES

1. Fisher B, Anderson S, Bryant J, et al. Twenty-year follow-up of a randomized trial comparing total for the treatment of invasive breast cancer. N Engl J Med 2002; 347(16):1233–41.
2. Veronesi U, Cascinelli N, Mariani L, et al. Twenty-year follow-up of a randomized study comparing breast-conserving surgery with radical mastectomy for early breast cancer. N Engl J Med 2002;347(16):1227–32.
3. van Dongen JA, Voogd AC, Fentiman IS, et al. Long-term results of a randomized trial comparing breast-conserving therapy with mastectomy: European Organization for Research and Treatment of Cancer 10801 trial. J Natl Cancer Inst 2000; 92(14):1143–50.
4. Overgaard M, Jensen MB, Overgaard J, et al. Postoperative radiotherapy in high-risk postmenopausal breast-cancer patients given adjuvant tamoxifen: Danish Breast Cancer Cooperative Group DBCG 82c randomised trial. Lancet 1999; 353(9165):1641–8.
5. Overgaard M, Hansen P, Overgaard J, et al. Postoperative radiotherapy in high-risk premenopausal women with breast cancer who receive adjuvant chemotherapy. Danish Breast Cancer Cooperative Group 82b Trial. N Engl J Med 1997;337(14):949–55.
6. Ragaz J, Olivotto IA, Spinelli JJ, et al. Locoregional radiation therapy in patients with high-risk breast cancer receiving adjuvant chemotherapy: 20-year results of the British Columbia randomized trial. J Natl Cancer Inst 2005;97(2):116–26.
7. Buchholz TA, Somerfield MR, Griggs JJ, et al. Margins for breast-conserving surgery with whole-breast irradiation in stage I and II invasive breast cancer: American Society of Clinical Oncology endorsement of the Society of Surgical Oncology/American Society for Radiation Oncology consensus guideline. J Clin Oncol 2014;32(14):1502–6.
8. Morrow M, Van Zee KJ, Solin LJ, et al. Society of Surgical Oncology–American Society for Radiation Oncology–American Society of Clinical Oncology Consensus

guideline on margins for breast-conserving surgery with whole-breast irradiation in ductal carcinoma in situ. Pract Radiat Oncol 2016;6(5):287–95.
9. Correa C, Harris EE, Leonardi MC, et al. Accelerated partial breast irradiation: executive summary for the update of an ASTRO evidence-based consensus statement. Pract Radiat Oncol 2016. http://dx.doi.org/10.1016/j.prro.2016.09.007.
10. Recht A, Comen EA, Fine RE, et al. Postmastectomy radiotherapy: an American Society of Clinical Oncology, American Society for Radiation Oncology, and Society of Surgical Oncology Focused Guideline Update. Pract Radiat Oncol 2016;6(6):e219–34.
11. Whelan TJ, Pignol J-P, Levine MN, et al. Long-term results of hypofractionated radiation therapy for breast cancer. N Engl J Med 2010;362(11):513–20.
12. Bijker N, Meijnen P, Peterse JL, et al. Breast-conserving treatment with or without radiotherapy in ductal carcinoma-in-situ: ten-year results of European Organisation for Research and Treatment of Cancer randomized phase III trial 10853–a study by the EORTC Breast Cancer Cooperative Group and. J Clin Oncol 2006;24(21):3381–7.
13. Houghton J. Radiotherapy and tamoxifen in women with completely excised ductal carcinoma in situ of the breast in the UK, Australia, and New Zealand: randomised controlled trial. Lancet 2003;362(9378):95–102.
14. Darby S, McGale P, Correa C, et al. Effect of radiotherapy after breast-conserving surgery on 10-year recurrence and 15-year breast cancer death: meta-analysis of individual patient data for 10,801 women in 17 randomised trials. Lancet 2011; 378(9804):1707–16.
15. Shah C, Vicini F, Wazer DE, et al. The American Brachytherapy Society consensus statement for accelerated partial breast irradiation. Brachytherapy 2013. http://dx.doi.org/10.1016/j.brachy.2013.02.001.
16. Manoharan SR, Rodriguez RR, Bobba VS, et al. Dosimetry evaluation of SAVI-based HDR brachytherapy for partial breast irradiation. J Med Phys 2010;353: 131–6.
17. Yashar CM, Scanderbeg D, Kuske R, et al. Initial clinical experience with the Strut-Adjusted Volume Implant (SAVI) breast brachytherapy device for accelerated partial-breast irradiation (APBI): first 100 patients with more than 1 year of follow-up. Int J Radiat Oncol Biol Phys 2011;80(3):765–70.
18. Scanderbeg D, Yashar C, White G, et al. Evaluation of three APBI techniques under NSABP B-39 guidelines. J Appl Clin Med Phys 2009;11(1):3021.
19. Shah C, Badiyan S, Ben Wilkinson J, et al. Treatment efficacy with accelerated partial breast irradiation (APBI): final analysis of the American Society of Breast Surgeons MammoSite(®) Breast Brachytherapy Registry Trial. Ann Surg Oncol 2013;20(10):3279–85.
20. Yashar C, Attai D, Butler E, et al. Strut-based accelerated partial breast irradiation: report of treatment results for 250 consecutive patients at 5 years from a multicenter retrospective study. Brachytherapy 2016;15(6):780–7.
21. White J, Winter K, Kuske RR, et al. Long-term cancer outcomes from study NRG Oncology/RTOG 9517: a phase 2 study of accelerated partial breast irradiation with multicatheter brachytherapy after lumpectomy for early-stage breast cancer. Int J Radiat Oncol Biol Phys 2016;95(5):1460–5.
22. Vicini F, Shah C, Ben Wilkinson J, et al. Should ductal carcinoma-in-situ (DCIS) be removed from the ASTRO consensus panel cautionary group for off-protocol use of accelerated partial breast irradiation (APBI)? A pooled analysis of outcomes for 300 patients with DCIS treated with APBI. Ann Surg Oncol 2013;20(4):1275–81.

23. Vaidya JS, Wenz F, Bulsara M, et al. Risk-adapted targeted intraoperative radiotherapy versus whole-breast radiotherapy for breast cancer: 5-year results for local control and overall survival from the TARGIT-A randomised trial. Lancet 2014;383(9917):603–13.
24. Veronesi U, Orecchia R, Maisonneuve P, et al. Intraoperative radiotherapy versus external radiotherapy for early breast cancer (ELIOT): a randomised controlled equivalence trial. Lancet Oncol 2013. http://dx.doi.org/10.1016/S1470-2045(13)70497-2.
25. Silverstein MJ, Fastner G, Maluta S, et al. Intraoperative radiation therapy: a critical analysis of the ELIOT and TARGIT trials. Part 1–ELIOT. Ann Surg Oncol 2014;21(12):3787–92.
26. Silverstein MJ, Fastner G, Maluta S, et al. Intraoperative radiation therapy: a critical analysis of the ELIOT and TARGIT trials. Part 2–TARGIT. Ann Surg Oncol 2014;21(12):3793–9.
27. Cuaron JJ, MacDonald SM, Cahlon O. Novel applications of proton therapy in breast carcinoma. Chin Clin Oncol 2016;5(4):52.
28. Hepel JT, Tokita M, MacAusland SG, et al. Toxicity of three-dimensional conformal radiotherapy for accelerated partial breast irradiation. Int J Radiat Oncol Biol Phys 2009;75(5):1290–6.
29. Obayomi-Davies O, Kole TP, Oppong B, et al. Stereotactic accelerated partial breast irradiation for early-stage breast cancer: rationale, feasibility, and early experience using the CyberKnife radiosurgery delivery platform. Front Oncol 2016;6:129.
30. Bentzen SM, Agrawal RK, Aird EGA, et al. The UK Standardisation of Breast Radiotherapy (START) Trial A of radiotherapy hypofractionation for treatment of early breast cancer: a randomised trial. Lancet Oncol 2008;9(4):331–41.
31. Bentzen SM, Agrawal RK, Aird EGA, et al. The UK Standardisation of Breast Radiotherapy (START) Trial B of radiotherapy hypofractionation for treatment of early breast cancer: a randomised trial. Lancet 2008;371(9618):1098–107.
32. Giuliano AE, Hunt KK, Ballman KV, et al. Axillary dissection vs no axillary dissection in women with invasive breast cancer and sentinel node metastasis: a randomized clinical trial. JAMA 2011;305(6):569–75.
33. Lucci A, McCall LM, Beitsch PD, et al. Surgical complications associated with sentinel lymph node dissection (SLND) plus axillary lymph node dissection compared with SLND alone in the American College of Surgeons Oncology Group Trial Z0011. J Clin Oncol 2007;25(24):3657–63.
34. Jagsi R, Chadha M, Moni J, et al. Radiation field design in the ACOSOG Z0011 (Alliance) trial. J Clin Oncol 2014. http://dx.doi.org/10.1200/JCO.2014.56.5838.
35. Whelan TJ, Olivotto IA, Parulekar WR, et al. Regional nodal irradiation in early-stage breast cancer. N Engl J Med 2015;373(4):307–16.
36. Poortmans PM, Collette S, Kirkove C, et al. Internal mammary and medial supraclavicular irradiation in breast cancer. N Engl J Med 2015;373(4):317–27.
37. Thorsen LBJ, Offersen BV, Dano H, et al. DBCG-IMN: a population-based cohort study on the effect of internal mammary node irradiation in early node-positive breast cancer. J Clin Oncol 2016;34(4):314–20.
38. Hennequin C, Bossard N, Servagi-Vernat S, et al. Ten-year survival results of a randomized trial of irradiation of internal mammary nodes after mastectomy. Int J Radiat Oncol Biol Phys 2013. http://dx.doi.org/10.1016/j.ijrobp.2013.03.021.
39. Darby SC, Ewertz M, McGale P, et al. Risk of ischemic heart disease in women after radiotherapy for breast cancer. N Engl J Med 2013;368(11):987–98.

40. Patt DA, Goodwin JS, Kuo Y-F, et al. Cardiac morbidity of adjuvant radiotherapy for breast cancer. J Clin Oncol 2005;23(30):7475–82.
41. Recht A, Edge SB, Solin LJ, et al. Postmastectomy radiotherapy: clinical practice guidelines of the American Society of Clinical Oncology. J Clin Oncol 2001;19(5): 1539–69.
42. McGale P, Taylor C, Correa C, et al. Effect of radiotherapy after mastectomy and axillary surgery on 10-year recurrence and 20-year breast cancer mortality: meta-analysis of individual patient data for 8135 women in 22 randomised trials. Lancet 2014;383(9935):2127–35.
43. Recht A, Houlihan MJ. Axillary lymph nodes and breast cancer: a review. Cancer 1995;76(9):1491–512.

Updates in Postmastectomy Radiation

Jean L. Wright, MD*, Arti Parekh, MD

KEYWORDS

- Mastectomy • Postmastectomy • Radiation • Clinical risk factors
- Locoregional failure

KEY POINTS

- Locoregional failure rates after postmastectomy radiation have decreased in the modern era because of multiple factors.
- In patients with 1 to 3 positive nodes, additional clinical and pathologic risk factors must be considered when recommending treatment.
- Postmastectomy radiation is recommended in certain patients with node-negative disease who have high-risk features.
- Increased use of neoadjuvant chemotherapy in early breast cancer creates clinical challenges in patient selection for postmastectomy radiation, and increasing data suggest that response to treatment may be used to tailor locoregional therapy recommendations in selected patients.

Radiation therapy has been used for decades to eradicate occult microscopic disease in the postmastectomy chest wall and draining regional nodal basins, thereby decreasing locoregional failure (LRF) and even improving survival end points in select patients.

Many of the historic data clinicians use to guide the use of postmastectomy radiation therapy (PMRT) includes patients treated in the 1970s and 1980s, an era in which LRF was substantially higher than it is now. Since the publication of the landmark randomized studies showing the benefits of PMRT, there has been a marked decrease in LRF among patients with breast cancer after mastectomy because of multiple factors.[1–4] These factors include improved diagnostic and staging tools, earlier stage at diagnosis, improved surgical techniques, and increasingly effective systemic therapies. In light of this, this article provides updates on recommendations regarding PMRT based on contemporary data.

Disclosure: The authors have nothing to disclose
Department of Radiation Oncology and Molecular Radiation Sciences, Johns Hopkins University, Suite 1440, 401 North Broadway, Baltimore, MD 21231, USA
* Corresponding author.
E-mail address: jwrigh71@jhmi.edu

Surg Oncol Clin N Am 26 (2017) 383–392
http://dx.doi.org/10.1016/j.soc.2017.01.010
surgonc.theclinics.com

PMRT FOR 1 TO 3 POSITIVE NODES

The use of PMRT in the setting of 4 or more positive lymph nodes has been broadly accepted because of the high risk of LRF in this population; however, controversy remains regarding the utility of PMRT in patients with 1 to 3 positive nodes. The Early Breast Cancer Trialists' Collaborative Group (EBCTCG) updated their meta-analysis on the role of PMRT in 2014.[1] The meta-analysis included 22 trials and 8135 patients with breast cancer between 1964 and 1986 who were randomly assigned to receive chest wall and regional nodal radiotherapy after mastectomy and axillary dissection. A subset analysis of 1133 patients with 1 to 3 positive nodes who had received systemic therapy showed a LRF rate of 21% without irradiation and 4.3% with PMRT at 10 years ($P<.001$). The 10-year rate for any recurrence, either local or distant, was 45.5% without radiation and 33.8% with radiation ($P<.001$). Moreover, breast cancer mortalities were 49.4% and 41.5% ($P = .01$) without radiation and with radiation, respectively. These data support the benefit of PMRT in preventing both LRF and overall recurrence, as well as improving breast cancer mortality. Although these numbers are clearly supportive of the benefits of PMRT, most patients included in the EBCTCG analysis were included in randomized trials conducted in the 1970s and 1980s and broadly grouped patients by nodal stage but not other more recently elucidated risk factors for recurrence such as receptor status, age, lymphovascular invasion (LVI), grade, and other pathologic features.[2–4] In the current era, rates of LRF seem to be considerably lower than the rates mentioned earlier, and are understood to vary substantially with risk factors for recurrence. The trend toward lower rates of LRF in more recent years is highlighted in a study from the MD Anderson Cancer Center in which a cohort of 1027 patients with T1 to T2 breast cancer with 1 to 3 positive lymph nodes treated with mastectomy and systemic therapy with or without PMRT were analyzed by treatment era.[5] Specifically, those treated in an early era (1978–1997) were compared with those treated in a later era (2000–2007). In the early cohort, PMRT was observed to decrease 5-year rates of LRF from 9.5% to 3.4% ($P = .028$). However in the later cohort, PMRT did not seem to significantly decrease rates of LRF, and 5-year rates of LRF without PMRT were only 2.8%. Overall in modern series, rates of LRF in patients treated with mastectomy and systemic therapy without radiation generally range from 4% to 23% (with most studies ranging from 4% to 10%) depending on risk factors.[5–8]

Several contemporary retrospective studies have highlighted the significance of specific risk factors for recurrence in determining the utility of PMRT in patients with 1 to 3 positive nodes. Moo and colleagues[9] published a retrospective analysis of 1331 patients with T1 to T2 tumors with 1 to 3 positive nodes who underwent mastectomy with or without PMRT. The overall rate of LRF in the no-PMRT group was 4.3%. On a multivariate analysis of patients in the no-PMRT group, both age less than or equal to 50 years and lymphovascular invasion (LVI) were significantly associated with increased risk of LRF, suggesting that these factors warrant consideration of PMRT in this cohort. Similarly, Yildirim and Berberoglu[8] published a study of patients with T1 to T2 tumors with 1 to 3 positive nodes who were observed without PMRT, and the overall rate of LRF was 4.3% at a median follow-up time of 70 months. On multivariate analysis, age less than or equal to 35 years, LVI, and ratio of positive nodes greater than 15% were the most important prognostic factors for LRF. Moreover, patients with 2 or 3 of the risk factors mentioned earlier had a LRF rate of 23%, compared with 2.7% among those who had only 1 risk factor. Both these studies highlight the importance of individual clinical-pathologic risk factors when evaluating the benefit of PMRT in patients with 1 to 3 positive nodes.

In 2008, Kyndi and colleagues[10] published an analysis of a cohort of patients from the Danish Breast Cancer Cooperative Group (DBCG) protocol trials 82b and 82c in whom receptor status had been retrospectively analyzed, examining the impact of receptor status on benefit from PMRT. Although a locoregional control benefit was seen in all subgroups with the addition of PMRT, the greatest benefit was seen in patients with estrogen-receptor (ER)–positive disease, and the least in ER-negative disease. Improvement in overall survival with the addition of PMRT was seen in ER-positive and progesterone receptor (PR)–positive disease but not ER-negative and PR-negative disease. This study predated the era of HER2 targeted therapy and is thus not useful in assessing the impact of PMRT in HER2-positive disease in the current era. However, a recent analysis of the National Comprehensive Cancer Center Breast Outcomes Database again showed the highest risk of LRF and the least reduction in LRF with PMRT in the setting of triple-negative disease, as well as a very low risk of LRF in HER2-positive disease in the setting of HER2 targeted therapy with or without PMRT.[11] Triple-negative receptor status in particular has emerged as a significant risk factor for LRF, and although the risk reduction with PMRT is smallest in this group, the benefit remains significant and triple-negative receptor status is generally considered an indication for PMRT in the setting of 1 to 3 positive nodes. With increasing data showing a locoregional control benefit with HER2 targeted therapy, there is no clear consensus on HER2 status as an indication for PMRT.[12]

The most recent randomized data informing our PMRT decisions stems from the recent MA.20 and European Organisation for Research and Treatment of Cancer (EORTC) studies, which assessed the benefit of regional nodal irradiation (RNI) in addition to standard whole-breast irradiation.[13,14] Although both studies included primarily women undergoing breast-conserving surgery, the benefit of RNI can be extrapolated to PMRT in node-positive patients, given that PMRT has historically included RNI. In MA.20, patients with either node-positive or high-risk node-negative disease were randomized to whole-breast irradiation (WBI) alone or with RNI (including internal mammary nodes, supraclavicular and level III axillary nodes). Most patients (85%) had 1 to 3 positive nodes. Although no difference in overall survival was observed, RNI conferred a significant improvement in both locoregional and distant disease-free survival. At 10 years, the incidence of LRF and distant metastasis (DM), respectively, was 4.5% and 12.9% for the WBI plus RNI group, compared with 7.2% and 16.5% for the WBI-alone group. Similarly, in the EORTC 22922 study reported by Poortmans and colleagues[14] 4004 women with either medially located tumors (regardless of nodal involvement) or tumors in any part of the breast with axillary node positivity were randomized to WBI alone or with RNI. As in MA.20, no overall survival benefit was seen; however, LRF, distant disease-free survival, and breast cancer mortality were all significantly improved. Rates of LRF and DM in the WBI group, respectively, were 9.5% and 19.6%, compared with 8.3% and 15.9% in the WBI plus RNI group. Although these studies primarily included patients treated with breast conservation, and LRF outcomes may therefore not correlate with the PMRT setting, they are relevant because they allow clinicians to extrapolate a potential DM and disease-free survival benefit with PMRT/RNI even in the modern era. Most editorials discussing the impact of these key studies suggest consideration of risk factors and individual patient characteristics in estimating the benefit of PMRT/RNI, but generally support the conclusion that overall recurrence and disease-free survival benefits may be observed in addition to locoregional control in selected patients.[15,16]

Current National Comprehensive Cancer Network guidelines suggest that, in patients who have undergone total mastectomy with axillary staging and have 1 to 3 positive nodes, PMRT to the chest wall and comprehensive nodal regions should be "strongly considered." New American Society of Clinical Oncology (ASCO), American Society for Radiation Oncology (ASTRO), Society of Surgical Oncology (SSO) guidelines for PMRT recently addressed this cohort and issued consensus recommendations to evaluate the need for PMRT in a multidisciplinary setting and to consider a multitude of factors, including life expectancy, tumor size, biological characteristics, and plans for systemic therapy, in weighing the risks and benefits of radiation.[17] In addition, smaller institutional series support strong consideration of PMRT in patients with T1, T2 disease and 1 to 3 positive nodes who are also younger ($\leq$50 years), have LVI, triple-negative disease, skin or nipple invasion, or several of these factors.[5,9]

Another challenge for clinicians that has become more common after the publication of American College of Surgeons Oncology Group (ACOSOG) Z-11 and the AMAROS trial (After mapping of the axilla: radiotherapy or surgery) is determining the role of PMRT in patients who have had a positive sentinel node biopsy without axillary dissection (ALND).[18,19] In patients who undergo mastectomy and have a positive sentinel node biopsy and do not proceed to ALND, the joint ASCO-ASTRO-SSO panel has recommended to proceed with PMRT only if there is sufficient evidence to recommend adjuvant radiation with the available clinical and pathologic information, and without further information from an ALND.[17] Otherwise, ALND is recommended. There remains substantial debate about which sentinel node–positive patients, if any, can forego both ALND and PMRT, because there are few data to guide clinicians in this area. Data from the International Breast Cancer Study Group 23-01 trial suggest no increase in LRF with the omission of PMRT in the setting of micrometastatic sentinel node–positive disease only, and thus it is reasonable to consider omission of PMRT in this setting, weighing additional risk factors for recurrence in the decision.[20]

NODE-NEGATIVE DISEASE WITH HIGH-RISK FEATURES

Another debated area regarding appropriateness for PMRT is node-negative patients with large tumors (>5 cm) or other high-risk features. In the older and historically referenced Danish 82b and 82c studies, outcomes supported the role of radiotherapy for both node-positive and node-negative patients with large primary tumors.[2,4] For example, for those 135 node-negative patients with large primary tumors included in the 82b randomized trial, LRF was 3% among patients treated with chemotherapy and radiation and 17% in those treated with chemotherapy alone. Similarly, in the 82c trial, among 132 node-negative patients, LRF occurred in 6% of patients treated with radiation and tamoxifen and in 23% of those who received tamoxifen alone. However, contemporary series again show lower rates of locoregional recurrence in patients with large node-negative tumors compared with the Danish studies.[7,21–23] For example, in a retrospective series of 877 node-negative postmastectomy patients treated at Massachusetts General Hospital, the overall cumulative incidence of LRF was 6%; however, many risk factors were identified that could be used to predict higher rates of LRF. These risk factors included premenopausal status, margins less than 2 mm, LVI, and tumor greater than 2 cm.[24] Similarly, in a series of 1505 patients with T1-2N0 breast cancer and mastectomy alone in British Columbia, an overall LRF rate of 7.8% was observed, with higher rates in patients with LVI, higher tumor stage and grade, and lack of systemic therapy.[23] Receptor status is also an important consideration in assessing risk of LRF in this population, as it is in the node-positive population. Tseng and colleagues[11] evaluated 5637 patients with stage I to III breast cancer who underwent mastectomy with or without PMRT and found that those with triple-negative disease had the highest rate of LRF at 5.25%.

The role of PMRT in the context of close or positive margins has also been debated. Several retrospective studies have explored this question, including a large study from Massachusetts General Hospital that analyzed 877 node-negative patients who did not receive PMRT. Patients with negative margins had a 10-year LRF of 5.1%, compared with 22% in patients with close margins and 21% in patients with positive margins ($P<.001$).[24] In another study of 397 women who underwent observation after mastectomy for invasive breast cancer diagnosed between 1998 and 2005, margins status was also significantly associated with LRF.[23] Patients with positive margins had a 5-year LRF of 6.2%, whereas patients with close and negative margins had 5-year LRF of 1.5% and 1.9%, respectively. In summary, PMRT can be considered for patients with node-negative disease in the setting of multiple adverse clinical and pathologic risk factors, including large tumor size (>5 cm), positive margins, age less than 50 years, higher grade, and adverse biological subtype as discussed earlier.

CONSIDERATIONS FOR POSTMASTECTOMY RADIATION AFTER NEOADJUVANT CHEMOTHERAPY

The data discussed thus far regarding PMRT in breast cancer management have included patients who received up-front surgery with or without systemic therapy. However, administration of neoadjuvant chemotherapy (NAC) before surgery has gained popularity in breast cancer because of its ability to increase the likelihood of breast conservation, the prognostic value of response to NAC, and the potential to use response to tailor locoregional therapy recommendations, including radiation. Although historically reserved for only the highest risk or inoperable patients, NAC is increasingly used in earlier-stage disease, such as triple-negative tumors or HER2-positive tumors larger than 2 cm with or without nodal involvement.[25] At the same time, the number of women who opt for mastectomy has also increased over the last decade.[26] These trends make an understanding of the role of PMRT after NAC increasingly important in the current era.

Key data regarding use of PMRT in the setting of NAC include those from MD Anderson Cancer Center. Early publications from this group evaluating primarily patients with stage II and III disease established that those with pathologic complete response (pCR) had lower rates of LRF compared with those without, but that overall the risk of LRF was high (19%–33%) in the setting of pCR when PMRT was omitted.[27,28] These publications led to an early conclusion that decisions about the use of PMRT should be made from presenting stage rather than response to treatment. However, subsequent series elucidated specific characteristics that predict for the risk of LRF in patients treated with NAC, laying the groundwork for the current understanding that response to treatment may be used to inform decisions regarding PMRT.[5,28] In a series of 106 patients with stage I to II disease with pCR after NAC, the 10-year rate of LRR was 0% at 10 years in patients with stage I or II disease, regardless of the use of PMRT. However, among patients with stage III disease at presentation, LRR rates decreased from 33.3% to 7.3% with the addition of PMRT ($P = .040$). This finding has led to the general recommendation for PMRT in patients with stage III disease, regardless of pathologic response, but called into question the need for PMRT in patients with earlier stages in the setting of pCR. There are also data to support the tailoring of PMRT after NAC and mastectomy based on age. In a study by Garg and colleagues[29] both locoregional control and overall survival were significantly better among all patients less than 35 years of age who received PMRT after NAC and mastectomy, supporting this demographic feature as a key consideration in determining the utility of PMRT.

Additional insight regarding the role of PMRT in patients receiving NAC comes from the National Surgical Adjuvant Breast and Bowel Project (NSABP) B-18 and B-27 trials of NAC.[30] Patients with cT1-3N0-1M0 breast cancer were randomly assigned to 1 of 2 NAC regimens; most patients were stage I and II. Those who underwent mastectomy did not receive PMRT, offering a unique opportunity to study recurrence rates in this setting. For patients who achieved pCR in both the nodes and breast, LRR rates were less than 10% after mastectomy alone. In contrast, for those with pathologically positive nodes after chemotherapy, LRR rates were higher, with the highest rates seen in those patients who were clinically node positive, in whom rates were closer to 20%. These trials do not include receptor status data, which are increasingly understood to have a significant impact on response to NAC and on risk of recurrence after NAC. In a pooled analysis of more than 6000 patients, von Minkwitz and colleagues[31] showed that response to NAC varies significantly with receptor subtype, and that response to treatment is also highly prognostic for disease-free-survival in the chemosensitive subtypes, including triple negative, HER2 positive, and luminal B, but not luminal A. Similar data for the impact of pCR on locoregional outcomes with respect to receptor subtype in patients who do not receive PMRT have been lacking, but it is likely that response to NAC is more prognostic for locoregional outcomes in chemosensitive subtypes compared with others, as it is for disease-free survival.

Thus, at this time it remains standard to recommend PMRT for patients presenting with stage III disease, regardless of response to NAC, and for those who have residual node-positive disease after NAC. The data also support omission of PMRT for those patients presenting with stage II disease who do have pCR. However, there are many patients in whom the data are less clear, including younger patients, particularly those less than 35 years old, and those who do not have pCR but do not have chemosensitive histologies, such as luminal A. Current national clinical trials have been developed and are currently accruing to attempt to answer these questions.

Two such active trials are the NSABP B51/RTOG 1304 and Alliance A011202. The theme of both of these trials is to determine whether less aggressive locoregional therapy can be used in patients treated with NAC. NSABP B51 specifically addresses the omission of RNI in patients with a nodal pCR after NAC. This trail enrolls women with cT1-3N1 disease who have pathologic confirmation of axillary nodal involvement at diagnosis and receive NAC with nodal pCR at the time of surgery. Patients who have mastectomy are randomized to no radiotherapy or to PMRT including the chest wall and comprehensive RNI. Patients are stratified by key risk factors, including receptor status. Alliance A011202 asks whether more aggressive axillary surgery can be avoided in favor of axillary irradiation (which has a lower rate of lymphedema compared with axillary dissection) in patients with a positive sentinel node after NAC.[19] Patients are randomly assigned to completion ALND plus RNI or RNI (including the full axilla) alone without ALND. Both of these trials evaluate invasive breast cancer recurrence-free interval as the primary end point. These studies will provide important insight onto optimal management of node-positive patients who undergo NAC, with the ultimate goal of less aggressive locoregional therapies based on response to NAC.

TARGET VOLUMES

The clinical decision regarding which specific nodal regions (axillary, supraclavicular, infraclavicular, internal mammary) should be included in addition to the chest wall is a complex and controversial one. Since nodal involvement is the most common indication for PMRT, and most studies evaluating the benefit of PMRT have included RNI, the most widely accepted approach to PMRT is inclusion of the chest wall, axilla, supraclavicular nodes, and internal mammary (IM) nodes on a case-by-case basis. As a general principle, in those patients who have had an ALND, the full axilla is not irradiated given the low risk of recurrence in already dissected areas. However, in some circumstances, the entire axilla is included if it was not explored or if extensive nodal involvement was found.

Perhaps the most controversial aspect of RNI is the decision to include the IM nodes in the radiation volume.[16] Treatment of these nodes can increase exposure to critical organs such as the heart, lungs, and contralateral breast and thus potential toxicities must be weighed against clinical benefit. As discussed earlier, 2 studies were published in the *New England Journal of Medicine* in 2015 showing a disease-free survival benefit to the addition of RNI to WBI. In both of these studies, RNI included the undissected axilla, supraclavicular nodes, and IM nodes. The most recently published guideline update for PMRT also advocates comprehensive RNI including the IM nodes.[17] Thus, there is increasing support for inclusion of the IM when RNI/PMRT is used. However, as with every clinical decision, the potential benefit of including the IM nodes should be weighed against the potential toxicity in the individual patient, including risk factors for recurrence, anatomy, and risk factors for cardiac morbidity.

POSTMASTECTOMY RADIATION THERAPY TECHNIQUES

Modern PMRT techniques involve three-dimensional planning to achieve adequate coverage of the intended target volumes. Patients are placed in the supine position with ipsilateral arm above the head and externally rotated. A computed tomography (CT) scan is obtained using a CT simulator, on which the target volumes and beams can be defined and placed.

Tangent photon beams are used to target the chest wall and any nodes below the superior border of the tangents, and are generated by a megavoltage linear accelerator. If the supraclavicular and infraclavicular/high axillary areas are to be included, a single anterior photon beam is routinely used at a slight medial angle to avoid the spinal cord. When the full axilla is being covered, an additional posterior boost beam may be considered to adequately deliver dose to the deeper nodes in this region. If the IM nodes are to be included, several approaches are possible. One is to use partially wide tangents by extending the medial border and placing the posterior beam edge more deeply to include the first 3 intercostal spaces, with appropriate heart and lung blocking below this level. If normal tissue constraints cannot be met using this approach, a separate medial electron beam may be matched to the photon tangents to target the IM volume at a shallow depth. Intensity modulated radiation therapy (IMRT)/volumetric modulated arc therapy (VMAT) and proton therapy are two techniques that may also offer dosimetric advantages in selected cases, although VMAT should be approached with caution because the heart is generally exposed to a larger low-dose bath compared with conventional techniques. Protons allow minimal radiation exposure to the heart and lungs because of the Bragg peak and lack of exit dose. Protons are currently being compared with conventional photon or photon/electron radiation techniques for treatment of the breast or chest wall with RNI inclusive of the IM nodes in a randomized trial, RADCOMP (Pragmatic Randomized Trial of Proton vs Photon Therapy for Patients With Non-Metastatic Breast Cancer: A Radiotherapy Comparative Effectiveness Consortium Trial), with cardiotoxicity as the primary end point. This trial hopes to answer the question of whether the dosimetric benefits of proton therapy will translate into clinical gains. As in all clinical decisions regarding PMRT, the optimal technique for a given patient depends on multiple factors, including patient anatomy, planned target volume, available technology, and the technical expertise of the treatment team.

REFERENCES

1. EBCTCG (Early Breast Cancer Trialists' Collaborative Group), McGale P, Taylor C, Correa C, et al. Effect of radiotherapy after mastectomy and axillary surgery on 10-year recurrence and 20-year breast cancer mortality: meta-analysis of individual patient data for 8135 women in 22 randomised trials. Lancet 2014;383(9935): 2127–35.
2. Overgaard M, Jensen MB, Overgaard J, et al. Postoperative radiotherapy in high-risk postmenopausal breast-cancer patients given adjuvant tamoxifen: Danish Breast Cancer Cooperative Group DBCG 82c randomised trial. Lancet 1999; 353(9165):1641–8.
3. Ragaz J, Jackson SM, Le N, et al. Adjuvant radiotherapy and chemotherapy in node-positive premenopausal women with breast cancer. N Engl J Med 1997; 337(14):956–62.
4. Overgaard M, Hansen PS, Overgaard J, et al. Postoperative radiotherapy in high-risk premenopausal women with breast cancer who receive adjuvant chemotherapy. Danish Breast Cancer Cooperative Group 82b trial. N Engl J Med 1997;337(14):949–55.
5. McBride A, Allen P, Woodward W, et al. Locoregional recurrence risk for patients with T1,2 breast cancer with 1-3 positive lymph nodes treated with mastectomy and systemic treatment. Int J Radiat Oncol Biol Phys 2014;89(2):392–8.
6. Recht A, Gray R, Davidson NE, et al. Locoregional failure 10 years after mastectomy and adjuvant chemotherapy with or without tamoxifen without irradiation: experience of the Eastern Cooperative Oncology Group. J Clin Oncol 1999; 17(6):1689–700.
7. Taghian AG, Jeong JH, Mamounas EP, et al. Low locoregional recurrence rate among node-negative breast cancer patients with tumors 5 cm or larger treated by mastectomy, with or without adjuvant systemic therapy and without radiotherapy: results from five national surgical adjuvant breast and bowel project randomized clinical trials. J Clin Oncol 2006;24(24):3927–32.
8. Yildirim E, Berberoglu U. Local recurrence in breast carcinoma patients with T(1-2) and 1-3 positive nodes: indications for radiotherapy. Eur J Surg Oncol 2007; 33(1):28–32.
9. Moo TA, McMillan R, Lee M, et al. Selection criteria for postmastectomy radiotherapy in t1-t2 tumors with 1 to 3 positive lymph nodes. Ann Surg Oncol 2013; 20(10):3169–74.
10. Kyndi M, Sorensen FB, Knudsen H, et al. Estrogen receptor, progesterone receptor, HER-2, and response to postmastectomy radiotherapy in high-risk breast cancer: the Danish Breast Cancer Cooperative Group. J Clin Oncol 2008;26(9):1419–26.
11. Tseng YD, Uno H, Hughes ME, et al. Biological subtype predicts risk of locoregional recurrence after mastectomy and impact of postmastectomy radiation in a large national database. Int J Radiat Oncol Biol Phys 2015;93(3):622–30.
12. Lanning RM, Morrow M, Riaz N, et al. The effect of adjuvant trastuzumab on locoregional recurrence of human epidermal growth factor receptor 2-positive breast cancer treated with mastectomy. Ann Surg Oncol 2015;22(8):2517–25.
13. Whelan TJ, Olivotto IA, Levine MN. Regional nodal irradiation in early-stage breast cancer. N Engl J Med 2015;373(19):1878–9.

14. Poortmans PM, Collette S, Kirkove C, et al. Internal mammary and medial supraclavicular irradiation in breast cancer. N Engl J Med 2015;373(4):317–27.
15. Burstein HJ, Morrow M. Nodal irradiation after breast-cancer surgery in the era of effective adjuvant therapy. N Engl J Med 2015;373(4):379–81.
16. Haffty BG, Whelan T, Poortmans PM. Radiation of the internal mammary nodes: is there a benefit? J Clin Oncol 2016;34(4):297–9.
17. Recht A, Comen EA, Fine RE, et al. Postmastectomy radiotherapy: an American Society of Clinical Oncology, American Society for Radiation Oncology, and Society of Surgical Oncology focused guideline update. Pract Radiat Oncol 2016; 6(6):e219–34.
18. Giuliano AE, Hunt KK, Ballman KV, et al. Axillary dissection vs no axillary dissection in women with invasive breast cancer and sentinel node metastasis: a randomized clinical trial. JAMA 2011;305(6):569–75.
19. Donker M, van Tienhoven G, Straver ME, et al. Radiotherapy or surgery of the axilla after a positive sentinel node in breast cancer (EORTC 10981-22023 AMAROS): a randomised, multicentre, open-label, phase 3 non-inferiority trial. Lancet Oncol 2014;15(12):1303–10.
20. Galimberti V, Cole BF, Zurrida S, et al. Axillary dissection versus no axillary dissection in patients with sentinel-node micrometastases (IBCSG 23-01): a phase 3 randomised controlled trial. Lancet Oncol 2013;14(4):297–305.
21. Jagsi R. Postmastectomy radiation therapy: an overview for the practicing surgeon. ISRN Surg 2013;2013:212979.
22. Wallgren A, Bonetti M, Gelber RD, et al. Risk factors for locoregional recurrence among breast cancer patients: results from international breast cancer study group trials I through VII. J Clin Oncol 2003;21(7):1205–13.
23. Truong PT, Sadek BT, Lesperance MF, et al. Is biological subtype prognostic of locoregional recurrence risk in women with pT1-2N0 breast cancer treated with mastectomy? Int J Radiat Oncol Biol Phys 2014;88(1):57–64.
24. Jagsi R, Raad RA, Goldberg S, et al. Locoregional recurrence rates and prognostic factors for failure in node-negative patients treated with mastectomy: implications for postmastectomy radiation. Int J Radiat Oncol Biol Phys 2005;62(4): 1035–9.
25. Gianni L, Pienkowski T, Im YH, et al. Efficacy and safety of neoadjuvant pertuzumab and trastuzumab in women with locally advanced, inflammatory, or early HER2-positive breast cancer (NeoSphere): a randomised multicentre, open-label, phase 2 trial. Lancet Oncol 2012;13(1):25–32.
26. Yao K, Stewart AK, Winchester DJ, et al. Trends in contralateral prophylactic mastectomy for unilateral cancer: a report from the National Cancer Data Base, 1998-2007. Ann Surg Oncol 2010;17(10):2554–62.
27. Buchholz TA, Tucker SL, Masullo L, et al. Predictors of local-regional recurrence after neoadjuvant chemotherapy and mastectomy without radiation. J Clin Oncol 2002;20(1):17–23.
28. Huang EH, Tucker SL, Strom EA, et al. Postmastectomy radiation improves local-regional control and survival for selected patients with locally advanced breast cancer treated with neoadjuvant chemotherapy and mastectomy. J Clin Oncol 2004;22(23):4691–9.
29. Garg AK, Oh JL, Oswald MJ, et al. Effect of postmastectomy radiotherapy in patients. Int J Radiat Oncol Biol Phys 2007;69(5):1478–83.
30. Mamounas EP, Anderson SJ, Dignam JJ, et al. Predictors of locoregional recurrence after neoadjuvant chemotherapy: results from combined analysis of

national surgical adjuvant breast and bowel project B-18 and B-27. J Clin Oncol 2012;30(32):3960–6.
31. von Minckwitz G, Untch M, Blohmer JU, et al. Definition and impact of pathologic complete response on prognosis after neoadjuvant chemotherapy in various intrinsic breast cancer subtypes. J Clin Oncol 2012;30(15):1796–804.

Management of Stage I Lung Cancer with Stereotactic Ablative Radiation Therapy

Tu Dan, MD[a,*], Noelle L. Williams, MD[b]

KEYWORDS

• SBRT • SABR • SRS • Stereotactic • Ablative • Hypofractionation • Lung cancer

KEY POINTS

- The incidence of early stage lung cancer is increasing owing to the adoption of lung cancer screening guidelines.
- Although surgery has been considered the historical standard for early stage disease, there is no level I evidence supporting its use over modern radiation therapy.
- Stereotactic ablative radiation therapy (SABR) is an emerging treatment option for patients with early stage disease that is distinctly different that conventional radiation therapy in both conduct and radiobiologic effect.
- Although unable to successfully accrue in the past, current studies are attempting to directly compare SABR versus surgery in operable patients.

INTRODUCTION

Early stage non–small cell lung cancer (NSCLC) is a growing clinical entity with evolving standards of care. As a whole, NSCLC is the second most common malignancy in men and women, with 224,390 new cases and 158,080 deaths predicted in 2016.[1] It remains the leading cause of death from cancer, with a 5-year overall survival of approximately 21%.[2] Deaths attributable from lung cancer are driven primarily from advanced disease, with early stage disease considered potentially curable. Although most patients have traditionally presented with late stage disease, the population of patients with early stage lung cancer is now expected to increase significantly due to improvements in diagnostic modalities and the widespread adoption of lung cancer screening programs.[3]

The authors have nothing to disclose.
[a] Department of Radiation Oncology, UT Southwestern, 5323 Harry Hines Boulevard, Dallas, TX 75390, USA; [b] Department of Radiation Oncology, Thomas Jefferson University, 111 South 11th Street, Philadelphia, PA 19107, USA
* Corresponding author.
E-mail address: Tu.Dan@utsouthwestern.edu

Surg Oncol Clin N Am 26 (2017) 393–403
http://dx.doi.org/10.1016/j.soc.2017.01.005 surgonc.theclinics.com

In 2014, lung cancer screening with low-dose chest computed tomography (CT) was recommended for high-risk individuals by the US Preventive Services Task Force based on several large, population-based studies.[4] The largest US-based trial was the National Lung Screening Trial, a national study accruing more than 50,000 patients demonstrating reduced lung cancer mortality with low-dose CT screening. In this study of high-risk individuals with 30 or more pack-year smoking history between the ages of 55 to 74 years of age, the relative risk of mortality from lung cancer decreased by one-fifth. Based on these results, several societies and national organizations have endorsed guidelines for lung cancer screening.[5–7] The adoption of lung cancer screening guidelines is expected to significantly increase the detection of early stage disease. As the incidence of early stage lung cancer increases, it will be critical to better define appropriate treatment options for patients in this population.

TREATMENT OPTIONS FOR EARLY STAGE NON–SMALL CELL LUNG CANCER

For decades, the historical standard for early stage NSCLC was surgical extirpation. Similar to early treatment paradigms for breast cancer, the best chance of cure was thought to be achieved through radical surgery. As a result, the standard of care endorsed by nearly all oncologic and surgical societies was centered around surgery as the cornerstone of treatment.[8] To date, surgery remains the favored approach, as current National Comprehensive Cancer Network guidelines recommend complete surgical resection as the preferred therapy for localized disease in patients who can tolerate the procedure.[9]

However, the role of surgery as the de facto definitive approach has increasingly come under inquiry as the evidence has not yet been established through randomized trials. Three randomized phase 3 trials have been attempted to directly compare surgery versus radiation, but all have prematurely closed due to poor accrual.[10,11] Consequently, there continues to be considerable debate as to what constitutes standard treatment options. The evidence for the use of surgery primarily relies on principles of oncologic management and early outcome data from selected groups of patients in surgical series.[12] Furthermore, for many years, the only viable treatment option to address gross disease was limited to surgery. Historical delivery of radiation often yielded poor outcomes using conventional fractionated radiotherapy. The use of large treatment fields due to targeting uncertainty limited the ability to deliver truly therapeutic doses, resulting in toxic treatment with poor local control rates.[13] Similar to data demonstrating potential harm in postoperative lung patients, the delivery of antiquated thoracic radiation has traditionally resulted in an unfavorable therapeutic ratio.[14] Consequently, radiation was primarily reserved in the cases of palliation. However, as technological advances rapidly came into adoption and radiation treatment techniques became more sophisticated, effective local control of disease became increasingly achievable. As the population of early stage NSCLC continues to grow, elucidating the role of radiation therapy in the definite management of early stage disease will become a more salient issue.

DEVELOPMENT OF STEREOTACTIC ABLATIVE RADIATION THERAPY

The development of key techniques in stereotactic delivery has transformed the treatment of early stage lung cancer over the past 2 decades. Beginning in the late 1980s, several investigators across the globe began experimenting with the use of larger and more targeted doses of radiation to extracranial targets based on techniques implemented from intracranial radiosurgery. Initially deriving its nomenclature from these intracranial techniques, the original term stereotactic body radiation therapy (SBRT) refers to the use of *stereotaxy* to improve treatment targeting by linking orthogonal Cartesian coordinates in an external reference frame to internal cross-sectional anatomy.[15] By doing so, the spatial accuracy and reliability of treatment delivery is substantially increased. One of the first experiences using stereotactic treatment was published from the Karolinska Hospital, where the Gamma knife radiosurgery platform was first successfully used. Data from Blomgren and colleagues[16] first demonstrated the safety and feasibility of extracranial high-dose stereotactic treatment. In this initial experience, 31 patients with extracranial solitary tumors of the liver, retroperitoneal space, and lung were treated with stereotactic radiotherapy with doses ranging from 7.7 to 30 Gy per fraction with highly inhomogeneous, conformal treatments. Local control rates were higher than expected, with no evidence of local progressive disease in 80% of treated lesions during a relatively short follow-up period of 1.5 to 38 months. Impressively, half of the treated tumors were noted to regress or disappear. In parallel fashion, investigators at the National Defense Medical College in Japan began to investigate similar techniques. In order to account for extracranial motion, Uematsu and colleagues[17] developed a prototype fusion of CT and linear accelerator so that positioning and targeting could be confirmed before each treatment session. Using this setup, investigators delivered high-dose stereotactic treatment to 45 patients with primary or oligometastatic primary tumors of the lung. The ranges of doses in this study were much higher than those delivered in the Karolinska experience, with Uematsu and colleagues[18] using doses ranging from 30 to 75 Gy in 5 to 15 fractions. Given the higher doses delivered, researchers were able to achieve very high local control rates, with local progression only occurring in 2 of 66 treated lesions.

The excellent clinical outcomes from these series suggested the feasibility and rational use of stereotactic radiation as a definitive treatment option for well-circumscribed extracranial targets. In addition, given that local control rates were higher than expected based on historical radiobiological models, there was suggestion that there was unique biology occurring with significantly larger fraction sizes.

BIOLOGIC RATIONALE FOR STEREOTACTIC ABLATIVE RADIATION THERAPY

Traditionally, the effects of fractionated radiation therapy have been attempted to be modeled for decades using a mathematical formula described as the linear-quadratic formula. By historical convention, the typical doses to produce this model often range from 1.8 to 8.0 Gy, with limited data incorporating the higher doses used in modern stereotactic treatments. This model was empirically derived based on in vitro data beginning in the early 1950s.[19] Since then, experimental evidence has suggested that the predictive value of this model decreases as dose increases, with poor estimation of effects from doses delivered in the stereotactic and radiosurgical ranges.[20] With stereotactic delivery, the goals of treatment biologically differ from that of conventional radiation therapy. Conventional fractionated radiation therapy is often delivered daily over a protracted course, relying on the cumulative differential damage of tumor tissue unable to repair damage at the same rate of normal tissue. In this manner, large amounts of normal tissue can be included in the treated field owing to potential repair mechanisms. In contrast, the goal of Stereotactic Ablative Radiation Therapy (SABR) is to ablate the targeted tissue while minimizing the normal tissue included, effectively ignoring the differential effect of radiation on normal and tumor tissue. These biologic differences are manifested in the size and dose of radiation delivered. Although conventional radiation is intended to cover large areas of normal tissue to account for subclinical disease, SABR is focused on solely gross tumor with minimal margins minimizing exposure to normal tissues.

Vascular Effects

In addition to the direct tumoricidal effects of radiation, there is compelling evidence that the vascular disrupting properties of high-dose radiation may contribute to the clinical effectiveness of stereotactic treatment. It is well known that one of the earliest uses of stereotactic treatment is in the setting of arteriovenous malformations.[21] Histopathologically, blood vessels following exposure to high-dose radiation demonstrate narrowing or obliteration of lumens, with the prime target appearing to be damage to endothelial cells. This phenomenon has been recapitulated with demonstration of significant radiation-induced vascular damage occurring in tumors. Irradiation of tumor xenografts with 5 to 10 Gy per fraction causes relatively mild vascular damages, but increasing the dose to higher than 10 Gy per fraction induces severe vascular damage, resulting in significantly reduced blood perfusion.[22]

Accelerated Repopulation

Given the relatively brief treatments of SABR, a typical treatment course is completed in 2 weeks or less, and may even be delivered as a single fraction.[23] The total duration of SABR is thus shorter than what is thought to be the average starting time for accelerated repopulation in tumors, typically thought to be in the 3- to 5-week range for squamous tumors. It is thought that a dose increase of about 0.6 Gy per day is required to compensate repopulation using conventional fractionated treatment.[24] By shortening treatment significantly, SABR effectively bypasses the issue of repopulation, leading to improved control rates.

Dose Escalation

The optimum dose and fractionation for curative intent for NSCLC remains uncertain. It was on this basis that the Radiation Therapy Oncology Group (RTOG) 0617 trial was conducted.[25] The biologic effective dose (BED) for SABR is typically much higher than the standard 60 to 66 Gy given for conventional therapy. However, despite indirect evidence that increasing dose is correlated with superior local control, this has not been demonstrated in a prospective fashion.[26] It has been suggested that in trials with concurrent chemotherapy, higher radiation therapy doses resulted in poorer survival, possibly due to high levels of toxicity.[27] In contrast, because of the smaller treatment volumes and higher fraction sizes used in SABR, dose escalation can be safely achieved. This increase in delivered BED has been linked to local control benefit.[28]

Systemic Effects

Although the prime intention of SABR is to maximize local tumor control in the treated field, there have been reported cases of nontargeted effects of radiation on distant tumor sites, often called the *abscopal* effect.[29] In the era of immune therapy, this out of the field treatment effect will increasingly become more important. In the setting of clinically localized lung disease, the systemic effects of radiation have been poorly characterized. However, there are some data to suggest that the relatively low rates of nodal failure in the treatment of early stage NSCLC may be in part due to an immunologic response.[30]

CLINICAL SERIES

Because of the historical preference of surgical therapy as the definitive therapy for early stage lung cancer, most data regarding the use of radiation have been in the inoperable or not medically fit population. As a result, survival in these series may be limited due to a negative selection bias of patients with more comorbid conditions. However, as adoption of this technology has increased, its use has become more ubiquitous.

The first North American experience using SABR was established by Timmerman and colleagues[31,32] at Indiana University in a series of phase 1 and 2 trials. In the initial phase 1 dose escalation toxicity, 47 patients with inoperable early stage NSCLC were immobilized in a stereotactic body frame and treated in escalating doses of radiotherapy beginning at 24 Gy total (3 $\times$ 8 Gy fractions) and cohorts dose escalated by 6.0 Gy total. Local control in this series was excellent with minimal toxicity reported. In the phase 2 trial using the established dosing from the phase 1 study, local control remained excellent with 95% control at 17.5 months. However, it was noted that 6 patients had treatment-related deaths, possibly due to central airway necrosis from treatment.

Based on this initial experience, the multi-institutional RTOG 0236 accrued 59 patients with inoperable early stage, peripheral tumors.[33] In this study, only 1 patient had a primary tumor failure with an estimated 3-year primary tumor control rate of 97.6%. The median overall survival was 48.1 months, which compared very favorably to historical surgery and radiation controls. No grade 5 treatment-related adverse events were reported, and no central lesions were included on this trial.

Since that time, the RTOG (now NRG Oncology) has investigated the use of SABR in several different settings for early stage patients. In RTOG 0915, investigators compared 2 treatment schedules in medically inoperable patients to determine the toxicity rate of different fractionation schemes. Patients were randomized to receive either 34 Gy in 1 fraction (arm 1) or 48 Gy in 4 consecutive daily fractions (arm 2). The 1-year local control rate was 97.0% (95% confidence interval [CI] 84.2%–99.9%) for arm 1 and 92.7% (95% CI 80.1%–98.5%) for arm 2, with no differences in toxicity in either group.[23] In RTOG 0618, investigators studied the use of SABR in operable patients as determined by an independent thoracic surgeon using specific criteria. Although only published in abstract form, this small study of 26 patients demonstrated a 2-year local and lobar failure rate of 19%, which was higher than expected.[34]

Surgery versus Stereotactic Ablative Radiation Therapy

Given the enthusiasm from favorable results in the inoperable setting, several attempts have been made to directly compare surgery and SABR in the operable or borderline operable setting. The RTOG 1021/ACOSOG Z4099 trial attempted to answer this question, but was prematurely closed due to poor accrual. Similarly, 2 other studies, the STARS and ROSEL trials, both failed to accrue to their projected number of patients. In an unplanned exploratory analysis, investigators suggested some evidence of the relative equipoise between the 2 modalities. In the pooled comparison of these incompletely accrued trials, investigators found overall survival at 3 years was 95% in patients receiving radiation versus 79% in the surgery group (hazard ratio, 0.14; $P<.037$), primarily owing to postoperative complications related to surgery.[11] The rates of local control were similar in both groups, with 3-year local control of 96% in the radiation group versus 100% in the surgery group. As the number of patients in this study and the nature of the pooled results were suboptimal, interpretations from this study have varied widely between surgeons and radiation oncologists. Since then, 2 new trials have recently been opened to attempt to answer this longstanding clinical question: the Joint Lung Cancer Trialist's Coalition STABLEMATES trial and the UK SABRTooth feasibility trial.[35,36]

TECHNICAL CONSIDERATIONS

Nomenclature

In the report of American Association of Physicists in Medicine Task Group 101, SABR is referred to as the "delivery of large doses in a few fractions, which results in a high biological effective dose (BED)."[37] Similarly, the American College of Radiology and the American Society for Radiation Oncology have defined SABR as "an external beam radiation therapy method used to very precisely deliver a high dose of radiation to an extracranial target within the body, using either a single dose or a small number of fractions."[38] After the development of SABR, several interchangeable terms have been used to describe SABR delivery, resulting in unnecessary confusion. These terms include "stereotactic radiotherapy," "fractionated stereotactic radiosurgery," "hypofractionated stereotactic radiosurgery," and more recently, "stereotactic ablative body radiotherapy (SABR)." Some practitioners have advocated for the adoption of SABR because of its incorporation of the term "ablation," which better designates the intention of treatment—the destruction of both tumor and normal tissue encompassed in the high-dose target.[39] Currently, consensus does not exist for defining SABR with respect to the appropriate number of radiation fractions, dose per fraction, or the maximum number and diameter of lesions to be treated. In the United States, SBRT/SABR is currently limited to 5 fractions or less as defined by Centers for Medicare and Medicaid Services.

Technical Requirements

Although there is no single requirement that encompasses every SABR case, stereotactic treatment is more appropriately defined by the conduct in which is it performed. Because of the high doses of radiation used and precision requirement, the practice of SABR requires an extreme level of confidence in the treatment delivery in comparison to standard approaches. In addition, smaller margins are used to exclude as much normal tissue as possible, increasing the possibility of marginal misses if proper measures are not in place. In order to achieve this, several technologies must be used to account for increased accuracy in target delineation and motion.

Motion Management

Moving targets represent a formidable obstacle in the accurate delivery of high doses while minimizing exposure to normal tissue. To account for tumor motion, several strategies have been used. First, estimating the extent of tumor motion must be accounted for. If the tumor can be well visualized using 2-dimensional imaging, practitioners may use fluoroscopic guidance to assess real-time motion. Alternatively, some vendors have developed orthogonal kilovoltage imaging stations using mounted detectors such those used by Cyberknife- and Exactrac-based systems. These systems are often supplemented using implanted fiducial markers that display more prominently under kilovoltage imaging than soft tissues. More recently, the usage of 4-dimensional (4D) CT scanning has been commonplace in radiation oncology departments. Using 4D CT scans, targets of interests are scanned under CT with respiratory surrogates corresponding to various phases of the respiratory cycle. Multiple 3-dimensional image sets are acquired, each corresponding to an associated breathing phase. Once a complete set of images has been acquired, they are reconstituted to produce a CT set that covers the entire breathing cycle with associated target motion.

Once target motion has been visualized, there are several strategies to account for and restrict excessive motion. Similar to their use in stereotactic radiosurgery, external frames can be used to rigidly align the patient in stereotactic space. Examples of external immobilization devices include body frames, vacuum molds, body fixes, and thermoplastics. In cases where target motion is excessive, abdominal compression can be used to limit diaphragmatic excursion, therefore reducing target motion.

To further limit breathing-associated motion, breath holding and respiratory gating techniques may be used. Breath-holding techniques may be more challenging due to a preponderance of patients with lung cancer with pulmonary comorbidities. However, in a motivated patient with adequate lung function, active breathing coordination devices may be used to synchronize beam-on time with specific phases of the respiratory cycle. In similar fashion, real-time assessment of respiratory motion can coregister with treatment delivery through the use of respiratory gating, which links beam-on time to a limited number of phases in the respiratory cycle. In this manner, explicit breath holding is not required; however, caution must be taken for patients with irregular breathing cycles, because this can lead to unreliable reconstruction of respiratory phases.

Advanced Image Guidance

In order to visualize targets immediately before and during treatment, several options are available. On board imaging with mounted cone-beam CTs is often used. As mentioned previously, orthogonal kilovoltage pairs may also be used. An advantage of mounted kilovoltage imaging is that it allows verification of target throughout treatment delivery. In the case of Cyberknife, real-time imaging can be used to create predicted motion paths for targets, allowing for the ability to track and adapt to target motion.

Planning Considerations

Unlike traditional radiation therapy planning, delivery of SABR often ignores the differential impact of ionizing radiation on normal tissues versus tumor. Instead, all targeted areas in SABR are expected to have locally destructive effects. Consequently, treatment planning for SABR requires consideration for smaller treatment margins and techniques that allow for increased conformality of high-dose radiation. For example, to increase the rate of dose fall-off outside of targeted structures, it is helpful to have inhomogeneous treatment plans where the center of targets receives a much higher dose than the prescription dose. In order to achieve this, beam arrangements often will include a multitude of non-coplanar beams or arc-based volumetric modulated arc therapy plans to lower entrance and exit doses and maintain high-dose gradients. As a result, homogeneity is often lost within the tissue, although this may be a clinical advantage if it is limited to gross tumor.

TOXICITY OF LUNG STEREOTACTIC ABLATIVE RADIATION THERAPY

Patients undergoing SABR for early stage lung cancer present a unique challenge when assessing treatment-related morbidity. As most of these patients suffer from multiple comorbid conditions making them ineligible for curative surgery, they are at baseline a high-risk population. In the absence of stereotactic treatment, local tumor progression is common, eventually leading to morbidity and death.[40] Conversely, although the use of SABR for early-stage lung cancer is often associated with generally low toxicity rates, without proper precautions, treatment-related side effects can be devastating.[41] These side effects can occur acutely following treatment, but may also have late presentations. In the phase 2 Indiana University experience, 6 patients experienced grade 5 toxicity, with a range of 0.6 to 19.5 months following completion of SABR treatment. On multivariate analysis, patients with perihilar/central tumors in trial had an 11-fold increased risk of experiencing severe toxicity compared with peripheral locations. Given these potentially fatal toxicities, caution must be exercised when treating central airway structures. In the RTOG 0813 protocol, dose-escalation was performed to determine a safe and effective dose for central lung tumors. In the most recently available abstract data, local control at 2 years in 71 patients treated with the 2 highest doses levels (11.5–12 Gy/fraction × 5 fractions) in this multicenter trial approached 90% with 3 grade 5 toxicities occurring in 71 patients.[42]

In addition to life-limiting toxicities, other treatment-related side effects may significantly contribute to quality of life. Several studies have attempted to characterize toxicities observed in organs near treated sites, such as the esophagus, brachial plexus, and chest wall. Esophageal toxicity is also associated with centrally located tumors, with side effects ranging from esophagitis to strictures and fistula formation.[43] In patients with superior sulcus tumors and tumors located in the apex of the lung, the risk of damage to the brachial plexus is not insignificant.[44]

One of the most common side effects of the treatment of peripheral lesions is the risk of rib fractures and persistent chest wall pain. Although the true mechanism underlying the mechanism of its development has not yet been established, chest wall toxicity is thought to be attributed to radiation-induced damage to the intercostal nerves, ribs, and muscles that make up the chest wall.[45] Other factors that may also increase the risk of post-treatment pain include younger patient age, weight, and continued smoking through treatment.[46]

SUMMARY

In the last decade, advances in image guidance, treatment planning systems, and improved spatial accuracy of treatment delivery have all converged to result in the successful use of SABR in the treatment of early stage lung cancer. This paradigm-shifting approach allows significant reduction of treatment volumes, facilitating the use of high-dose radiation and increased BEDs delivered to tumors. In addition, the use of SABR reduces overall treatment time for patients and is considered to be a nonmorbid, noninvasive treatment option. As improvements in these delivery techniques continue, there will be a growing need to establish the preferred management for early stage disease, particularly in the setting where patients may be eligible for multiple treatment modalities. Currently, there appears to be at least relative equipoise as the results of larger, confirmatory data are eagerly awaited.

REFERENCES

1. Siegel RL, Miller KD, Jemal A. Cancer statistics, 2016. CA Cancer J Clin 2016;66(1):7–30.
2. Miller KD, Siegel RL, Lin CC, et al. Cancer treatment and survivorship statistics, 2016. CA Cancer J Clin 2016;66(4):271–89.
3. Edwards JP, Datta I, Hunt JD, et al. Forecasting the impact of stereotactic ablative radiotherapy for early-stage lung cancer on the thoracic surgery workforce. Eur J Cardiothorac Surg 2016;49(6):1599–606.
4. Moyer VA. Screening for lung cancer: U.S. preventive services task force recommendation statement. Ann Intern Med 2014;160(5):330–8.
5. Jaklitsch MT, Jacobson FL, Austin JHM, et al. The American Association for Thoracic Surgery guidelines for lung cancer screening using low-dose computed tomography scans for lung cancer survivors and other high-risk groups. J Thorac Cardiovasc Surg 2012;144(1):33–8.

6. Bach PB, Mirkin JN, Oliver TK, et al. Benefits and harms of CT screening for lung cancer: a systematic review. JAMA 2012;307(22):2418–29.
7. Detterbeck FC, Mazzone PJ, Naidich DP, et al. Screening for lung cancer: diagnosis and management of lung cancer, 3rd ed: American College of Chest Physicians evidence-based clinical practice guidelines. Chest 2013;143(5 Suppl): e78S–92S.
8. Howington JA, Blum MG, Chang AC, et al. Treatment of stage I and II non-small cell lung cancer: diagnosis and management of lung cancer, 3rd ed: American College of Chest Physicians evidence-based clinical practice guidelines. Chest 2013;143(5 Suppl):e278S–313S.
9. Ettinger DS, Wood DE, Akerley W, et al. NCCN guidelines insights: non-small cell lung cancer, Version 4.2016. J Natl Compr Canc Netw 2016;14(3):255–64.
10. Fernando HC, Timmerman R. American College of Surgeons Oncology Group Z4099/Radiation Therapy Oncology Group 1021: a randomized study of sublobar resection compared with stereotactic body radiotherapy for high-risk stage I non-small cell lung cancer. J Thorac Cardiovasc Surg 2012;144(3):S35–8.
11. Chang JY, Senan S, Paul MA, et al. Stereotactic ablative radiotherapy versus lobectomy for operable stage I non-small-cell lung cancer: a pooled analysis of two randomised trials. Lancet Oncol 2015;16(6):630–7.
12. Churchill ED, Sweet RH, Soutter L, et al. The surgical management of carcinoma of the lung; a study of the cases treated at the Massachusetts General Hospital from 1930 to 1950. J Thorac Surg 1950;20(3):349–65.
13. Rowell NP, Williams CJ. Radical radiotherapy for stage I/II non-small cell lung cancer in patients not sufficiently fit for or declining surgery (medically inoperable): a systematic review. Thorax 2001;56(8):628–38.
14. PORT Meta-analysis Trialists Group. Postoperative radiotherapy for non-small cell lung cancer. Cochrane Database Syst Rev 2000;(2):CD002142.
15. Leksell L. The stereotaxic method and radiosurgery of the brain. Acta Chir Scand 1951;102(4):316–9.
16. Blomgren H, Lax I, Näslund I, et al. Stereotactic high dose fraction radiation therapy of extracranial tumors using an accelerator. Clinical experience of the first thirty-one patients. Acta Oncol 1995;34(6):861–70.
17. Uematsu M, Fukui T, Shioda A, et al. A dual computed tomography linear accelerator unit for stereotactic radiation therapy: a new approach without cranially fixated stereotactic frames. Int J Radiat Oncol Biol Phys 1996;35(3):587–92.
18. Uematsu M, Shioda A, Tahara K, et al. Focal, high dose, and fractionated modified stereotactic radiation therapy for lung carcinoma patients: a preliminary experience. Cancer 1998;82(6):1062–70.
19. Elkind MM, Sutton H. Radiation response of mammalian cells grown in culture. 1. Repair of X-ray damage in surviving Chinese hamster cells. Radiat Res 1960;13: 556–93.
20. Park C, Papiez L, Zhang S, et al. Universal survival curve and single fraction equivalent dose: useful tools in understanding potency of ablative radiotherapy. Int J Radiat Oncol 2008;70(3):847–52.
21. Schneider BF, Eberhard DA, Steiner LE. Histopathology of arteriovenous malformations after gamma knife radiosurgery. J Neurosurg 1997;87(3):352–7.
22. Park HJ, Griffin RJ, Hui S, et al. Radiation-induced vascular damage in tumors: implications of vascular damage in ablative hypofractionated radiotherapy (SBRT and SRS). Radiat Res 2012;177(3):311–27.
23. Videtic GMM, Hu C, Singh AK, et al. A randomized phase 2 study comparing 2 stereotactic body radiation therapy schedules for medically inoperable patients

with stage I peripheral non-small cell lung cancer: NRG Oncology RTOG 0915 (NCCTG N0927). Int J Radiat Oncol Biol Phys 2015;93(4):757–64.
24. Withers HR, Taylor JM, Maciejewski B. The hazard of accelerated tumor clonogen repopulation during radiotherapy. Acta Oncol 1988;27(2):131–46.
25. Bradley JD, Paulus R, Komaki R, et al. Standard-dose versus high-dose conformal radiotherapy with concurrent and consolidation carboplatin plus paclitaxel with or without cetuximab for patients with stage IIIA or IIIB non-small-cell lung cancer (RTOG 0617): a randomised, two-by-two factorial phase 3 study. Lancet Oncol 2015;16(2):187–99.
26. Mehta M, Scrimger R, Mackie R, et al. A new approach to dose escalation in non-small-cell lung cancer. Int J Radiat Oncol Biol Phys 2001;49(1):23–33.
27. Ramroth J, Cutter DJ, Darby SC, et al. Dose and fractionation in radiation therapy of curative intent for non-small cell lung cancer: meta-analysis of randomized trials. Int J Radiat Oncol Biol Phys 2016;96(4):736–47.
28. Onishi H, Araki T, Shirato H, et al. Stereotactic hypofractionated high-dose irradiation for stage I nonsmall cell lung carcinoma: clinical outcomes in 245 subjects in a Japanese multiinstitutional study. Cancer 2004;101(7):1623–31.
29. Siva S, Lobachevsky P, MacManus MP, et al. Radiotherapy for non-small cell lung cancer induces DNA damage response in both irradiated and out-of-field normal tissues. Clin Cancer Res 2016;22(19):4817–26.
30. Lee Y, Auh SL, Wang Y, et al. Therapeutic effects of ablative radiation on local tumor require CD8+ T cells: changing strategies for cancer treatment. Blood 2009; 114(3):589–95.
31. McGarry RC, Papiez L, Williams M, et al. Stereotactic body radiation therapy of early-stage non–small-cell lung carcinoma: phase I study. Int J Radiat Oncol 2005;63(4):1010–5.
32. Timmerman R, McGarry R, Yiannoutsos C, et al. Excessive toxicity when treating central tumors in a phase II study of stereotactic body radiation therapy for medically inoperable early-stage lung cancer. J Clin Oncol 2006;24(30):4833–9.
33. Timmerman R, Paulus R, Galvin J, et al. STereotactic body radiation therapy for inoperable early stage lung cancer. JAMA 2010;303(11):1070–6.
34. Timmerman RD, Paulus R, Pass HI, et al. RTOG 0618: stereotactic body radiation therapy (SBRT) to treat operable early-stage lung cancer patients. J Clin Oncol 2013;31(suppl) [abstract 7523]. Available at: http://meetinglibrary.asco.org/content/111599-132. Accessed October 31, 2016.
35. JoLT-Ca Sublobar Resection (SR) Versus Stereotactic Ablative Radiotherapy (SAbR) for Lung Cancer—Full Text View—ClinicalTrials.gov. Available at: https://clinicaltrials.gov/ct2/show/NCT02468024. Accessed October 31, 2016.
36. Snee MP, McParland L, Collinson F, et al. The SABRTooth feasibility trial protocol: a study to determine the feasibility and acceptability of conducting a phase III randomised controlled trial comparing stereotactic ablative radiotherapy (SABR) with surgery in patients with peripheral stage I non-small cell lung cancer (NSCLC) considered to be at higher risk of complications from surgical resection. Pilot Feasibility Stud 2016;2:5.
37. Benedict SH, Yenice KM, Followill D, et al. Stereotactic body radiation therapy: the report of AAPM Task Group 101. Med Phys 2010;37(8):4078–101.
38. Solberg TD, Balter JM, Benedict SH, et al. Quality and safety considerations in stereotactic radiosurgery and stereotactic body radiation therapy: executive summary. Pract Radiat Oncol 2012;2(1):2–9.
39. Loo BW Jr, Chang JY, Dawson LA, et al. Stereotactic ablative radiotherapy: what's in a name? Pract Radiat Oncol 2011;1(1):38–9.

40. McGarry RC, Song G, des Rosiers P, et al. Observation-only management of early stage, medically inoperable lung cancer: poor outcome. Chest 2002;121(4):1155–8.
41. Corradetti MN, Haas AR, Rengan R. Central-airway necrosis after stereotactic body-radiation therapy. N Engl J Med 2012;366(24):2327–9.
42. Bezjak A, Paulus R, Gaspar LE, et al. Efficacy and toxicity analysis of NRG oncology/RTOG 0813 trial of stereotactic body radiation therapy (SBRT) for centrally located non-small cell lung cancer (NSCLC). Int J Radiat Oncol Biol Phys 2016;96(2):S8.
43. Onimaru R, Shirato H, Shimizu S, et al. Tolerance of organs at risk in small-volume, hypofractionated, image-guided radiotherapy for primary and metastatic lung cancers. Int J Radiat Oncol Biol Phys 2003;56(1):126–35.
44. Forquer JA, Fakiris AJ, Timmerman RD, et al. Brachial plexopathy from stereotactic body radiotherapy in early-stage NSCLC: dose-limiting toxicity in apical tumor sites. Radiother Oncol 2009;93(3):408–13.
45. Mutter RW, Liu F, Abreu A, et al. Dose-volume parameters predict for the development of chest wall pain after stereotactic body radiation for lung cancer. Int J Radiat Oncol Biol Phys 2012;82(5):1783–90.
46. Stephans KL, Djemil T, Tendulkar RD, et al. Prediction of chest wall toxicity from lung stereotactic body radiotherapy (SBRT). Int J Radiat Oncol Biol Phys 2012;82(2):974–80.

Optimal Use of Combined Modality Therapy in the Treatment of Esophageal Cancer

Talha Shaikh, MD, Joshua E. Meyer, MD, Eric M. Horwitz, MD*

KEYWORDS

- Esophageal cancer • Chemoradiation • Trimodality • IMRT • Esophagectomy

KEY POINTS

- Esophageal cancer continues to be associated with poor treatment outcomes despite significant advances in treatment technique.
- There has been an increasing incidence of esophageal adenocarcinoma and decreasing esophageal squamous cell carcinoma owing to changes in diet and lifestyle factors.
- Owing to the adoption of endoscopic surveillance, there has been an increasing incidence of early stage esophageal cancer with potential treatment options including endomucosal therapy, esophagectomy, or chemoradiation.
- Trimodality therapy consisting of neoadjuvant chemoradiation followed by esophagectomy is the preferred treatment option for patients with locally advanced esophageal cancer.

EPIDEMIOLOGY

Esophageal cancer is the sixth most common cancer diagnosis in the world with more than 450,000 patients diagnosed each year.[1] Although squamous cell carcinoma is the most common histology globally, adenocarcinoma is the most common histologic diagnosis in the United States. Despite significant advances in treatment techniques as well as the introduction of newer chemotherapy and targeted biologic agents, prognosis remains poor with 5-year survival rates of approximately 15% to 20%.[2,3] When examining outcomes according to stage, patients with clinically localized disease have a 5-year survival of nearly 40% versus only 4% in patients with metastatic disease. Over the past decade, the use of endoscopic screening has increased the number of early stage cancers diagnosed each year, yet approximately one-third of patients are still diagnosed with advanced disease.[3]

Disclosure Statement: The authors have nothing to disclose.
Department of Radiation Oncology, Fox Chase Cancer Center, 333 Cottman Avenue, Philadelphia, PA 19111, USA
* Corresponding author.
E-mail address: eric.horwitz@fccc.edu

Surg Oncol Clin N Am 26 (2017) 405–429
http://dx.doi.org/10.1016/j.soc.2017.01.009
surgonc.theclinics.com

RISK FACTORS

Risk factors for the development of esophageal cancer are provided in **Table 1**. Esophageal cancer peaks in late adulthood (60–70 years of age), and the incidence varies greatly according to gender, geography, and ethnicity. In general, esophageal cancer is diagnosed more commonly in males, although the patterns in diagnosis vary by geographic area. When examining histology, squamous cell carcinoma is far more common in black patients, and adenocarcinomas are more commonly seen in white patients.

The incidence of esophageal adenocarcinoma has increased dramatically in the United States over the past several decades, while the incidence of squamous cell carcinoma has been decreasing (**Fig. 1**).[4–6] The increase in esophageal adenocarcinoma has been attributed to changes in diet, with increased intake of high-fat foods and a decrease in fruit and vegetable consumption.[7] Gastroesophageal reflux disease has been linked to esophageal adenocarcinoma (but not esophageal squamous cell carcinoma) in multiple population-based series.[8,9] A large metaanalysis suggested that weekly symptoms of gastroesophageal reflux disease resulted in a dramatic increase in the risk for esophageal adenocarcinoma (odds ratio, 4.92; 95% confidence interval, 3.90–6.22) compared with asymptomatic controls.[10] The decrease in squamous cell carcinoma incidence is likely owing to decreasing rates of smoking and alcohol use.

Barrett's esophagus is defined as a change in the normal squamous epithelium of the distal esophagus to a columnar type, with the classic appearance of a salmon-colored mucosa and the presence of goblet cells. These changes are thought to occur owing to a chronic inflammatory state that increases the risk for the development of esophageal adenocarcinoma. Patients diagnosed with Barrett's esophagus have 11 times the risk of developing esophageal cancer versus those without Barrett's. A large series from the Netherlands examined a cohort of 42,207 patients and found a risk of 0.4% of developing esophageal cancer with a history of Barrett's.[11] This study clearly illustrates that, although the risk of esophageal cancer in patients with Barrett's is high relative to the general population, it is still relatively low.

Patients found to have Barrett's esophagus typically undergo surveillance esophagogastroduodenoscopy owing to the increased risk of esophageal cancer. Typically, it is recommended that patients with Barrett's undergo esophagogastroduodenoscopy every 3 to 5 years with standardized sampling and methodological documentation of the extent of disease. When a high-grade dysplastic lesion is identified, patients may undergo either endoscopic mucosal resection (EMR) or surgical resection. There is wide variation in the incidence of esophageal adenocarcinoma in this setting, ranging from 0% to 3.5% per year.[12]

Table 1
Risk factors associated with development esophageal cancer

Adenocarcinoma	Squamous Cell Carcinoma
Obesity	Socioeconomic class
Smoking	Nitrosamine
Gastroesophageal reflux disease	Polyaromatic hydrocarbons
Barrett's esophagus	Tobacco smoking
Family history	Poor oral hyenine
	Family history
	Alcohol

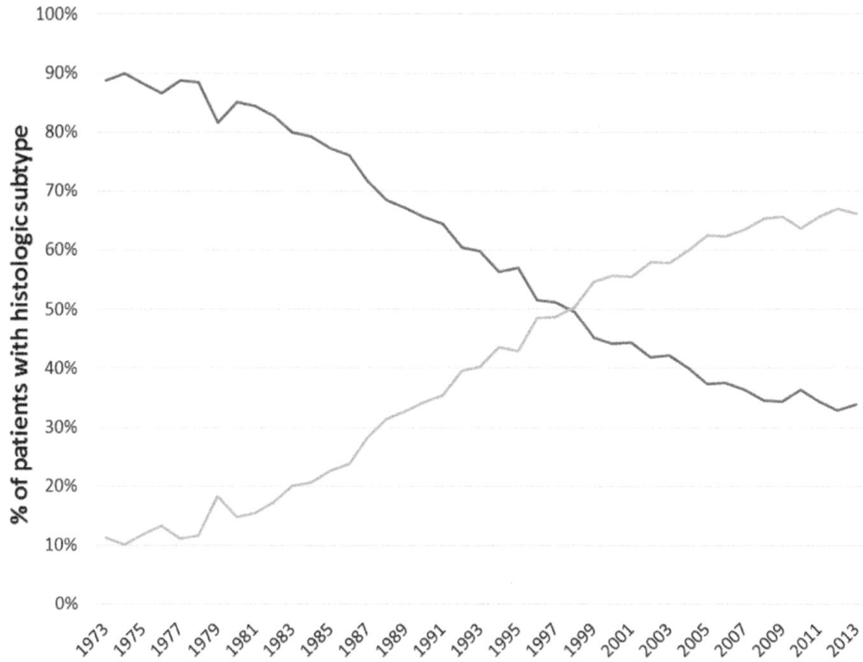

Fig. 1. Incidence esophageal adenocarcinoma (green) and squamous cell carcinoma (blue) in the United States.

ANATOMY

The esophagus is a hollow, viscus organ that extends inferiorly from the cricoid cartilage at the cricopharyngeus muscle to the gastroesophageal junction (**Fig. 2**). The esophagus is further subdivided into cervical (15–18 cm from the incisors), upper thoracic (18–24 cm), middle thoracic (24–32 cm), and lower thoracic (32–40 cm) esophagus. Keratinizing squamous epithelium lines nearly the entire length of the esophagus, although the squamous epithelium can be replaced by intestinal-type glandular epithelium (Barrett's esophagus). Beneath the epithelial layer of the esophagus is the basement membrane followed by the lamina propria, muscularis mucosa, submucosa, muscularis propria, and adventitia. Unlike other parts of the gastrointestinal tract, the esophagus lacks a true serosa and thus esophageal tumors have the ability to spread to adjacent organs and distal nodal regions relatively unhindered, without having to traverse a serosal layer.

The esophagus has a rich lymphatic system, with potential metastatic disease dependent on tumor location. Furthermore, because the submucosal lymphatics may traverse long distances along the length of the esophagus, radiation volumes are generally long to encompass these at-risk regions. The cervical esophagus may drain to cervical neck nodes and supraclavicular nodes. The upper thoracic esophagus drains to lymph nodes along the innominate artery and ligamentum arteriosium, in addition to paraesophageal and paratracheal nodes. The middle thoracic esophagus drains to the tracheobronchial, paraesophageal, and pulmonary hilar nodes. The gastroesophageal junction drains to nodes along the left gastric artery, celiac axis, common hepatic artery, splenic artery, lesser curvature of the stomach, and paracardial region. Although the potential nodal drainage patterns are extensive in

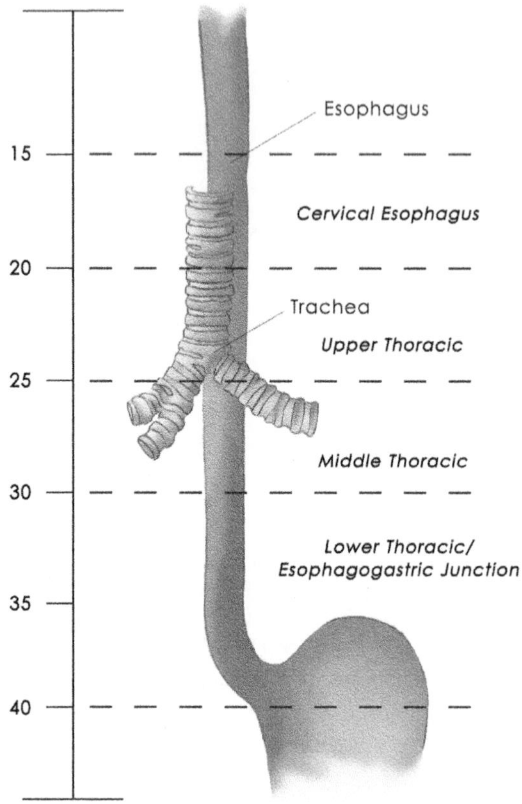

Fig. 2. Anatomy of the esophagus. (*Courtesy of* May Ayad, BA, Clarion, PA.)

patients with esophageal cancer, radiotherapy fields do not routinely prophylactically encompass all at risk nodal regions.

STAGING AND WORKUP

Patients diagnosed with esophageal cancer most commonly present with symptoms of progressive dysphagia or odynophagia and weight loss. Other symptoms such as chest pain are less common, but may suggest involvement of adjacent mediastinal structures. Even less common are insidious findings such as anemia, lymphadenopathy, or hoarseness, suggesting recurrent laryngeal nerve involvement.

The American Joint Committee on Cancer TNM classification and staging has been directly linked to outcomes in patients diagnosed and treated for esophageal cancer. The most recent seventh edition has several important changes from the previous version of the staging manual.[13] In particular, the American Joint Committee on Cancer TNM staging now separates squamous cell carcinoma from adenocarcinoma, reflecting the increasing understanding that these are 2 separate entities with substantially different outcomes and prognosis. Other changes in the seventh edition include the subclassification of T4 tumors into resectable (T4a) or unresectable (T4b) disease. Furthermore, the staging system adds location and grade into the classification system. The nodal classification was also altered; the current system uses the number of lymph nodes positive instead of location of the disease. In addition, celiac lymph node involvement, previously considered metastatic disease, is now classified as regional. **Table 2** details the stage groupings according to the American Joint Committee on Cancer TNM seventh edition.

Accurate staging is essential in esophageal cancer, because the treatment modality of choice varies greatly according to the extent of disease. The initial diagnostic method is typically an endoscopy with biopsy, providing a histologic diagnosis and demonstrating the extent of disease. The use of endoscopic ultrasound provides the depth of infiltration and has 60% to 90% accuracy for T staging and 50% to 90% accuracy for nodal staging (**Fig. 3**). In patients with proximal esophageal cancers, tracheobronchoscopy is indicated with biopsies and brushings to rule out tumor infiltration into the trachea or mainstem bronchus. Patients with tumors adherent to the mediastinum are typically considered unresectable.

In addition to locoregional staging, computed tomography (CT) of the chest and abdomen allow for the evaluation of distant metastatic disease as well as infiltration of adjacent organs. More recently, PET has become a critical component in the staging workup for esophageal cancers, because 15% of patients may have distant metastasis not otherwise detected.[14] Before proceeding with multimodality therapy, all patients should undergo a PET/CT scan to evaluate for potential distant metastatic disease (**Fig. 4**). The role of PET/CT in an adaptive treatment strategy is an area of active investigation. The role of laparoscopy in preoperative staging is based on institutional preference. Although many institutions have moved away from routine laparoscopies in these patients, pretreatment surgical staging has been shown to be more accurate versus imaging techniques. In a study conducted by the Cancer and Leukemia Group B, invasive staging more accurately identified lymph node positivity or advanced locoregional disease, although it should be noted that this study was conducted in the pre-PET/CT era.[15]

TREATMENT MODALITIES

Treatment of esophageal cancer necessitates maximizing survival while offering symptomatic improvement, because a significant number of patients present with dysphagia or related symptoms. Although surgery alone may be curative in select patients with early disease (cT1N0), a combined approach is indicated typically for most patients with locally advanced disease. Endoscopic procedures for superficial mucosal lesions can be curative, although patients with more invasive lymph node negative tumors may require esophagectomy as well as chemotherapy with or without radiation. Historically, the appropriate management for locally advanced esophageal cancers has been controversial, with potential options including esophagectomy, chemotherapy followed by esophagectomy, chemoradiation followed by esophagectomy, or esophagectomy alone. More recently, a trimodality approach consisting of chemoradiation followed by surgery has been increasingly accepted as the preferred treatment option for these patients.

Surgery

The majority of patients diagnosed with esophageal cancer have penetration of the submucosal tissue and surgical evaluation is recommended. In general, surgery consists of a transthoracic en bloc esophagectomy and lymphadenectomy. The resected esophagus is replaced by a conduit and anastomosed to the remaining esophagus. There are several methods of esophagectomy described in the literature. Each one differs by the site of anastomosis and may be preferred according to the site of the tumor.

Table 2
American Joint Committee on Cancer staging for esophageal cancer

	Description
Primary tumor	
TX	Primary tumor cannot be assessed
T0	No evidence of primary tumor
Tis	High-grade dysplasia
T1	Tumor invades lamina propria, muscularis mucosae, or submucosa
T1a	Tumor invades lamina propria or muscularis mucosae
T1b	Tumor invades submucosa
T2	Tumor invades muscularis propria
T3	Tumor invades adventitia
T4	Tumor invades adjacent structures
T4a	Resectable tumor invading pleura, pericardium, or diaphragm
T4b	Unresectable tumor invading other adjacent structures, such as aorta, vertebral body or trachea
Regional lymph nodes	
NX	Regional nodes not assessed
N0	No regional lymph node metastasis
N1	Metastasis in 1–2 regional lymph nodes*
N2	Metastasis in 3–6 regional lymph nodes*
N3	Metastasis in 7 or more regional lymph nodes
Distant metastasis	
MX	Distant metastasis cannot be assessed
M0	No distant metastasis
M1	Distant metastasis
Stage grouping (adenocarcinoma)	
Stage 0	Tis, N0, M0, grade 1 or X
Stage IA	T1, N0, M0, grade 1–2 or X
Stage IB	T1, N0, M0, grade 3 T2, N0, M0, grade 1–2 or X
Stage IIA	T2, N0, M0, grade 3
Stage IIB	T3, N0, M0, any grade T1-2, N1, M0, any grade
Stage IIIA	T1-2, N2, M0, any grade T3, N1, M0, any grade T4a, N0, M0, any grade
Stage IIIB	T3, N2, M0, any grade
Stage IIIC	T4a, N1-2, M0, any grade T4b, any N, M0, any grade Any T, N3, M0, any grade
Stage IV	Any T, any N, M1, any grade
Stage grouping (squamous cell carcinoma)	
Stage 0	Tis, N0, M0, grade 1 or X, any location
Stage IA	T1, N0, M0, grade 1 or X, any location

(*continued on next page*)

Table 2 (*continued*)	
	Description
Stage IB	T1, N0, M0, grade 2 or 3, any location T2-3, N0, M0, grade 1 or X, lower esophagus or X
Stage IIA	T2-3, N0, M0, grade 1 or X, upper and middle esophagus T2-3, N0, M0, grade 2 or 3, lower esophagus or X
Stage IIB	Stage IIB T2-3, N0, M0, grade 2 or 3, upper and middle esophagus T1-2, N1, M0, any grade, any location
Stage IIIA	T1-2, N2, M0, any grade, any location T3, N1, M0, any grade, any location T4a, N0, M0, any grade, any location
Stage IIIB	T3, N2, M0, any grade, any location
Stage IIIC	T4a, N1-2, M0, any grade, any location T4b, any N, M0, any grade, any location Any T, N3, M0, any grade, any location
Stage IV	Any T, any N, M1, any grade, any location

* Regional lymph nodes extend from cervical nodes to celiac nodes.

A transhiatal esophagectomy consists of dissecting the upper portion of the esophagus using a cervical approach along with an abdominal incision; this procedure does not require a thoracotomy. A blunt dissection technique is used to minimize risk of injury to the esophagus or surrounding tissue, and a cervical esophagogastrostomy anastomosis is performed in the left neck. Owing to the location of the left recurrent laryngeal nerve, care must be taken to minimize the risk of injury. A transthoracic (Ivor-Lewis) approach is the most commonly used method, consisting of a right thoracotomy and a laparotomy. This approach allows good access to middle and distal esophageal lesions. The transhiatal approach allows for a more thorough dissection of the paraesophageal lymph nodes owing to better visualization. A disadvantage of this approach is that there is a potential for an anastomotic leak into the thorax or a thoracic duct leak, either of which can be significant complications. The McKeown or "3-field" esophagectomy consists of all 3 incisions (cervical, right thoracotomy, and laparotomy) and has resulted in similar outcomes compared with the other approaches.[16] Recent advances in technology have also allowed for the adoption of minimally invasive techniques that consist of a combination of laparoscopic, thoracoscopic, and robotic approaches. Early series examining minimally invasive esophagectomy have demonstrated excellent clinical outcomes.[17–19]

In patients undergoing esophagectomy, there are data suggesting that an increased lymph node harvest during surgery improves treatment outcomes. Greenstein and colleagues[20] retrospectively reviewed a cohort of 972 patients and found a stepwise increase in 5-year disease-specific survival with increasing lymph nodes dissected; 55% with less than 11, 66% with 11 to 17, and 75% with 18 or more. Other series have also demonstrated an association between number of lymph nodes removed and treatment outcomes.[21–23] Current guidelines suggest at least 15 lymph nodes dissected at the time of esophagectomy, and the location of these lymph nodes varies by tumor site.[24] Upper and middle esophageal lesions typically require a dissection of the lymph nodes in the surrounding adventitia, whereas distal esophageal lesions require a dissection of paraesophageal nodes along the paracardiac and gastrohepatic ligament and along the left gastric artery.

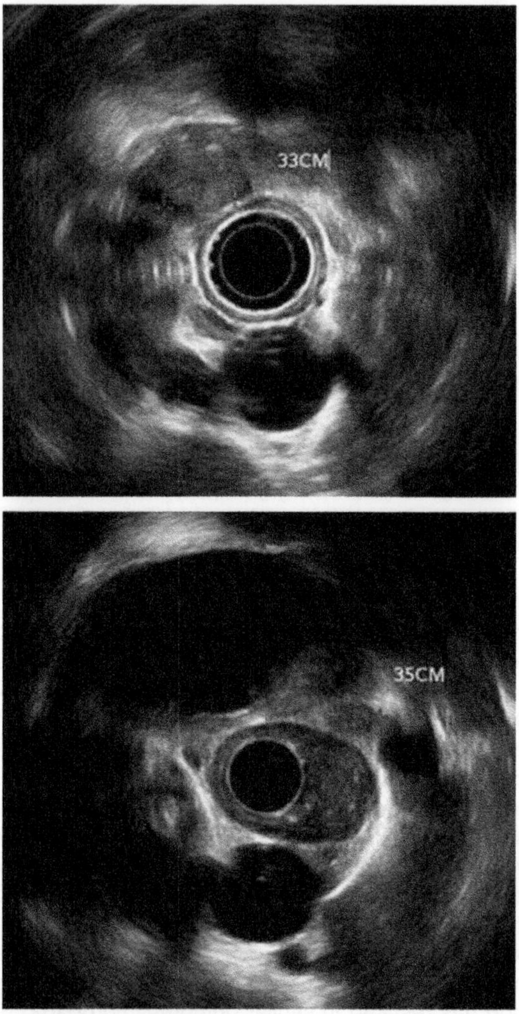

Fig. 3. Patient with a T3N1 esophageal adenocarcinoma of the lower esophagus.

Surgical resection margin status is a key driver of tumor recurrence, and safely obtaining negative margins is crucial when planning surgery. In concept, there are 3 margins that must be assessed at the time of surgery, the proximal tumor margin, the distal tumor margin, and the circumferential tumor margin. The proximal and distal tumor margins should generally be at least 4 to 5 cm and the circumferential tumor margin should be 1 mm or greater. A recent metaanalysis of 14 studies found significantly higher mortality rates in patients with positive circumferential resection margins and found a survival advantage with a resection margin of more than 1 mm.[25]

Esophagectomy continues to be one of the most morbid procedures in oncology, although mortality rates have improved from 10% in the 1970s to 3% in the 1990s.[26] Data has suggested that high-volume centers having significantly improved treatment outcomes. A recent metaanalysis demonstrated that overall mortality is decreased in treatment centers performing a high number of esophagectomy cases.[27]

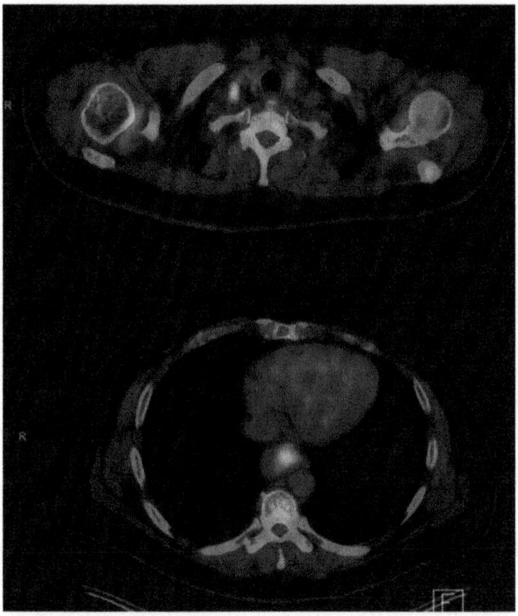

Fig. 4. PET/computed tomography image of patients with distal esophageal cancer and supraclavicular lymph node involvement.

Patients who will undergo an esophagectomy should be referred to a high-volume center owing to improved outcomes.

Systemic Therapy

Systemic therapy plays an important role in the management of patients with both localized and metastatic disease. Although surgical resection alone may be an acceptable treatment approach for patients with early stage (Tis or T1) esophageal cancer, patients with locally advanced disease generally require multimodality therapy. The dual role of cytotoxic chemotherapy is to sterilize micrometastatic disease owing to the high rates of distant failure as well as to potentiate the effectiveness of radiotherapy in patients receiving chemoradiation.[28] In the landmark Herskovic study, patients randomized to chemotherapy and radiation had a significant survival advantage of 12.5 months versus 8.9 months in the radiation alone arm.[29]

Chemotherapy for metastatic esophageal and gastroesophageal cancers has evolved significantly over the past several decades. Whereas historical treatment approaches consisted of single agents, more recent treatment approaches involve at least doublets with improved overall survival with dual therapy. A large metaanalysis demonstrated a significant survival benefit with combination chemotherapy versus single-agent chemotherapy (hazard ratio, 0.82; 95% confidence interval, 0.74–0.90).[30]

Recent advances have also allowed for the recognition of targetable mutations in the management of metastatic esophageal cancer. In particular, approximately 20% of esophageal cancers have overexpression of HER2, a transmembrane tyrosine kinase receptor. Trastuzumab, a humanized monoclonal antibody that binds to the extracellular domain of HER2, has been found to improve overall survival in patients with metastatic HER-2–positive gastroesophageal junction or gastric adenocarcinoma.[31] Other ongoing research efforts are examining targetable epidermal growth factor receptor, cMET, and other mutations in esophageal cancer.

Radiotherapy

Radiotherapy is part of the curative treatment approach in patients with locally advanced esophageal cancer. Radiotherapy can also be used for palliation in patients with metastatic disease. In patients with nonmetastatic disease, radiotherapy may be used in conjunction with chemotherapy as definitive treatment or preoperatively with chemotherapy before esophagectomy. In general, patients with nonmetastatic disease receiving radiotherapy should also receive systemic therapy owing to the poor outcomes in patients receiving radiation alone. In Radiation Therapy Oncology Group (RTOG) 85-01, there were no 5-year survivors after radiotherapy alone versus a 5-year survival of 27% after chemoradiation. Therefore, concurrent chemoradiation is the preferred treatment approach in patients receiving definitive treatment.[29]

Multimodality therapy consisting of chemoradiation followed by surgery has been increasingly adopted in the management of esophageal cancer. There are 7 randomized trials that have examined preoperative chemoradiation versus surgical resection. The trials have demonstrated mixed results, with some series demonstrating a benefit from neoadjuvant therapy while others demonstrated no difference. Most recently, the landmark CROSS trial (Chemoradiotherapy for Oesophageal Cancer Followed by Surgery Study) randomized 366 patients to neoadjuvant chemoradiation with carboplatin and paclitaxel or surgery alone. The results demonstrated a significant survival advantage in patients receiving trimodality therapy (median survival: 24 vs 49 months). Because this trial was well-powered, used modern surgery and chemotherapy, and treated a contemporary mix of patients, trimodality therapy consisting of chemoradiation followed by esophagectomy has become the preferred treatment option for patients with locally advanced esophageal cancer.[24]

The role of surgery in patients with locally advanced esophageal cancer has also been tested with the theory that an organ preservation approach may result in similar outcomes without subjecting patients to surgical morbidity. Two trials conducted in Europe addressed the role for surgery after chemoradiation in squamous cell carcinoma patients. Stahl and colleagues[32] randomized patients who had received induction chemotherapy to either definitive chemoradiation or chemoradiation followed by surgery. The Federation Francophone de Cancerologie Digestive randomized patients who responded to chemoradiation to either observation or surgery.[33] Neither trial demonstrated a difference in overall survival, although there were higher rates of treatment-related mortality in the surgical arms. In patients with adenocarcinoma, pathologic complete response rates are substantially lower (23% vs 49% in the CROSS trial) and, therefore, the risk of persistent disease is much greater. Given the decline in surgical morbidity and mortality, trimodality therapy remains a commonly used strategy.[34]

Another investigational approach is reservation of surgery as a salvage option, in an effort to better select those patients who will benefit from surgery. RTOG 0246 tested chemoradiation consisting of induction 5-fluoracil (5-FU), cisplatin, and paclitaxel, followed by concurrent chemoradiation with 50.4 Gy and 5-FU, and cisplatin with surgical salvage for patients with residual or recurrent disease without systemic disease.[35] The 1-year survival (71%) did not achieve the trial's prespecified endpoint of 1-year survival of 77.5%, although this may have owing to the higher than expected neoadjuvant treatment-related mortality.

Because persistent or recurrent local disease is still relatively common after definitive chemoradiation, dose-escalated radiotherapy has been tested to examine whether local control and survival can be improved with an increasing dose to the tumor volume. In the Intergroup 0123 trial, patients were randomized to either 64.8 Gy or

50.4 Gy with concurrent cisplatin and 5-FU. There was no difference in overall survival (13 months vs 18.1 months) or locoregional failure (56% vs 52%) with high-dose radiation.[36] Another attempt at dose escalation was via a brachytherapy boost in RTOG 9207, where patients received concurrent chemoradiation followed by intraluminal brachytherapy along with concurrent 5-FU.[37] Unfortunately, owing to a high rate of treatment-related morbidity, this technique is not recommended typically.

In patients diagnosed with cervical esophageal cancer, the surgery required to remove the tumor adequately is comprehensive and can lead to significant morbidity and mortality. As a result, the tumor is commonly treated similarly to a primary head and neck cancer with definitive chemoradiation being the treatment modality of choice. Definitive chemoradiation allows for organ preservation while resulting in similar treatment efficacy. Unfortunately, there are relatively few data in this realm. In a series of 34 patients treated with concurrent chemoradiation with cisplatin and 5-FU, the local control rate was 88%, although 2 patients died from treatment-related toxicity.[38] Similar outcomes have been demonstrated by other institutions, although higher doses were used in these series.[39–41]

Although radiotherapy is an effective treatment modality, dose delivery to surrounding structures can lead to a significant risk for toxicity.[42,43] Over the past decade, there have been significant technological advances in the realm of radiotherapy that allow for image-guided radiotherapy and intensity-modulated radiotherapy. Image-guided radiotherapy integrates imaging to allow for anatomic visualization of the tumor and surrounding structures to improve the accuracy and precision of radiation delivery. The use of 4-dimensional planning also allows for more accurate target delineation by creating an internal target volume that accounts for respiratory motion and allows for more conformal treatment planning volumes. Intensity-modulated radiotherapy consists of modulating the intensity of each radiation beam to improve target volume coverage while minimizing dose to organs at risk (**Fig. 5**). Several series have suggested that intensity-modulated radiotherapy is safe and effective and will likely be increasingly adopted in the coming years.[44–47] Similarly, proton therapy has the theoretic advantage of further improving dose distribution owing with a sharp dose falloff provided that clinical trials demonstrate either improved overall survival or reduced toxicity. As a result, proton therapy may allow for a further decrease in the dose to the surrounding structures. Additional data are necessary to establish the efficacy and toxicity benefit of proton therapy treatment for esophageal cancer.

TREATMENT

Early Stage Disease

With the adoption of routine endoscopic surveillance, there has been an increasing incidence of esophageal cancer detected at an early stage.[48] Whereas esophagectomy has historically been the preferred treatment option even in patients with high-grade dysplasia or early esophageal cancer, endoscopic techniques have been adopted increasingly. Ideally, endoscopic approaches are only considered for a select group of patients who are at low risk for lymph node involvement (**Box 1**). When evaluating patients who may be candidates for an endoscopic procedure, the depth of tumor invasion into the wall of the esophagus is crucial to identify the potential for nodal metastasis. Although endoscopic ultrasound imaging is a noninvasive diagnostic methodology, its accuracy in early stage patients is controversial with a large metaanalysis demonstrating a T-stage concordance with pathologic staging of 65%.[49]

For patients with esophageal cancer that extends no further than the lamina propria or muscularis mucosa (Tis, T1a), endomucosal therapy or definitive chemoradiation

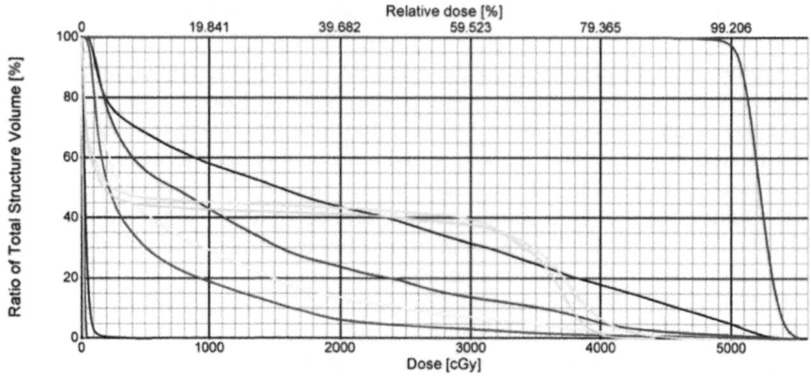

	Structure	Structure Status	Coverage [%/%]	Volume	Min Dose	Max Dose	Mean Dose	Modal Dose	Median Dose	Std Dev
	scord	Approved	100.0 / 100.2	51.6 cm³	0.0 cGy	4418.1 cGy	1525.4 cGy	0.3 cGy	179.9 cGy	1708.0 cGy
	scord+3mm	Approved	100.0 / 100.0	118.1 cm³	0.0 cGy	4895.7 cGy	1639.6 cGy	0.4 cGy	242.3 cGy	1760.3 cGy
	right kidney	Approved	100.0 / 100.1	122.6 cm³	0.0 cGy	26.0 cGy	9.3 cGy	0.4 cGy	9.2 cGy	6.5 cGy
	left kidney	Approved	100.0 / 100.0	162.2 cm³	0.0 cGy	47.4 cGy	15.2 cGy	0.4 cGy	14.8 cGy	10.5 cGy
	heart	Approved	100.0 / 100.0	767.8 cm³	46.1 cGy	5584.0 cGy	1972.8 cGy	101.0 cGy	1534.2 cGy	1714.4 cGy
	Lung_L	Approved	100.0 / 100.1	1394.9 cm³	0.0 cGy	5468.8 cGy	1257.1 cGy	142.2 cGy	720.2 cGy	1315.4 cGy
	liver	Approved	100.0 / 100.0	1479.2 cm³	0.0 cGy	546.4 cGy	33.8 cGy	11.5 cGy	25.5 cGy	32.8 cGy
	Lung_R	Approved	100.0 / 100.0	1677.7 cm³	20.5 cGy	5524.9 cGy	584.9 cGy	98.5 cGy	216.8 cGy	827.3 cGy

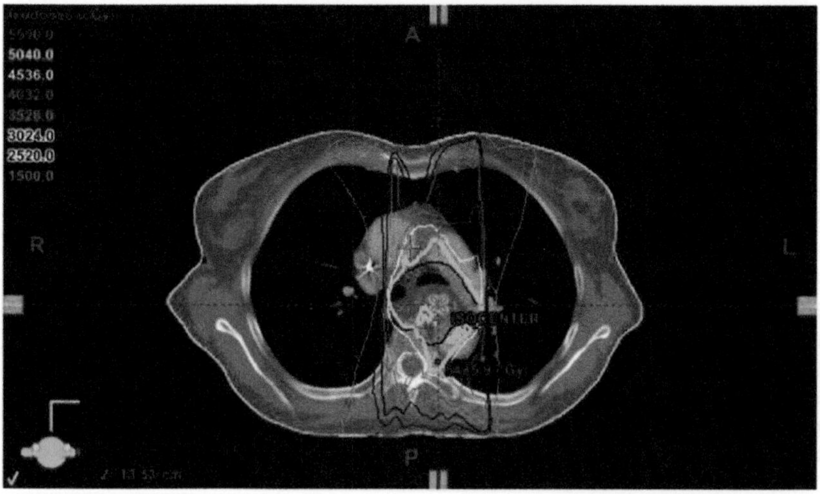

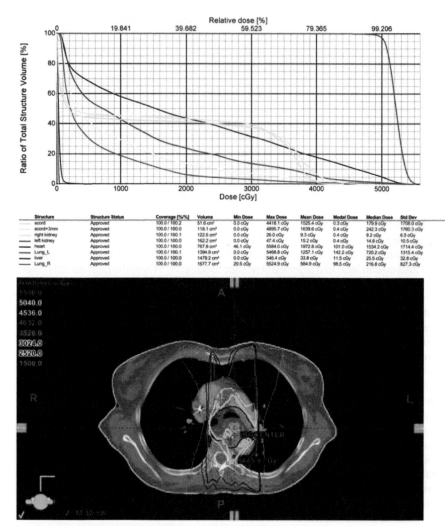

Fig. 5. Dose distribution of treatment plan for intensity modulated radiation.

Box 1 **Criteria for endoscopic mucosal resection**
T1a tumor (restricted to mucosal layer)
Tumor diameter ≤2 cm
Grade 1 or grade 2
No lymphovascular invasion
No ulceration

may be appropriate options. Potential endomucosal options for early stage disease include EMR, photodynamic therapy, and radiofrequency ablation. The most commonly used method, EMR, consists of lifting the mucosa and resecting the superficial lesion. The advantage of EMR over ablative techniques is that it allows for the pathologic confirmation of the depth of invasion thus allowing for evaluation of completeness of therapy. Recent data demonstrate an increase in the use of endoscopic resection in the management of early stage esophageal cancer.[50]

For patients with stage I esophageal cancer invading the muscularis propria, esophagectomy is the recommended treatment approach owing to an increased risk of nodal metastasis and the potential for inadequate treatment of deeper penetrating tumors with endomucosal therapies. In addition, patients who demonstrate recurrence or persistently positive margins after endoscopic therapy are typically recommended to undergo esophagectomy. In addition to the therapeutic gain of surgery, esophagectomy also allows for better pathologic evaluation and thus can help to dictate whether adjuvant therapy is needed.

Definitive chemoradiotherapy is a potential treatment option for patients with Tis or T1a disease who are not candidates for endoscopic procedures or esophagectomy. In a series reported by Motoori and colleagues,[51] 102 patients underwent esophagectomy versus 71 patients receiving definitive chemoradiotherapy for T1b esophageal cancer. At a median follow-up of approximately 5 years, there was no difference in overall survival, with a 3-year overall survival of 87% in the surgery arm versus 78% in the chemoradiation arm. These results suggest that in patients who may not be candidates for surgery, chemoradiation may be a reasonable alternative.

Surgical Multimodality Options: Neoadjuvant Therapy

Neoadjuvant chemotherapy or combination chemoradiation can potentially sterilize subclinical distant disease while also treating the primary tumor. There have been several series examining both chemotherapy and chemoradiation in patients with locally advanced esophageal cancer with conflicting outcomes across series.

There is a limited role for neoadjuvant radiotherapy alone in patients with locally advanced esophageal cancer. Several randomized trials conducted in the 1970s and 1980s examined preoperative radiotherapy followed by esophagectomy.[52–56] None of these trials found an improvement in outcomes with the addition of radiotherapy. Although these series were conducted in an era of antiquated treatment techniques, the use of systemic therapy has effectively eliminated bimodal therapy consisting of radiotherapy followed by surgery as a treatment approach.

Although there are no positive trials in favor of radiotherapy followed by esophagectomy, there are conflicting data in favor of chemotherapy followed by surgery. One of the largest trials examining neoadjuvant chemotherapy was conducted by the Medical Research Council in which 802 patients were randomized to either neoadjuvant chemotherapy with 2 cycles of 5-FU and cisplatin followed by surgery versus surgery alone.[57] This study found an improved overall survival (hazard ratio, 0.79; 95% confidence interval, 0.68–0.93) with the addition of chemotherapy. At 3 years, the overall survival in the bimodality arm was 43% versus 34% in the surgery alone arm. In contrast, the Intergroup 113 trial similarly randomized 467 patients to neoadjuvant chemotherapy with 3 cycles of 5-FU and cisplatin and found no difference in overall survival between patient groups, although R1 resections were more common in patients receiving surgery alone.[58] One reason for the difference in outcomes between the 2 studies may be a higher chemotherapy dose in the Intergroup trial, resulting in increased toxicity. Other trials have demonstrated similarly conflicting results regarding neoadjuvant chemotherapy.[52,58–61] A metaanalysis examining 9 trials that compared neoadjuvant chemotherapy followed by surgery versus surgery alone demonstrated a survival benefit with the addition of neoadjuvant chemotherapy to esophagectomy, with a hazard ratio for death of 0.87.[62] Overall, the pathologic complete response rates in these trials range from 0% to 4%.

Trimodality therapy consisting of neoadjuvant chemotherapy and radiation followed by surgery has been increasingly adopted over the past decade. The rationale behind this approach is that radiotherapy can help to sterilize the surgical field while chemotherapy can potentiate the radiation in addition to sterilizing distant disease. Similar to the trials examining neoadjuvant chemotherapy, the trials examining chemoradiation have had conflicting results; however, the recently published CROSS trial has affirmed the superiority of trimodality therapy versus surgery alone.

Three randomized trials have demonstrated an overall survival advantage from the addition of preoperative chemoradiation over esophagectomy alone. Walsh and colleagues[63] examined a cohort of 103 patients with esophageal adenocarcinoma of the distal esophagus or gastroesophageal junction who were randomized to neoadjuvant chemoradiation consisting of cisplatin and 5-FU versus surgery alone. There was a significant survival advantage with the use of trimodality therapy with a 3-year survival of 32% versus 6% in patients receiving surgery alone. There was significant downstaging in the preoperative chemoradiation arm. Similarly, Tepper and colleagues[64] randomized patients to cisplatin and 5-FU with concurrent radiotherapy followed by surgery versus surgery alone. Although this trial closed early owing to poor accrual, the addition of chemoradiation provided a significant survival advantage (5-year overall survival of 39% vs 16%) (**Table 3**).

Table 3
Select randomized trials examining preoperative chemoradiation

Author (Year)	N	Chemotherapy	3-Year Overall Survival (%)	*P* Value
Urba et al,[65] 2001	50	Chemoradiation (cisplatin, fluorouracil, vinblastine) + radiation (45 Gy)	30	.15
	50	Surgery alone	16	
Tepper et al,[64] 2008	30	Chemoradiation (cisplatin, fluorouracil) + radiation (50.4 Gy)	39 (5-y)	.002
	26	Surgery alone	16 (5-y)	
Burmeister et al,[66] 2002	128	Chemoradiation (cisplatin, fluorouracil) + radiation (35 Gy)	19	.38
	128	Surgery alone	22	
Walsh et al,[63] 1996	58	Chemoradiation (cisplatin, fluorouracil) + radiation (40 Gy)	26	.01
	55	Surgery alone	20	
Mariette et al,[67] 2010	97	Chemoradiation (cisplatin, fluorouracil) + radiation (45 Gy)	29	.68
	98	Surgery alone	55	
Van Hagen et al,[68] 2012	175	Chemoradiation (carboplatin, paclitaxel) + radiation (45 Gy)	59	.011
	188	Surgery alone	44	

The most contemporary and definitive study examining trimodality therapy was the CROSS trial, which randomized 368 patients to either surgery alone or chemoradiation consisting of carboplatin and paclitaxel followed by surgery.[68,69] Patients receiving trimodality therapy had a significant survival benefit, with a median overall survival of 49 months versus 24 months. Preoperative chemoradiation resulted in significant downstaging with 29% achieving a pathologic complete response. In addition, 92% of patients in the trimodality arm received margin-negative resections versus 69% in the surgery alone arm. In a subsequent analysis, chemoradiation significantly reduced locoregional failure from 34% to 14%, in addition to decreasing peritoneal and hematogenous spread.[70]

One of the theoretic concerns about trimodality therapy is the potential for increased morbidity after preoperative chemoradiation. It is reassuring to note that most published trials do not demonstrate an increase in surgical morbidity after trimodality therapy. The CROSS trial demonstrated similar morbidity and mortality in the trimodality and surgery alone arm.[68] There were no differences in pulmonary or cardiac complications or anastomotic leakage. The 30-day mortality was 6% in the trimodality arm versus 7% in the surgery alone arm. Based on these results, trimodality therapy consisting of chemoradiation followed by esophagectomy is the preferred treatment approach in patients with locally advanced esophageal cancer.

Pathologic complete response is an important predictor of treatment outcomes after neoadjuvant chemoradiation. Not surprisingly, multiple series have demonstrated that patients with no residual tumor on pathology have an improved survival versus those with residual disease.[71–74] Owing to the improved outcomes, multiple investigators have attempted to identify factors associated with a pathologic complete response. Most of the factors identified are not modifiable and typically include stage, tumor length, and histology.[75–77] Recent data suggest that a prolonged length between preoperative chemoradiation and esophagectomy may result in increased response rates. An analysis by Shaikh and colleagues[78] found a stepwise increase in pathologic complete response rates with increasing time between chemoradiation and surgery suggesting prolonging this interval may allow for tumor regression (**Fig. 6**). This has also been demonstrated in other series.[79,80]

Surgical Multimodality Options: Adjuvant Therapy

The role of adjuvant radiation therapy in patients with locally advanced esophageal cancer is controversial after several randomized trials have demonstrated no apparent

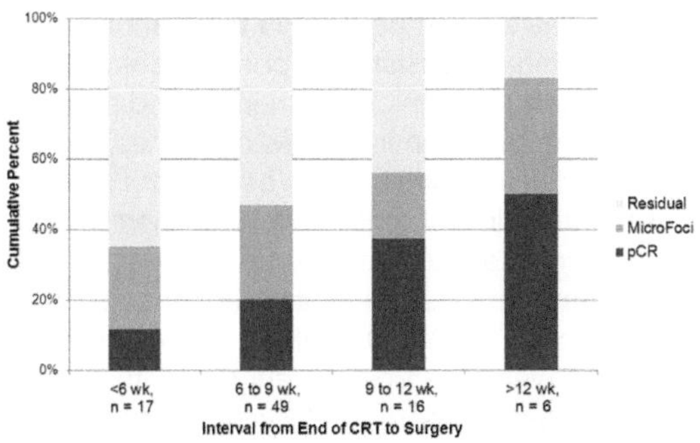

Fig. 6. Pathologic response by interval from end of chemoradiation therapy (CRT) to surgery. pCR, pathologic complete response. (*From* Shaikh T, Ruth K, Scott WJ, et al. Increased time from neoadjuvant chemoradiation to surgery is associated with higher pathologic complete response rates in esophageal cancer. Annals Thoracic Surgery 2015;99(1):273; with permission.)

benefit.[81,82] In addition, postoperative treatment may lead to an increased risk of complications after surgery. In a randomized trial comparing surgery with surgery followed by adjuvant radiotherapy, 37% of patients receiving radiotherapy developed postoperative complications versus 6% in the surgery alone arm.

The Intergroup 0116 trial is the only published randomized trial demonstrating a survival benefit with the addition of postoperative chemoradiation.[83] This trial randomized patients with either gastric or gastroesophageal junction adenocarcinoma to either postoperative chemoradiation with 5-FU and leucovorin or observation after surgical resection. The authors found a survival advantage to postoperative multimodality therapy with a median overall survival of 36 months versus 27 months in the surgery alone arm. Although the majority of patients on this trial had gastric adenocarcinoma, this trial suggests there may be a role for postoperative chemoradiation in select gastroesophageal junction cancers.

Although there is a limited role for postoperative treatment in patients with esophageal cancer, those who have a clinical early stage tumor but are upstaged at the time of surgery may benefit from postoperative therapy. An analysis of the National Cancer Database by Wong and colleagues[84] found improved overall survival with the addition of postoperative radiation in patients with lymph node–positive disease or positive margins. Other smaller retrospective series have also suggested a benefit from adjuvant radiotherapy in patients with residual disease or lymph node positivity.[85,86]

Nonsurgical Multimodality Options: Definitive Chemoradiation

Combination chemotherapy and radiotherapy without surgery has also been studied extensively. In general, chemotherapy consists of cytotoxic agents such as 5-FU and platinum, although other agents have been used as well. There is no particular doublet combination that has been found to be superior in terms of a pathologic complete response, R0 resection, or overall survival.[87,88] RTOG 0436 is a randomized phase III trial evaluating the addition of cetuximab to standard doublet chemotherapy in patients with esophageal cancer undergoing definitive chemoradiation. Current guidelines typically recommend concurrent chemotherapy and radiotherapy rather than sequential regimens because there are limited data supporting the use of sequential treatment.

In patients who are not surgical candidates, the preferred treatment approach is concurrent chemoradiation, typically with a platinum-based regimen. Multiple trials have demonstrated the superiority of chemoradiation over radiotherapy alone. Herskovic and colleagues[29] randomized 121 patients to either radiotherapy alone of 64 Gy or concurrent chemoradiotherapy with 5-FU and cisplatin and 50.4 Gy of radiation. The 5-year survival was 27% in patients in the combined modality arm. Other older series have demonstrated consistently poor outcomes in patients receiving radiotherapy alone versus combination chemotherapy and radiation.[89–91]

Although concurrent chemoradiation improves outcomes, as many as 20% of patients still have a component of local failure after treatment.[29] These high rates of local failure prompted investigation into intensifying local therapy in patients receiving definitive treatment. As discussed, the Intergroup 0123 study did not demonstrate an improvement in outcomes with dose escalated radiotherapy in patients with locally advanced esophageal cancer.[36] A recent analysis of the National Cancer Database also demonstrated no improvement in overall survival with dose escalation beyond 50.4 Gy. Current guidelines recommend the delivery of approximately 50.4 Gy in patients receiving definitive therapy.[92]

Owing to the comparable efficacy of definitive chemoradiation versus trimodality therapy, there has been an increasing interest in potentially omitting upfront esophagectomy and reserving it for the salvage setting, particularly in patients with squamous cell carcinoma owing to the high response rates. Bedenne and colleagues[33] randomized 259 patients to either induction chemotherapy with 5-FU and cisplatin with radiotherapy (standard or split course) followed by esophagectomy or completion of chemoradiation to a total dose of 61 Gy. They found no difference in the 2-year overall survival, with 34% of patients alive in the trimodality arm versus 40% in the chemoradiation arm. Similarly, Stahl and colleagues[32] randomized 172 patients with squamous cell carcinoma of the esophagus to induction chemotherapy followed by chemoradiation (40 Gy) and surgery or definitive chemoradiation (64 Gy). They also found no difference in overall survival, although patients in the surgery arm had improved local progression-free survival.

In general, emerging data suggest that, in select patients with squamous cell carcinoma of the esophagus, definitive chemoradiation may result in similar treatment outcomes to patients receiving trimodality therapy. Proponents of definitive chemoradiation suggest that the addition of surgery may not improve cure while increasing the risk of surgical morbidity. In particular, patients who have a clinical complete response generally have excellent outcomes and adding surgery may not be a beneficial intervention. Meanwhile, patients who have a partial response or no response are those who may benefit from surgical intervention. A retrospective series by Markar and colleagues[93] reported on outcomes of patients undergoing definitive chemoradiation followed by salvage esophagectomy versus those undergoing a planned esophagectomy. At 3 years, there was no difference in overall survival (43% vs 40%) or disease-free survival (39% vs 33%) between the 2 groups, although patients in the salvage esophagectomy arm had higher rates of anastomotic leaks and surgical site infections.

One of the challenges in pursuing a nonsurgical treatment approach is identifying recurrence or persistent disease. Unlike in the pretreatment setting, traditional imaging techniques are often of limited value when assessing treatment response. In addition, response to chemoradiation may increase the likelihood of sampling error, causing biopsies to seem to be negative despite minimal residual disease. Functional imaging using PET may be more valuable in the evaluation of residual disease or recurrence in patients undergoing chemoradiation. Current guidelines suggest that in select patients with no evidence of disease on endoscopy or biopsy after chemoradiation, surveillance may be a potentially acceptable approach, whereas patients with persistent local disease should undergo surgical resection.[24]

Metastatic Disease

The goal of treatment in patients with metastatic disease is to palliate symptoms and thus improve quality of life, while also attempting to prolong survival. As discussed, patients diagnosed with esophageal cancer most commonly present with symptoms of dysphagia and thus often have weight loss and poor nutritional status. As a result, in patients with metastatic disease local treatment can potentially improve swallowing function and improve overall performance status.

Although there have been trials examining systemic therapy in the management of esophageal cancer (**Fig. 7**), there is no consensus on the best approach. In general, combination chemotherapy is preferred, although the agents of choice may vary by institution. Most commonly, a platinum-based and fluoropyrimidine-based agent are preferred for patients without HER2 overexpression.[94] Patients with HER2 overexpression have been found to have an overall survival benefit with the addition of trastuzumab. For patients presenting with metastatic disease, we recommend enrolling in a clinical trial owing to the limited data in this setting.

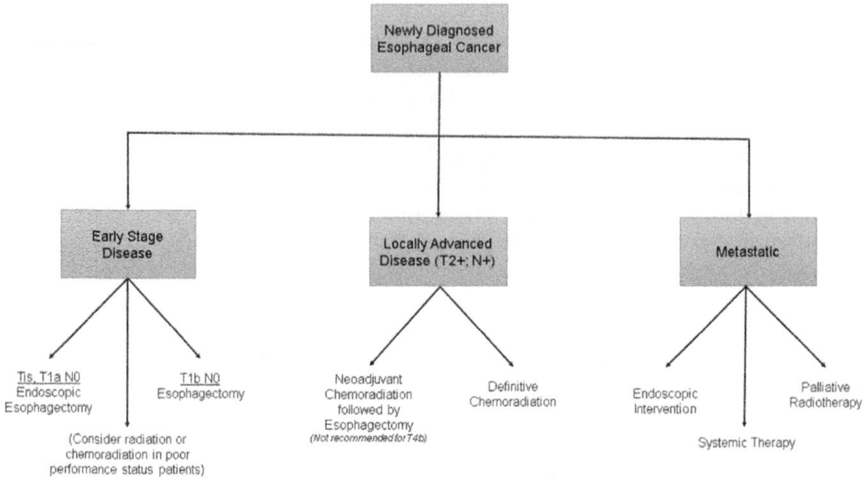

Fig. 7. Proposed algorithm for the management of esophageal cancer.

In patients requiring palliation, nonsurgical techniques are preferred owing to the potential morbidity associated with surgical interventions. Most commonly, endoscopic procedures or radiotherapy are used with excellent outcomes and significant improvement in symptoms. Endoscopic procedures used to improve esophageal symptoms include dilation and stent placement as well as ablation (laser, cryotherapy, photodynamic therapy). The main benefit of endoscopic intervention for palliation is that symptom improvement may be immediate. However, an analysis by Shenfine and colleagues[95] found that 35% of patients undergoing stent placement require reintervention. Similarly, another analysis found that 19% of patients experience tumor overgrowth within a median of 97 days after stent placement.[96] A metaanalysis by the Cochrane Collaborate Group found that self-expanding metal stents are quicker in palliating dysphagia versus other treatment modalities, although they may require reintervention.[97]

Owing to the high rates of reobstruction followed by these endoscopic procedures, radiotherapy is often recommended because of the potential to prolong the symptom-free interval. Homs and colleagues[98] randomized 209 patients to either stent placement or high-dose rate brachytherapy with a single-dose of 12 Gy. Although stent placement resulted in faster dysphagia relief, it resulted in higher complication rates and lower quality of life scores. In a series of 103 patients receiving external beam radiotherapy alone, 89% had an improvement in symptoms with 66% of patients having palliation for at least 2 months.[99] Although concurrent radiation may be delivered with palliative chemotherapy, in a recent trial by the Trans-Tasman Radiation Oncology Group patients were randomized to either palliative radiation alone or with chemotherapy.[100] The investigators found no difference in dysphagia response between either groups, but patients receiving chemotherapy did have higher rates of toxicity.

SUMMARY

Although long-term survival for patients with esophageal cancer has historically been poor, recent data suggest that multimodality care can potentially offer patients a significant chance for cure, particularly in localized disease. Although single-modality therapy may be appropriate in select patients with early stage disease, trimodality therapy consisting of neoadjuvant chemoradiation followed by esophagectomy is the preferred treatment approach in patients with locally advanced esophageal cancer. In patients who are not surgical candidates, definitive chemoradiotherapy also leads to good treatment outcomes with relatively little morbidity or mortality. All patients with newly diagnosed esophageal cancer should be evaluated in the multidisciplinary setting by a surgeon, radiation oncologist, and medical oncologist owing to the importance of each specialty in the management of these patients.

Although survival rates for esophageal cancer have increased, there remains significant room for improvement. Advances in surgical techniques and procedures will allow for less invasive methods of esophagectomy, thus decreasing the potential for morbidity and mortality. In addition, selective salvage esophagectomy is an area of active investigation, and organ preservation may become a potential option in high-volume centers. Furthermore, advances in radiotherapy technique will further allow for better tumor coverage while minimizing surrounding radiotherapy dose. Finally, advances in targeted compounds and systemic therapy and possibly immunotherapy are imperative to improve eradication of distant disease and potentiation of local therapy. Future trials will further optimize the multidisciplinary care of these patients.

REFERENCES

1. Jemal A, Bray F, Center MM, et al. Global cancer statistics. CA Cancer J Clin 2011;61(2):69–90.
2. Dubecz A, Gall I, Solymosi N, et al. Temporal trends in long-term survival and cure rates in esophageal cancer: a SEER database analysis. J Thorac Oncol 2012;7(2):443–7.
3. Siegel RL, Miller KD, Jemal A. Cancer statistics, 2015. CA Cancer J Clin 2015; 65(1):5–29.
4. Steevens J, Botterweck AA, Dirx MJ, et al. Trends in incidence of oesophageal and stomach cancer subtypes in Europe. Eur J Gastroenterol Hepatol 2010; 22(6):669–78.
5. Vizcaino AP, Moreno V, Lambert R, et al. Time trends incidence of both major histologic types of esophageal carcinomas in selected countries, 1973-1995. Int J Cancer 2002;99(6):860–8.
6. Blot WJ, Devesa SS, Kneller RW, et al. Rising incidence of adenocarcinoma of the esophagus and gastric cardia. JAMA 1991;265(10):1287–9.
7. Steevens J, Schouten LJ, Goldbohm RA, et al. Vegetables and fruits consumption and risk of esophageal and gastric cancer subtypes in the Netherlands Cohort Study. Int J Cancer 2011;129(11):2681–93.
8. Lagergren J, Bergstrom R, Lindgren A, et al. Symptomatic gastroesophageal reflux as a risk factor for esophageal adenocarcinoma. N Engl J Med 1999; 340(11):825–31.
9. Hvid-Jensen F, Pedersen L, Drewes AM, et al. Incidence of adenocarcinoma among patients with Barrett's esophagus. N Engl J Med 2011;365(15):1375–83.
10. Rubenstein JH, Taylor JB. Meta-analysis: the association of oesophageal adenocarcinoma with symptoms of gastro-oesophageal reflux. Aliment Pharmacol Ther 2010;32(10):1222–7.
11. de Jonge PJ, van Blankenstein M, Looman CW, et al. Risk of malignant progression in patients with Barrett's oesophagus: a Dutch nationwide cohort study. Gut 2010;59(8):1030–6.

12. Yousef F, Cardwell C, Cantwell MM, et al. The incidence of esophageal cancer and high-grade dysplasia in Barrett's esophagus: a systematic review and meta-analysis. Am J Epidemiol 2008;168(3):237–49.
13. Edge SB, American Joint Committee on Cancer, American Cancer Society. AJCC cancer staging handbook: from the AJCC cancer staging manual. 7th edition. New York: Springer; 2010.
14. Flamen P, Lerut A, Van Cutsem E, et al. Utility of positron emission tomography for the staging of patients with potentially operable esophageal carcinoma. J Clin Oncol 2000;18(18):3202–10.
15. Krasna MJ, Reed CE, Nedzwiecki D, et al. CALGB 9380: a prospective trial of the feasibility of thoracoscopy/laparoscopy in staging esophageal cancer. Ann Thorac Surg 2001;71(4):1073–9.
16. McKeown KC. Total three-stage oesophagectomy for cancer of the oesophagus. Br J Surg 1976;63(4):259–62.
17. Zhou C, Zhang L, Wang H, et al. Superiority of minimally invasive oesophagectomy in reducing in-hospital mortality of patients with resectable oesophageal cancer: a meta-analysis. PLoS One 2015;10(7):e0132889.
18. Luketich JD, Pennathur A, Awais O, et al. Outcomes after minimally invasive esophagectomy: review of over 1000 patients. Ann Surg 2012;256(1):95–103.
19. Biere SS, van Berge Henegouwen MI, Maas KW, et al. Minimally invasive versus open oesophagectomy for patients with oesophageal cancer: a multicentre, open-label, randomised controlled trial. Lancet 2012;379(9829):1887–92.
20. Greenstein AJ, Litle VR, Swanson SJ, et al. Effect of the number of lymph nodes sampled on postoperative survival of lymph node-negative esophageal cancer. Cancer 2008;112(6):1239–46.
21. Schwarz RE, Smith DD. Clinical impact of lymphadenectomy extent in resectable esophageal cancer. J Gastrointest Surg 2007;11(11):1384–93 [discussion: 1393–4].
22. Peyre CG, Hagen JA, DeMeester SR, et al. The number of lymph nodes removed predicts survival in esophageal cancer: an international study on the impact of extent of surgical resection. Ann Surg 2008;248(4):549–56.
23. Rizk NP, Ishwaran H, Rice TW, et al. Optimum lymphadenectomy for esophageal cancer. Ann Surg 2010;251(1):46–50.
24. Ajani JA, D'Amico TA, Almhanna K, et al. Esophageal and esophagogastric junction cancers, version 1.2015. J Natl Compr Canc Netw 2015;13(2):194–227.
25. Chan DS, Reid TD, Howell I, et al. Systematic review and meta-analysis of the influence of circumferential resection margin involvement on survival in patients with operable oesophageal cancer. Br J Surg 2013;100(4):456–64.
26. Swisher SG, Hunt KK, Holmes EC, et al. Changes in the surgical management of esophageal cancer from 1970 to 1993. Am J Surg 1995;169(6):609–14.
27. Markar SR, Karthikesalingam A, Thrumurthy S, et al. Volume-outcome relationship in surgery for esophageal malignancy: systematic review and meta-analysis 2000-2011. J Gastrointest Surg 2012;16(5):1055–63.
28. Shaikh T, Zaki MA, Dominello MM, et al. Patterns and predictors of failure following tri-modality therapy for locally advanced esophageal cancer. Acta Oncol 2016;55(3):303–8.
29. Herskovic A, Martz K, al-Sarraf M, et al. Combined chemotherapy and radiotherapy compared with radiotherapy alone in patients with cancer of the esophagus. N Engl J Med 1992;326(24):1593–8.
30. Wagner AD, Unverzagt S, Grothe W, et al. Chemotherapy for advanced gastric cancer. Cochrane Database Syst Rev 2010;(3):CD004064.

31. Bang YJ, Van Cutsem E, Feyereislova A, et al. Trastuzumab in combination with chemotherapy versus chemotherapy alone for treatment of HER2-positive advanced gastric or gastro-oesophageal junction cancer (ToGA): a phase 3, open-label, randomised controlled trial. Lancet 2010;376(9742):687–97.
32. Stahl M, Stuschke M, Lehmann N, et al. Chemoradiation with and without surgery in patients with locally advanced squamous cell carcinoma of the esophagus. J Clin Oncol 2005;23(10):2310–7.
33. Bedenne L, Michel P, Bouche O, et al. Chemoradiation followed by surgery compared with chemoradiation alone in squamous cancer of the esophagus: FFCD 9102. J Clin Oncol 2007;25(10):1160–8.
34. Paul S, Altorki N. Outcomes in the management of esophageal cancer. J Surg Oncol 2014;110(5):599–610.
35. Swisher SG, Winter KA, Komaki RU, et al. A Phase II study of a paclitaxel-based chemoradiation regimen with selective surgical salvage for resectable locoregionally advanced esophageal cancer: initial reporting of RTOG 0246. Int J Radiat Oncol Biol Phys 2012;82(5):1967–72.
36. Minsky BD, Pajak TF, Ginsberg RJ, et al. INT 0123 (Radiation Therapy Oncology Group 94-05) phase III trial of combined-modality therapy for esophageal cancer: high-dose versus standard-dose radiation therapy. J Clin Oncol 2002;20(5): 1167–74.
37. Gaspar LE, Winter K, Kocha WI, et al. A phase I/II study of external beam radiation, brachytherapy, and concurrent chemotherapy for patients with localized carcinoma of the esophagus (Radiation Therapy Oncology Group Study 9207): final report. Cancer 2000;88(5):988–95.
38. Burmeister BH, Dickie G, Smithers BM, et al. Thirty-four patients with carcinoma of the cervical esophagus treated with chemoradiation therapy. Arch Otolaryngol Head Neck Surg 2000;126(2):205–8.
39. Wang S, Liao Z, Chen Y, et al. Esophageal cancer located at the neck and upper thorax treated with concurrent chemoradiation: a single-institution experience. J Thorac Oncol 2006;1(3):252–9.
40. Uno T, Isobe K, Kawakami H, et al. Concurrent chemoradiation for patients with squamous cell carcinoma of the cervical esophagus. Dis Esophagus 2007; 20(1):12–8.
41. Buckstein MR, Rhome RM, Ohri N. Neoadjuvant chemoradiation dose and outcomes in esophageal cancers, a national cancer data base study. Int J Radiat Oncol Biol Phys 2016;96(2):S190.
42. Shaikh T, Churilla TM, Monpara P, et al. Risk of radiation pneumonitis in patients receiving taxane-based trimodality therapy for locally advanced esophageal cancer. Pract Radiat Oncol 2016;6(6):388–94.
43. Tait LM, Meyer JE, McSpadden E, et al. Women at increased risk for cardiac toxicity following chemoradiation therapy for esophageal carcinoma. Pract Radiat Oncol 2013;3(4):e149–55.
44. La TH, Minn AY, Su Z, et al. Multimodality treatment with intensity modulated radiation therapy for esophageal cancer. Dis Esophagus 2010;23(4):300–8.
45. Nutting CM, Bedford JL, Cosgrove VP, et al. A comparison of conformal and intensity-modulated techniques for oesophageal radiotherapy. Radiother Oncol 2001;61(2):157–63.
46. Kole TP, Aghayere O, Kwah J, et al. Comparison of heart and coronary artery doses associated with intensity-modulated radiotherapy versus three-dimensional conformal radiotherapy for distal esophageal cancer. Int J Radiat Oncol Biol Phys 2012;83(5):1580–6.

47. Lin SH, Wang L, Myles B, et al. Propensity score-based comparison of long-term outcomes with 3-dimensional conformal radiotherapy vs intensity-modulated radiotherapy for esophageal cancer. Int J Radiat Oncol Biol Phys 2012;84(5): 1078–85.
48. Brown LM, Devesa SS. Epidemiologic trends in esophageal and gastric cancer in the United States. Surg Oncol Clin N Am 2002;11(2):235–56.
49. Young PE, Gentry AB, Acosta RD, et al. Endoscopic ultrasound does not accurately stage early adenocarcinoma or high-grade dysplasia of the esophagus. Clin Gastroenterol Hepatol 2010;8(12):1037–41.
50. Merkow RP, Bilimoria KY, Keswani RN, et al. Treatment trends, risk of lymph node metastasis, and outcomes for localized esophageal cancer. J Natl Cancer Inst 2014;106(7).
51. Motoori M, Yano M, Ishihara R, et al. Comparison between radical esophagectomy and definitive chemoradiotherapy in patients with clinical T1bN0M0 esophageal cancer. Ann Surg Oncol 2012;19(7):2135–41.
52. Nygaard K, Hagen S, Hansen HS, et al. Pre-operative radiotherapy prolongs survival in operable esophageal carcinoma: a randomized, multicenter study of pre-operative radiotherapy and chemotherapy. The second Scandinavian trial in esophageal cancer. World J Surg 1992;16(6):1104–9 [discussion: 1110].
53. Arnott SJ, Duncan W, Kerr GR, et al. Low dose preoperative radiotherapy for carcinoma of the oesophagus: results of a randomized clinical trial. Radiother Oncol 1992;24(2):108–13.
54. Wang M, Gu XZ, Yin WB, et al. Randomized clinical trial on the combination of preoperative irradiation and surgery in the treatment of esophageal carcinoma: report on 206 patients. Int J Radiat Oncol Biol Phys 1989;16(2):325–7.
55. Gignoux M, Roussel A, Paillot B, et al. The value of preoperative radiotherapy in esophageal cancer: results of a study of the E.O.R.T.C. World J Surg 1987; 11(4):426–32.
56. Launois B, Delarue D, Campion JP, et al. Preoperative radiotherapy for carcinoma of the esophagus. Surg Gynecol Obstet 1981;153(5):690–2.
57. Medical Research Council Oesophageal Cancer Working Group. Surgical resection with or without preoperative chemotherapy in oesophageal cancer: a randomised controlled trial. Lancet 2002;359(9319):1727–33.
58. Kelsen DP, Winter KA, Gunderson LL, et al. Long-term results of RTOG trial 8911 (USA Intergroup 113): a random assignment trial comparison of chemotherapy followed by surgery compared with surgery alone for esophageal cancer. J Clin Oncol 2007;25(24):3719–25.
59. Schlag PM. Randomized trial of preoperative chemotherapy for squamous cell cancer of the esophagus. The Chirurgische Arbeitsgemeinschaft Fuer Onkologie der Deutschen Gesellschaft Fuer Chirurgie Study Group. Arch Surg 1992; 127(12):1446–50.
60. Allum WH, Stenning SP, Bancewicz J, et al. Long-term results of a randomized trial of surgery with or without preoperative chemotherapy in esophageal cancer. J Clin Oncol 2009;27(30):5062–7.
61. Law S, Fok M, Chow S, et al. Preoperative chemotherapy versus surgical therapy alone for squamous cell carcinoma of the esophagus: a prospective randomized trial. J Thorac Cardiovasc Surg 1997;114(2):210–7.
62. Sjoquist KM, Burmeister BH, Smithers BM, et al. Survival after neoadjuvant chemotherapy or chemoradiotherapy for resectable oesophageal carcinoma: an updated meta-analysis. Lancet Oncol 2011;12(7):681–92.

63. Walsh TN, Noonan N, Hollywood D, et al. A comparison of multimodal therapy and surgery for esophageal adenocarcinoma. N Engl J Med 1996;335(7):462–7.
64. Tepper J, Krasna MJ, Niedzwiecki D, et al. Phase III trial of trimodality therapy with cisplatin, fluorouracil, radiotherapy, and surgery compared with surgery alone for esophageal cancer: CALGB 9781. J Clin Oncol 2008;26(7):1086–92.
65. Urba SG, Orringer MB, Turrisi A, et al. Randomized trial of preoperative chemoradiation versus surgery alone in patients with locoregional esophageal carcinoma. J Clin Oncol 2001;19(2):305–13.
66. Burmeister BH, Smithers BM, Gebski V, et al. Surgery alone versus chemoradiotherapy followed by surgery for resectable cancer of the oesophagus: a randomised controlled phase III trial. Lancet Oncol 2005;6(9):659–68.
67. Mariette C, Dahan L, Mornex F, et al. Surgery alone versus chemoradiotherapy followed by surgery for stage I and II esophageal cancer: final analysis of randomized controlled phase III trial FFCD 9901. J Clin Oncol 2014;32(23):2416–22.
68. van Hagen P, Hulshof MC, van Lanschot JJ, et al. Preoperative chemoradiotherapy for esophageal or junctional cancer. N Engl J Med 2012;366(22):2074–84.
69. Shapiro J, van Lanschot JJ, Hulshof MC, et al. Neoadjuvant chemoradiotherapy plus surgery versus surgery alone for oesophageal or junctional cancer (CROSS): long-term results of a randomised controlled trial. Lancet Oncol 2015;16(9):1090–8.
70. Oppedijk V, van der Gaast A, van Lanschot JJ, et al. Patterns of recurrence after surgery alone versus preoperative chemoradiotherapy and surgery in the CROSS trials. J Clin Oncol 2014;32(5):385–91.
71. Donahue JM, Nichols FC, Li Z, et al. Complete pathologic response after neoadjuvant chemoradiotherapy for esophageal cancer is associated with enhanced survival. Ann Thorac Surg 2009;87(2):392–8 [discussion: 398–9].
72. Darnton SJ, Archer VR, Stocken DD, et al. Preoperative mitomycin, ifosfamide, and cisplatin followed by esophagectomy in squamous cell carcinoma of the esophagus: pathologic complete response induced by chemotherapy leads to long-term survival. J Clin Oncol 2003;21(21):4009–15.
73. Steiger Z, Franklin R, Wilson RF, et al. Complete eradication of squamous cell carcinoma of the esophagus with combined chemotherapy and radiotherapy. Am Surg 1981;47(3):95–8.
74. Berger AC, Farma J, Scott WJ, et al. Complete response to neoadjuvant chemoradiotherapy in esophageal carcinoma is associated with significantly improved survival. J Clin Oncol 2005;23(19):4330–7.
75. Huang RW, Chao YK, Wen YW, et al. Predictors of pathological complete response to neoadjuvant chemoradiotherapy for esophageal squamous cell carcinoma. World J Surg Oncol 2014;12:170.
76. Chao YK, Tseng CK, Wen YW, et al. Using pretreatment tumor depth and length to select esophageal squamous cell carcinoma patients for nonoperative treatment after neoadjuvant chemoradiotherapy. Ann Surg Oncol 2013;20(9):3000–8.
77. Ajani JA, Correa AM, Hofstetter WL, et al. Clinical parameters model for predicting pathologic complete response following preoperative chemoradiation in patients with esophageal cancer. Ann Oncol 2012;23(10):2638–42.
78. Shaikh T, Ruth K, Scott WJ, et al. Increased time from neoadjuvant chemoradiation to surgery is associated with higher pathologic complete response rates in esophageal cancer. Ann Thorac Surg 2015;99(1):270–6.

79. Lee A, Wong AT, Schwartz D, et al. Is there a benefit to prolonging the interval between neoadjuvant chemoradiation and esophagectomy in esophageal cancer? Ann Thorac Surg 2016;102(2):433–8.
80. Shapiro J, van Hagen P, Lingsma HF, et al. Prolonged time to surgery after neoadjuvant chemoradiotherapy increases histopathological response without affecting survival in patients with esophageal or junctional cancer. Ann Surg 2014;260(5):807–13 [discussion: 813–4].
81. Teniere P, Hay JM, Fingerhut A, et al. Postoperative radiation therapy does not increase survival after curative resection for squamous cell carcinoma of the middle and lower esophagus as shown by a multicenter controlled trial. French University Association for Surgical Research. Surg Gynecol Obstet 1991;173(2): 123–30.
82. Fok M, Sham JS, Choy D, et al. Postoperative radiotherapy for carcinoma of the esophagus: a prospective, randomized controlled study. Surgery 1993;113(2): 138–47.
83. Macdonald JS, Smalley SR, Benedetti J, et al. Chemoradiotherapy after surgery compared with surgery alone for adenocarcinoma of the stomach or gastroesophageal junction. N Engl J Med 2001;345(10):725–30.
84. Wong AT, Shao M, Rineer J, et al. The impact of adjuvant postoperative radiation therapy and chemotherapy on survival after esophagectomy for esophageal carcinoma. Ann Surg 2016. [Epub ahead of print].
85. Rice TW, Adelstein DJ, Chidel MA, et al. Benefit of postoperative adjuvant chemoradiotherapy in locoregionally advanced esophageal carcinoma. J Thorac Cardiovasc Surg 2003;126(5):1590–6.
86. Hsu PK, Huang CS, Wang BY, et al. Survival benefits of postoperative chemoradiation for lymph node-positive esophageal squamous cell carcinoma. Ann Thorac Surg 2014;97(5):1734–41.
87. Tomblyn MB, Goldman BH, Thomas CR Jr, et al. Cetuximab plus cisplatin, irinotecan, and thoracic radiotherapy as definitive treatment for locally advanced, unresectable esophageal cancer: a phase-II study of the SWOG (S0414). J Thorac Oncol 2012;7(5):906–12.
88. Kleinberg LR, Eapen S, Hamilton S, et al. E1201: an Eastern Cooperative Oncology Group (ECOG) randomized phase II trial to measure response rate and toxicity of preoperative combined modality paclitaxel/cisplatin/RT or irinotecan/cisplatin/RT in adenocarcinoma of the esophagus. Int J Radiat Oncol Biol Phys 2006;66(3):S80.
89. Chan A, Wong A, Arthur K. Concomitant 5-fluorouracil infusion, mitomycin C and radical radiation therapy in esophageal squamous cell carcinoma. Int J Radiat Oncol Biol Phys 1989;16(1):59–65.
90. al-Sarraf M, Martz K, Herskovic A, et al. Progress report of combined chemoradiotherapy versus radiotherapy alone in patients with esophageal cancer: an intergroup study. J Clin Oncol 1997;15(1):277–84.
91. Conroy T, Galais MP, Raoul JL, et al. Definitive chemoradiotherapy with FOLFOX versus fluorouracil and cisplatin in patients with oesophageal cancer (PRODIGE5/ACCORD17): final results of a randomised, phase 2/3 trial. Lancet Oncol 2014;15(3):305–14.
92. Shao MS, Wong AT, Schwartz D, et al. Definitive or preoperative chemoradiation therapy for esophageal cancer: patterns of care and survival outcomes. Ann Thorac Surg 2016;101(6):2148–54.

93. Markar S, Gronnier C, Duhamel A, et al. Salvage surgery after chemoradiotherapy in the management of esophageal cancer: is it a viable therapeutic option? J Clin Oncol 2015;33(33):3866–73.
94. Shah MA. Update on metastatic gastric and esophageal cancers. J Clin Oncol 2015;33(16):1760–9.
95. Shenfine J, McNamee P, Steen N, et al. A randomized controlled clinical trial of palliative therapies for patients with inoperable esophageal cancer. Am J Gastroenterol 2009;104(7):1674–85.
96. Conio M, Repici A, Battaglia G, et al. A randomized prospective comparison of self-expandable plastic stents and partially covered self-expandable metal stents in the palliation of malignant esophageal dysphagia. Am J Gastroenterol 2007;102(12):2667–77.
97. Dai Y, Li C, Xie Y, et al. Interventions for dysphagia in oesophageal cancer. Cochrane Database Syst Rev 2014;(10):CD005048.
98. Homs MY, Steyerberg EW, Eijkenboom WM, et al. Single-dose brachytherapy versus metal stent placement for the palliation of dysphagia from oesophageal cancer: multicentre randomised trial. Lancet 2004;364(9444):1497–504.
99. Wara WM, Mauch PM, Thomas AN, et al. Palliation for carcinoma of the esophagus. Radiology 1976;121(3 Pt. 1):717–20.
100. Penniment MG, Harvey JA, Wong R, et al. Best practice in advanced esophageal cancer: a report on Trans-Tasman Radiation Oncology Group TROG 03.01 and NCIC CTG ES.2 multinational phase 3 study in advanced esophageal cancer (OC) comparing quality of life (QOL) and palliation of dysphagia in patients treated with radiation therapy (RT) or chemoradiation therapy (CRT). Int J Radiat Oncol Biol Phys 2014;90(1):S3.

The Role of Radiation Therapy for Pancreatic Cancer in the Adjuvant and Neoadjuvant Settings

Shahed N. Badiyan, MD[a,*], Jason K. Molitoris, MD, PhD[b], Michael D. Chuong, MD[c], William F. Regine, MD[a], Adeel Kaiser, MD[a]

KEYWORDS

• Pancreatic cancer • Pancreas cancer • Adjuvant • Neoadjuvant • Chemoradiation • Radiation therapy • Proton therapy • Stereotactic body radiotherapy

KEY POINTS

- The use of radiation therapy after resection of pancreatic cancer is controversial because of conflicting results in several clinical trials.
- Neoadjuvant radiation therapy for resectable or borderline resectable pancreatic cancer is frequently prescribed in combination with chemotherapy to improve margin-negative resection rates.
- Hypofractionated radiation therapy regimens via stereotactic body radiation therapy or particle therapy have become more commonly used in the neoadjuvant setting.
- The genetic profile of pancreatic cancers may enable physicians to select patients more likely to benefit from local therapies such as radiation.

INTRODUCTION

Pancreatic cancer is projected to be the third leading cause of cancer death in the United States in 2016 and is expected to be diagnosed in approximately 53,000 individuals.[1] Although treatment methods have advanced in the last 2 decades, outcomes remain poor, with 5-year survival rates of approximately 8% for patients with ductal

Disclosure: SN Badiyan has research funding from Astra Zeneca.

[a] Department of Radiation Oncology, University of Maryland School of Medicine, Baltimore, MD, USA; [b] Department of Radiation Oncology, University of Maryland Medical Center, Baltimore, MD, USA; [c] Department of Radiation Oncology, Miami Cancer Institute, Baptist Health South Florida, Miami, FL, USA

* Corresponding author. Department of Radiation Oncology, Maryland Proton Treatment Center, 850 West Baltimore Street, Office 273, Baltimore, MD 21201.
E-mail address: sbadiyan@umm.edu

Surg Oncol Clin N Am 26 (2017) 431–453
http://dx.doi.org/10.1016/j.soc.2017.01.012 surgonc.theclinics.com

carcinoma, the most common form of pancreatic cancer.[2] Most diagnoses of pancreatic cancer cannot be traced to a single identifiable cause; however, smoking tobacco, obesity, and diabetes mellitus are associated with increased risk. Germline mutations in genes such as BRCA1/2, CDKN2A, and PRSS1 have been linked to 5% to 10% of new diagnoses.[3,4]

Screening for pancreatic cancer may be effective in some high-risk populations, but the lack of an effective method of screening for the general population has contributed to poor outcomes.[3] Early-stage pancreatic cancer is frequently asymptomatic, resulting in most diagnoses occurring at advanced stages of disease. Surgery remains the only definitive cure; however, even in patients with resectable disease, outcomes are far from ideal, with 5-year overall survival (OS) rates of approximately 20%.[5,6] These dismal survival rates are the result of the high risk of both local and distant disease recurrence after surgery. Despite substantial risk of local progression, the high rate of distant metastases has dominated adjuvant therapy discussions and led many institutions to withhold radiation therapy (RT). A recent autopsy study of patients succumbing to pancreatic cancer provided evidence for the importance of primary tumor control in pancreatic cancer. The study found that 30% of patients died of local progression of primary tumors without evidence of metastatic disease,[7] suggesting the importance of RT to provide local control of primary tumors.

STAGING

Initial work-up and staging in pancreatic cancer centers on the ability to distinguish between those tumors that are likely to be resectable with clear margins (R0) and those that are likely to result in a positive margin (R1 or R2) after surgery alone. To that end, nonmetastatic pancreatic cancers are categorized into 3 groups: resectable pancreatic cancer (RPC; likely to be resected with R0 margins), borderline RPC (BRPC; likely to result in R1 margins), and locally advanced pancreatic cancer (LAPC; likely to result in R2 margins). American Joint Committee on Cancer staging can be used for prognostic information, and primary tumor (T) staging roughly corresponds with tumor resectability: RPC (T1 and T2), BRPC (T3), and LAPC (T4).

One of the challenges in initial diagnosis and staging of pancreatic cancer is detection of the true extent of disease. Computed tomography (CT) pancreas protocols include a high-resolution abdominal CT scan that captures images during 2 phases (portal venous and pancreatic) after administration of intravenous contrast and have become the standard test for local and distant tumor staging. However, nearly one-third of patients with locally advanced disease identified by CT are found to have occult metastases by staging laparoscopy.[8] Although ^{18}F-fluorodeoxyglucose PET/CT imaging has shown a sensitivity of 87% for detection of metastatic disease in patients with pancreatic cancer, National Comprehensive Cancer Network (NCCN) pancreatic cancer guidelines recommend that PET imaging be used only in high-risk patients to detect extrapancreatic metastases but not in place of high-quality, contrast-enhanced CT. MRI can be used in patients with severe allergies to iodinated contrast or when findings on pancreas protocol CT are unclear. Endoscopic ultrasonography is not recommended for routine staging but can be used to guide fine-needle aspiration biopsy of a pancreatic mass.[9]

Three organizations have produced definitions of resectability for pancreatic cancer to standardize and improve patient selection for surgery: (1) MD Anderson Cancer Center (MDACC)[10]; (2) a consortium of gastrointestinal (GI) surgery organizations, including the Americas Hepato-Pancreato-Biliary Association, the Society of Surgical Oncology, and the Society for the Surgery of the Alimentary Tract[11]; and (3) the

Intergroup, which is a consortium of 3 cooperative clinical trial groups, namely the Alliance for Clinical Trials in Oncology, Southwest Oncology Group (SWOG), and Eastern Cooperative Oncology Group (ECOG).[12] The most restrictive definition of BRPC tumors was that published by the Intergroup, in which the circumferential degree of contact between tumor and blood vessels is quantified rather than using a definition with more subjective terms such as impingement and abutment. The Intergroup definition of pancreatic tumor resectability has been endorsed by the NCCN and can be found in **Table 1**.

ADJUVANT RADIATION THERAPY FOR PANCREATIC CANCER

Although adjuvant chemotherapy clearly improves survival after surgery for pancreatic cancer, the role of RT has been contested for many years. This controversy stems from historical randomized trials showing a lack of consensus on benefits compared with adjuvant chemotherapy or surgery alone.

The Gastrointestinal Tumor Study Group 9173 trial was the first to evaluate adjuvant chemoradiation (CRT) in a randomized fashion.[13] A total of 43 patients with resected pancreatic cancer and negative margins were randomized to observation or CRT. RT was delivered to a dose of 40 Gy in 2-Gy fractions in split-course fashion (a 2-week break was planned after 20 Gy). Concurrent and maintenance 5-fluorouracil (5-FU) were given. Despite the trial closing early because of poor accrual, a significant survival benefit was found favoring the CRT arm. Thirty additional patients were later treated on a nonrandomized CRT arm, and their survival was similar to that of subjects in the randomized CRT arm.

Table 1
Intergroup definition of pancreatic tumor resectability endorsed by the National Comprehensive Cancer Network

	Resectable	Borderline Resectable	Locally Advanced
SMV/PV	Interface between tumor and vessel measuring <180° of circumference of vessel wall	Interface between tumor and vessel measuring ≥180° of circumference of vessel wall, and/or reconstructable[a] occlusion	Not reconstructable
SMA/hepatic	No contact	Interface between tumor and vessel measuring <180° of circumference of vessel wall	Interface between tumor and vessel measuring ≥180° of circumference of vessel wall
CHA	No contact	Reconstructable,[a] short-segment interface between tumor and vessel of any degree	Not reconstructable, or long-segment interface between tumor and vessel
Celiac trunk	No contact	Interface between tumor and vessel measuring <180° of circumference of vessel wall	Interface between tumor and vessel measuring ≥180° of circumference of vessel wall

Abbreviations: CHA, common hepatic artery; PV, portal vein; SMA, superior mesenteric artery; SMV, superior mesenteric vein.

[a] Normal vein or artery proximal and distal to site of suggested tumor-vessel involvement suitable for vascular reconstruction.

Conflicting conclusions were reported from several subsequent European randomized trials. In a randomized trial from the European Organization for Research and Treatment of Cancer (EORTC), patients were assigned to either surgery alone or surgery and adjuvant CRT.[14,15] The final analysis reported no statistically significant differences in survival between the study arms; however, it is important to recognize that almost 50% of the study population had more favorable periampullary tumors, 20% of patients randomized to receive CRT did not receive adjuvant therapy, and nearly 50% of patients did not receive chemotherapy per protocol. Moreover, had statistical analyses used a 1-sided and not 2-sided log rank test, the higher survival in the CRT arm would have reached statistical significance ($P = .049$).[16]

The largest prospective study to evaluate adjuvant therapy for patients with pancreatic cancer is the European Study for Pancreatic Cancer (ESPAC-1) trial, which randomized 254 patients to observation versus chemotherapy or observation versus CRT.[17] A 2 × 2 factorial randomization between observation, chemotherapy, CRT, and CRT with maintenance chemotherapy included 285 additional patients. Chemotherapy alone was associated with improved survival, but CRT was associated with worse survival than no CRT (10% and 20%, respectively; $P = .05$). These findings have been questioned, with investigators noting that physicians were allowed to choose the randomization; centralized review of RT was lacking, as were standardized RT dose and fields; background adjuvant therapy, consisting of chemotherapy or chemoradiotherapy before the patient entered the trial, was used in 42% of enrolled patients; and a longer interval to treatment initiation was seen in the CRT arm.[18,19] Despite the many flaws of the EORTC and ESPAC-1 trials, their results were used as justification for a shift away from adjuvant RT toward the use of adjuvant chemotherapy alone at many institutions, especially in Europe.

In contrast with historical trials that used antiquated radiation techniques and suboptimal split-course dosing, recent studies have suggested that modern treatment planning and higher doses of RT may increase the benefit of adjuvant CRT.[20–22] In a retrospective analysis from the Mayo Clinic and Johns Hopkins University (two very-high-volume centers with experienced pancreatic multidisciplinary teams), results from 1386 patients with resected pancreatic cancer who received adjuvant CRT to 50.4 Gy were compared with surgery alone. Patients who underwent adjuvant CRT had improved survival on propensity score analysis ($P<.001$).[23] Higher median survival favoring receipt of CRT was found on matched-pair analysis (21.9 vs 14.3 months; $P<.001$). High-quality RT was also shown to be critical in the Radiation Therapy Oncology Group (RTOG) 9704 trial, which randomized resected patients to CRT sandwiched between either gemcitabine or 5-FU.[5] This randomized trial was the first to require central quality assurance review of radiation fields and showed that treatment per protocol was significantly associated with improved survival.[24]

The results of the ongoing RTOG 0848 randomized trial are eagerly awaited for clarification of the role of adjuvant CRT. This trial is currently randomizing patients to adjuvant gemcitabine with or without adjuvant CRT. The trial design originally included an initial randomization to gemcitabine with or without erlotinib, but erlotinib has been removed based on recently reported results of a trial for LAPC in which no survival difference was found with the addition of erlotinib.[25]

NEOADJUVANT THERAPY RATIONALE: RESECTABLE PANCREATIC CANCER

Although surgical resection continues to be required for treatment of pancreatic cancer with curative intent, the rate of micrometastatic disease dissemination at the time of diagnosis remains high. As a result of surgical complications, detection of metastatic disease, and declining performance status, only two-thirds of patients receive adjuvant therapy with curative intent after resection.[26] In an effort to maximize treatment and minimize surgical morbidity, multiple groups have performed prospective trials of neoadjuvant CRT for RPC and BRPC.

Neoadjuvant therapy is now widely used in the treatment of GI malignancies. In addition to decreasing the use of surgery in patients unlikely to benefit, neoadjuvant therapy has several potential benefits. Postsurgical disruption of vasculature results in hypoxia in the tumor bed, decreasing both the effectiveness of radiation and delivery of chemotherapeutics. Neoadjuvant therapy can also increase the rate of R0 resections, which is known to be an important prognostic factor for survival.[27,28] Interpreting the relevant data is challenging, because most of the completed clinical trials for neoadjuvant therapy were small studies designed to assess safety and feasibility and because wide heterogeneity characterizes the RPC and BRPC populations. In addition, because distant metastatic disease continues to drive outcomes, advances showing the superiority of systemic therapy with gemcitabine[29] and later FOLFIRINOX (5FU, leucovorin, irinotecan, oxaliplatin)[30] in metastatic pancreatic cancer led to reevaluation of radiation safety and efficacy. Prospective clinical trials investigating adjuvant RT for pancreatic cancer are shown in **Table 2**.

NEOADJUVANT THERAPY: RESECTABLE PANCREATIC CANCER

Initial efforts to treat RPC with neoadjuvant therapy focused on safety and efficacy. Multiple trials at MDACC were performed on small patient numbers with infusional 5-FU and conventional fractionation (50.4 Gy in 28 fractions)[31] as well as hypofractionation (30 Gy in 10 fractions)[32] and paclitaxel-based CRT.[33] During the same period, ECOG completed a phase II trial of conventionally fractionated radiation with continuous infusional 5-FU and mitomycin. Of 53 patients enrolled, 41 (77%) underwent exploratory surgery, with only 24 (45%) ultimately undergoing resection. Median OS rates for all patients and the 24 who underwent resection were 9.7 and 15 months, respectively. The predominant pattern of failure in these patients remained distant disease dissemination.[34]

Subsequent trials transitioned to gemcitabine-based chemotherapy after demonstration of improved survival in locally advanced and metastatic disease.[29] Talamonti and colleagues[35] reported in 2006 on a small multi-institutional phase II trial of neoadjuvant full-dose gemcitabine chemotherapy with concurrent hypofractionated radiation (36 Gy over 15 daily fractions). Seventeen of the 20 patients enrolled underwent resection with a median OS of 26 months and 2-year OS of 61%. One grade 3 GI toxicity was reported with neoadjuvant therapy, and an R0 resection was reported in 94% of resected patients. Although small enrollment numbers limited the scope of the findings, this study showed the feasibility of neoadjuvant treatment with gemcitabine.

Evans and colleagues[36] reported on a phase I/II trial of 86 patients with RPC head/uncinate process adenocarcinoma treated with concurrent low-dose gemcitabine and radiation (30 Gy in 10 fractions). Median OS was almost 23 months for all patients and 34 months for the 74% of patients who underwent surgery. Five-year OS rates for resection and no resection were 36% and 0%, respectively. R1 resection rates were decreased from 20% in their institutional report on patients treated without neoadjuvant therapy[28] to 11% with concurrent low-dose gemcitabine and radiation.[28,36] Published concurrently, a phase II study by the same group incorporated cisplatin with gemcitabine before gemcitabine-based CRT. That study reported a similar survival benefit for the 66% of patients who underwent surgery (31 months) compared

Table 2
Prospective clinical trials of adjuvant radiation therapy for pancreatic cancer

Study, Report Year	N	Treatment Arms	R1 Resection Rate (%)	Any Grade ≥3 Toxicity (%)	Median Survival (mo)
GITSG,[13] 1985	22	Observation	—	0	10.9
	21	5-FU + 40 Gy split-course RT	—	14	20.0
EORTC,[14] 1999	54	Observation	—	0	12.6
	60	5-FU + 40 Gy split-course RT	—	2	17.1
Van Laethem et al,[88] 2003	22	Gem then gem + 40 Gy split-course RT	0	36 (heme) 32 (nonheme)	15.0
Wilkowski et al,[89] 2004	30	Gem + cis + 45-Gy RT then gem + cis	100	—	22.8
Allen et al,[90] 2004	32	Gem + 24–42-Gy RT then gem	25 (R1) 6 (R2)	—	16.5
ESPAC-1,[17] 2004	69	Observation	—	—	16.9
	75	5-FU	—	—	21.6
	73	5-FU + 20-Gy RT	—	—	13.9
	72	5-FU then 5-FU + 20-Gy RT	—	—	19.9
Demols et al,[91] 2005	30	Gem then gem + 45-Gy RT	0	33 (grade 3) 10 (grade 4)	19.0
Blackstock et al,[92] 2006	46	Gem + 50.4-Gy RT then gem	0	—	18.3

Brade et al,[93] 2007	32	Gem then gem + 35–52.5-Gy RT	25.0	48% during CRT	18.4
RTOG 9704,[5,48] 2008	230	5-FU then 5-FU + 50.4-Gy RT	33.0	9	16.9
	221	Gem then 5-FU + 50.4-Gy RT	35.0	58	20.5
Linehan et al,[94] 2008	53	5-FU + cis + IFNα + 50.4-Gy RT then gem	33.0	68	25
EORTC 40013/FFCD	45	Gem	2.0	0 (grade 4)	24.4
9203/GERCOR,[95] 2010	45	Gem + 50.4-Gy RT	4.0	4.7 (grade 4)	24.3
Morganti et al,[96] 2010	12	Cape + 50–55-Gy RT over 5 wk	—	0	—
Katz et al,[97] 2011	28	IFNα-2b + 5-FU/cis + 50.4-Gy RT then 5-FU	14.0	89	42.3
ACOSOG Z05031,[98] 2011	89	IFNα-2b + 5-FU/cis + 50.4-Gy RT then 5-FU	25.0	95	25.4
CapR1,[99] 2012	53	5-FU/cis + IFNα-2b + 50.4-Gy RT	45.0	85	26.5
	57	5-FU	34.0	16	28.5
Herman et al,[100] 2013	48	Erlotinib + cape + 50.4-Gy RT	16.7	33 (CRT) 43 (post-CRT)	24.4
Cho et al,[101] 2015	29	Gem and docetaxel then cape + 50.4-Gy RT	—	15[a]	17

Abbreviations: 5-FU, 5-fluorouracil; cape, capecitabine; cis, cisplatin; CRT, chemoradiation; gem, gemcitabine; Gy, gray; heme, hematologic; IFNα-2b, interferon alpha 2b; nonheme, nonhematologic; RT, radiation therapy.

[a] Included additional 21 patients with ampullary or biliary cancers.

with those who did not (10.5 months).[37] Local failure was reported in 25% of patients undergoing resection, with only 2 patients showing isolated local recurrence. Distant disease continued to predominate, with 42% developing distant disease and 31% showing peritoneal dissemination. The investigators also noted that outcomes with dual-agent therapy were not improved compared with gemcitabine-only CRT, suggesting that alternative approaches were required.

In an effort to shorten the duration of RT, Hong and colleagues[38] used proton therapy (PT) for phase I dose escalation from 30 Gy in 10 fractions to 5 Gy in 5 sequential fractions with concurrent capecitabine. They had previously performed dosimetric analyses showing decreased radiation exposure to surrounding organs with PT compared with intensity-modulated RT (IMRT). Initial results showed acceptable toxicity at all treatment levels.[39] A subsequent phase II study of 25 Gy given in 5 fractions reported that 37 of 48 patients (77%) underwent surgery. A median OS of 17.2 months was observed for all patients, which extended to 27 months for those completing resection. Thirty-one of 37 patients (84%) received postoperative gemcitabine chemotherapy; however, distant recurrence continued to dominate, with 35 of 48 patients (73%) failing distantly and only 8 of 48 patients (17%) failing locally.[39]

NEOADJUVANT THERAPY: BORDERLINE RESECTABLE PANCREATIC CANCER

The likelihood of R0 resection decreases in patients with evidence of tumor involvement of the peripancreatic vasculature. It is thought that R1 resections result in survival similar to that in patients with unresected LAPC and with increased morbidity,[22] so that neoadjuvant CRT may play a greater role in BRPC. An initial study by Mehta and colleagues[40] characterized BRPC as having portal vein, superior mesenteric vein, or superior mesenteric artery involvement. In that study, 15 patients completed CRT with infusional 5-FU and standard fractionated radiation (50.4–56 Gy) with a 60% resection rate and a median OS of 30 months for those who underwent resection. Since publication of that study in 2001, several prospective studies have evaluated the role of neoadjuvant therapy in patients with BRPC. However, because of the varying definitions used for BRPC, as well as multiple studies that combined BRPC and RPC, a large degree of heterogeneity characterized initial reports on neoadjuvant treatment outcomes.

Van Buren and colleagues[41] published a phase II trial including 59 patients with BRPC and RPC treated with full-dose gemcitabine and bevacizumab, a vascular endothelial growth factor inhibitor, followed by hypofractionated radiation (30 Gy in 10 fractions) and concurrent bevacizumab. Similar to prior reports, 73% of patients underwent resection with a median OS of 16.8 months for all patients and 19.7 months for those undergoing resection. R0 resection was attained in 88% and local control was 75%, both of which were similar to prior studies with only RPC. A study using similar chemotherapy and radiation schema with a median survival of 46 months was presented in 2012.[42]

After determination of safety in a phase I trial, a multi-institutional phase II clinical trial evaluated 68 patients with RPC, BRPC, or LAPC who were treated with full-dose gemcitabine and oxaliplatin with concurrent fractionated radiation (30 Gy in 15 fractions). Surgical resection was completed in 63% of the entire study population and 62% of patients with BRPC. Patients with BRPC had a median OS of 25.4 months. R0 resection was obtained in 84% of patients, for whom median OS was 34.6 months.[43] Although the trial failed to show an improvement in 2-year disease-free survival (26.1%) compared with the historical control of 35% from the Charité Onkologie 001 (CONKO 001) study of patients with RPC receiving adjuvant gemcitabine, the patients had more advanced tumors given the large proportion of BRPC.

Given the high rate of distant metastatic disease in BRPC, several groups have added induction systemic therapy before CRT as a method to increase systemic doses of chemotherapy. Pipas and colleagues[44] reported on a single-institutional phase II study of patients with RPC, BRPC, and LAPC with cetuximab, an epidermal growth factor receptor antibody, followed by concurrent gemcitabine and radiation. The median OS for resected patients was 24.3 months and for R0 resection was 92%, similar to prior trials. A study by Landry and colleagues[45] attempted to randomize patients between gemcitabine-based CRT and induction gemcitabine and cisplatin followed by 5-FU–based CRT. Only 21 patients (10 CRT and 11 induction chemotherapy followed by CRT) were enrolled, and the trial closed early as a result of poor accrual. The study was also challenging to interpret because of enrollment of both patients with LAPC and patients with BRPC.

Trials discussed thus far have used standard radiation fractionation schedules. More contemporary studies have also explored the use of hypofractionated regimens using stereotactic body RT (SBRT), particularly in the setting of BRPC. Shaib and colleagues[46] performed a single-institution phase I dose-escalation trial to determine the safety and efficacy of 3-fraction SBRT delivered after FOLFIRINOX. SBRT doses ranged from 30 Gy with a 2-Gy-per-fraction boost to the posterior margin of the tumor up to 36 Gy with a 3-Gy-per-fraction boost. In the 12 treated patients, no grade 3 or 4 toxicities were noted over a median follow-up of 18 months. Seven of the 12 patients treated with SBRT underwent resection, with one patient having in situ disease at the margin. Median OS was 11 months, although interpretation is challenging in a small cohort with poor prognostic factors, including nodal disease and increased levels of carbohydrate antigen 19-9.

Several planned or ongoing studies are evaluating SBRT for BRPC. Researchers at the University of Maryland School of Medicine are conducting a phase II trial of FOLFIRINOX followed by a 5-fraction SBRT regimen in BRPC (NCT01992705). Based on their recently published phase II trial of induction gemcitabine followed by SBRT in LAPC,[21] the Alliance for Clinical Trials in Oncology is performing a multi-institutional randomized phase II trial of FOLFIRINOX with or without SBRT or hypofractionated image-guided RT for BRPC. Prospective clinical trials of neoadjuvant CRT for RPC and BRPC are listed in **Table 3**.

RADIATION TECHNIQUES: FROM TWO-DIMENSIONAL TO INTENSITY-MODULATED RADIATION THERAPY

The evolution of pancreatic cancer therapy has coincided with considerable advances in the technology of radiation delivery. Initial pancreatic cancer trials from the 1980s used two-dimensional (2D) treatment planning approaches for dose calculation and normal tissue avoidance.[13] This strategy has now been supplanted by three-dimensional (3D) conformal RT (3DCRT), IMRT, SBRT, and PT techniques offering more conformal treatment. These modern approaches use newer beam delivery and software technology, permitting more accurate planning and dose delivery.

The transition from 2D to 3DCRT came with little resistance in the 1990s. Newer software allowed digital, CT-based reconstruction of internal tumor and normal tissue structures with startling clarity. A major advance with this technology was the ability to use beam's eye-view perspectives to examine patient anatomy from multiple angles to ensure target coverage and normal tissue sparing.[47] By the inception of the seminal

Table 3
Prospective clinical trials of neoadjuvant radiation therapy for resectable and borderline resectable pancreatic cancer

Study, Report Year	N	Resectability	Total RT Dose (Gy)	RT Dose per Fraction (Gy)	CRT Regimen	Any Grade ≥3 Toxicity (%)	Resection Rate (%)	R0 Resection Rate (%)	Median OS (mo)
3DCRT/IMRT									
Evans et al,[31] 1992	28	RPC	50.4	1.8	5-FU + RT	—	61	82	—
Yeung et al,[102] 1993	26	RPC/BRPC LAPC	50.4	1.8	5-FU + MMC + RT	—	46	—	10.0
Pisters et al,[32] 1998	35	RPC	30	3.0	5-FU + RT + IORT 10–15 Gy	9	57	90	25[e]
ECOG,[34] 1998	53	RPC/BRPC	50.4	1.8	5-FU + MMC + RT	—	45	33[a]	9.7
Mehta et al,[40] 2001	15	BRPC	50.4–56	1.8–2.0	5-FU + RT	0	60	100	30[e]
Pisters et al,[33] 2002	35	RPC	30	3.0	Paclitaxel + RT ± IORT	46	57	68	12
Joensuu et al,[103] 2004	28	BRPC	50.4	1.8	Gem + RT	6	75	—	25.0
Pipas et al,[104] 2005	24	RPC (17%) BRPC (29%) LAPC (54%)	50.4	1.8	Gem + docetaxel then gem + RT	—	71	76	14.0
SFRO-FFCD 97–04,[105] 2006	41	RPC/BRPC	50	2.0	5-FU + cis + RT	66	63	80	9.4
Talamonti et al,[35] 2006	20	RPC/BRPC	36	2.4	Gem then gem + RT	10	85	94	26[e]
Desai et al,[106] 2007	44	RPC/BRPC (27%) LAPC (66%) Met (7%)	27.0	1.8	Gem + oxali + RT	—	58[c]	100	12.5[d]

Macchia et al,[107] 2007	28	RPC/BRPC (32%) LAPC (68%)	39.6	1.8	5-FU + RT then surgery + IORT 10 Gy then 5-FU + doxo + MMC	10.7 during CRT	78 in RPC/BRPC 11 in LAPC	89	11.3
Evans et al,[36] 2008	86	RPC/BRPC	30.0	3.0	Gem + RT	—	74	89	22.7
Varadhachary et al,[37] 2008	79	RPC/BRPC	30.0	3.0	Gem + cis then gem + RT	—	66	96	17.4
Small et al,[108] 2008	39	RPC (41%) BRPC (23%) LAPC (36%)	36.0	2.4	Gem + RT	25.6 (nonheme related to treatment)	44	—	—
Landry et al,[45] 2010	10 11	BRPC BRPC	50.4 50.4	1.8	Gem + RT Gem/cis then 5-FU + RT	36 (grade 4) 18 (grade 4)	30 18	33 50	19.4 13.4
Turrini et al,[109] 2010	34	RPC	45	1.8	Docetaxel + RT	6	50	100	15.5
Small et al,[110] 2011	32	RPC/BRPC/LAPC	36	2.4	Gem + bev	79	18.8[b]	—	11.8
Leone et al,[111] 2013	39	BRPC (38%) LAPC (62%)	50.4	1.8	Gem + oxali then gem + RT	—	60 in BRPC 8 in LAPC	82	16.7
Pipas et al,[44] 2012	33	RPC (12%) BRPC (70%) LAPC (18%)	54	1.92	Gem + cetuximab + RT	—	78 in BRPC 50 in LAPC	92	17.3
Satoi et al,[112] 2012	34	BRPC/LAPC	50.4	1.8	S-1 + RT	—	88	93	—
Shroff et al,[42] 2012	11	RPC/BRPC	50.4	1.8	Gem + bev + RT	—	82	100	30.1
Van Buren et al,[41] 2013	59	BRPC/RPC	30	3.0	Gem + bev then RT + bev	—	73	88	16.8

(continued on next page)

Table 3
(continued)

Study, Report Year	N	Resectability	Total RT Dose (Gy)	RT Dose per Fraction (Gy)	CRT Regimen	Any Grade ≥3 Toxicity (%)	Resection Rate (%)	R0 Resection Rate (%)	Median OS (mo)
Kim et al,[43] 2013	39	RPC (34%) BRPC (57%) LAPC (9%)	30	2.0	Gem + oxali + RT	37 (heme grade 3) 18 (heme grade 4) 46 (nonheme grade 3) 1 (nonheme grade 4)	63	84	18.2
Jensen et al,[113] 2014	23	BRPC/LAPC	50.4	1.8	5-FU + cis + IFNα	82.6	30.4	85.7	11.5
Wo et al,[114] 2014	10	RPC	25–30	3–5	Cetuximab + RT	70 (grade 3) 10 (grade 4)	80	—	—
Esnaola et al,[115] 2014	13	BRPC/LAPC	54	1.8	Gem + oxali + cetuximab then cape + RT	29.7 during chemo; 9.5 during CRT	69.2	100	24.1
SBRT									
Shaib et al,[46] 2016	13	BRPC	36–45	12–15	mFOLFIRINOX then SBRT	0	62	100	11
PT									
Hong et al,[39] 2014	50	RPC	25 Gy RBE	5 Gy RBE	Cape + RT	—	77	84	17

Abbreviations: 3DCRT, three-dimensional conformal RT; 5-FU, 5-fluorouracil; bev, bevacizumab; cape, capecitabine; chemo, chemotherapy; cis, cisplatin; CRT, chemoradiation; doxo, doxorubicin; gem, gemcitabine; IORT, intraoperative radiation therapy; LAPC, locally advanced pancreatic cancer; mFOLFIRINOX, modified 5-FU, oxaliplatin, leucovorin, irinotecan; MMC, mitomycin-C; nonheme, nonhematologic; oxali, oxaliplatin; PT, proton therapy; RT, radiation therapy; S-1, tegafur/gimeracil/oteracil; SBRT, stereotactic body radiation therapy.

[a] Assessed in only 21 patients.
[b] Included patients with LAPC.
[c] Included only patients with RPC/BRPC.
[d] Included patients with LAPC and metastatic disease.
[e] Included only patients who completed preoperative therapy and underwent resection.

RTOG 97-04 trial in 1998, 3DCRT was firmly established as the new standard of care. This trial required target and normal tissue delineation to limit doses to the kidneys, liver, spinal cord, and small bowel, which could only be accomplished with CT-based tissue contouring.[48]

The benefits of 3DCRT were thought to be self-evident, with little demand for comparative analysis. However, with changes in the health care climate and the advent of IMRT, the next major advance in pancreatic cancer RT, rigorous dosimetric analyses were required before widespread adoption. Numerous studies have shown that IMRT achieves superior delivery of sharp dose gradients at the periphery of the target volume, thereby greatly limiting unwanted dose to nearby normal tissues.[49–52] This benefit may be further enhanced using noncoplanar beam strategies,[53] helical tomotherapy,[52,54] and/or dose painting.[55] In a study of 71 patients treated with adjuvant IMRT-based radiation, the incidence of acute nausea and vomiting was limited to 8%, with only 6% of patients experiencing late small bowel complications.[56] This trial also showed a low (19%) local-regional failure rate. The low rate of failure alleviated concerns that reductions in toxicity with IMRT would come at the expense of greater treatment failures.

The gradual evolution from 2D to 3D to IMRT techniques was accompanied with little change in tumor-dosing strategies. Both the published RTOG 97-04 trial and the active RTOG 0848 study used a 50.4-Gy dose prescription given in standard 1.8-Gy daily fractions over 5.5 weeks.[48,57] However, with recent advances in chemotherapy, the role of protracted radiation schedules for pancreatic cancer treatment has been called into question. Despite certain trial shortcomings, survival outcomes from the prospective LAP 07 and Fédération Francophone de Cancérologie Digestive/Société Francophone de Radiothérapie Oncologique trials showed similar or better outcomes with chemotherapy alone than CRT using standard fractionation radiation.[25,58] These trials have spurred interest in abbreviated radiation schedules using SBRT, which minimizes the interruption of full-dose systemic therapy. SBRT allows the delivery of large radiation doses in a highly conformal fashion to tumor tissue in 1 to 5 fractions. The magnitude of these doses is thought to have a more powerful biological effect than that of standard fractionated radiation.[59] In order to safely deliver high doses of radiation, several treatment planning techniques are used. Four-dimensional CT scans, which measure tumor motion, are used for planning in conjunction with motion-mitigation strategies, such as abdominal compression or active breathing control. In addition, volumetric imaging via onboard cone-beam CT is used for each SBRT fraction. Target tissues are restricted to gross disease without coverage of elective lymph nodes. In a recent review of published institutional series for LAPC, SBRT regimens showed a median survival of 14 to 15 months, 1-year local control rates of about 80%, and grade 3 toxicities less than 10%.[60] The utility of SBRT is being examined in resected patients,[61,62] and patients with BRPC[63] and RPC.[64]

PROTON THERAPY

Although IMRT and SBRT approaches permit delivery of highly conformal radiation to tumor targets, the physical properties of photon beams ultimately limit minimization of normal tissue dose. Therefore, efforts have been made to further improve radiation to the pancreas by integration of particle therapies, in particular PT, because of their unique beam characteristics.[65] Photon beams reach a dose maximum a few centimeters below the skin surface and then decrease exponentially with increasing tissue depth. This property is distinct from that of proton beams, which maintain a fairly constant depth dose until they reach the area of maximal energy deposition, known the

Bragg peak. There is no dose beyond the Bragg peak, and dose at this location has a stronger radiobiological effect than photon energy.[65] The lack of dose beyond the Bragg peak results in a decrease in normal tissue exposure to radiation. Thus, PT has the potential to result in clinically meaningful reductions in acute and long-term normal tissue toxicities. Dosimetric studies comparing PT with photon therapy in pancreatic cancer have provided evidence of the potential for an improved therapeutic ratio favoring PT.[66,67] One such study comparing the V20 Gy (the volume of an organ receiving at least 20 Gy) for PT and IMRT showed that proton plans offered significantly reduced median small bowel V20 Gy (15.4% vs 47.0%), median stomach V20 Gy (2.3% vs 20.0%), and median right kidney V18 Gy (27.3% vs 50.5%) doses.[68] Doses to the small bowel and stomach in this range have been found to correlate with acute nausea and vomiting during CRT for LAPC,[69] suggesting that PT may cause less acute GI toxicity than IMRT. Example IMRT and PT treatment plans for pancreatic cancer are shown in **Fig. 1**.

Although clinical data on PT are still maturing, initial experiences have shown great promise. A recently reported study from the Massachusetts General Hospital examining a preoperative PT regimen for pancreatic cancer of 25 Gy in 5 fractions showed only 4.1% grade 3 toxicities in the phase 1 portion and 16.2% local failure in the phase 2 portion.[39] Similarly, researchers from the University of Florida reported on a 22-patient study incorporating chemotherapy and conventionally fractioned PT to 50.4 Gy.[70] Minimal grade 1 to 2 and no grade 3 toxicities were reported. Future trials should further quantify and clarify the benefits of PT.

PERSONALIZED TREATMENT AND FUTURE DIRECTIONS

As the genetic underpinnings of pancreatic cancer are better elucidated, clinical trials are also incorporating treatment selection based on genomic factors. Activating KRAS mutations have been found in up to 90% of pancreatic cancers,[71,72] and recent studies have reported that human pancreatic cancers can be subdivided into 3 genetic subtypes (quasimesenchymal, classic, and exocrinelike) that vary based on prognosis and resistance to therapies targeting the RAS pathway.[73] These findings

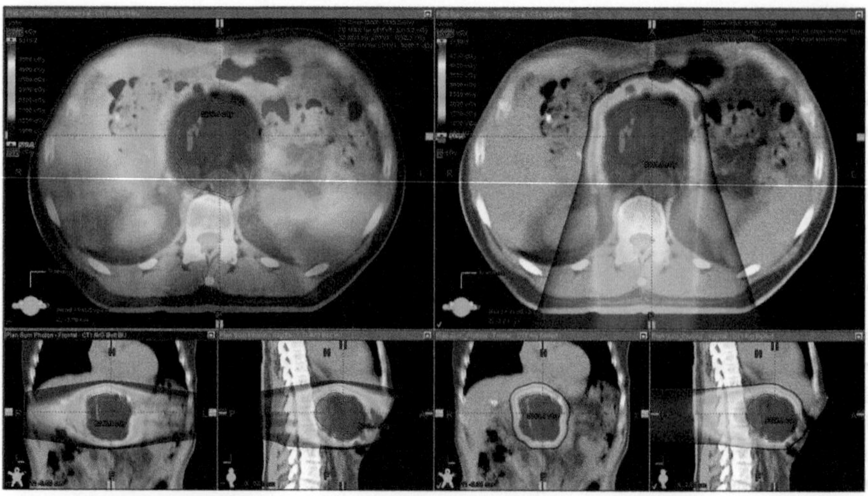

Fig. 1. Neoadjuvant IMRT plan (*left*) and a proton therapy plan (*right*) for a patient with pancreatic cancer.

suggest that future therapy for pancreatic cancer may be informed by the genetic profile of the malignancy.

An understanding of genetic profiles in pancreatic cancer may also help to predict patterns of tumor recurrence. Mutation of the DPC4 (SMAD4) tumor suppressor gene in pancreatic cancers has been correlated with patterns of failure in 2 institutional series.[7,74] Tumors with wild-type DPC4 have higher rates of local tumor progression than mutated DPC4 tumors. This promising finding may allow the selection of patients (wild-type DPC4) who are more likely to benefit from RT to the local tumor. DPC4 expression is currently being evaluated in several clinical trials investigating RT for treatment of pancreatic cancer (NCT02241551, NCT01972919).

Other targetable genes expressed by pancreatic cancers have been discovered. The secreted protein acidic and rich in cysteine (SPARC) gene has been associated with an adverse prognosis[75] and is a target of nab-paclitaxel, an albumin-bound formulation of paclitaxel that binds SPARC, allowing improved delivery of gemcitabine to tumor cells. This treatment results in improved efficacy of the combination compared with gemcitabine alone.[76] In addition to an increased risk of breast and ovarian cancers, patients with germline BRCA1/2 mutations have also shown higher rates of pancreatic cancers. Poly-ADP ribose polymerase (PARP) is an enzyme that is critical to base excision repair. Inhibition of the enzyme leads to cell death during DNA replication in patients with germline BRCA mutations.[77] A phase II study of the PARP inhibitor olaparib has shown promising results in patients with BRCA-mutated pancreatic cancer.[78]

The only prognostic biomarker for pancreatic cancer approved to date by the US Food and Drug Administration is CA19-9. Although not specific to pancreatic cancer, CA19-9 is a good diagnostic marker in symptomatic patients, with a sensitivity of ~80% and specificity up to 90%.[79] However, its low positive predictive value makes it a poor general screening tool in asymptomatic patients.[80] In the setting of biopsy-proven disease, a reduction in CA19-9 levels after resection has been associated with higher rates of survival.[80–82] Patients with postoperative CA19-9 levels less than 90 U/mL have been shown to be more likely to benefit from adjuvant chemotherapy.[83] Secondary analysis of RTOG 9704 found that postoperative CA19-9 levels were the only independent predictor of both local/regional recurrence and distant failure.[84] In addition, after CRT, normalization of CA19-9 levels has been associated with improvements in OS.[85] Future studies will need to develop predictor and prognostic biomarkers and discover targetable mutations in pancreatic cancer that can be used to improve outcomes.

IMMUNOTHERAPY

The immune system has long been known to play a critical role in cancer initiation and progression. Pancreatic cancer has been shown to harbor an immunosuppressive tumor microenvironment, enabling it to avoid detection by the immune system.[86] The development of immunotherapy, targeting the immune system for treatment of cancer, has opened an era of novel treatments for pancreatic cancer. Current immunotherapy approaches for pancreatic cancer include checkpoint modulators, vaccines, regulatory T cell (T_{reg}) depletion, cytokines, and adoptive T-cell transfer. RT has been shown to have profound effects in countering immunosuppressive tumor microenvironments by a variety of mechanisms. Thus, RT has been proposed as a treatment to improve the efficacy of immunotherapies such as checkpoint modulators.[87] At the University of Maryland School of Medicine, a clinical trial is underway exploring this new approach for treatment of metastatic pancreatic cancer (NCT02885727).

SUMMARY

The role of RT for RPC and BRPC has evolved from use predominantly in the adjuvant setting to more frequent use in the neoadjuvant setting. Although some older studies failed to show benefits with RT in pancreatic cancer because of high rates of distant metastases, more recent studies have shown that, in appropriately selected patients, RT can improve local control and rates of margin-negative resection. Future studies will explore the utility of novel RT strategies, such as SBRT and PT, and investigate the immune-modulating properties of RT in combination with immunotherapy.

REFERENCES

1. Siegel RL, Miller KD, Jemal A. Cancer statistics, 2016. CA Cancer J Clin 2016; 66(1):7–30.
2. Howlander N, Noone AM, Krapcho M, et al. SEER cancer statistics review, 1975-2013. Bethesda (MD): National Cancer Institute; 2016. SEER data submission, posted to the SEER Web site, April 2016. Available at: https://seer.cancer.gov/statfacts/html/pancreas.html. Accessed April 2016.
3. Vasen H, Ibrahim I, Ponce CG, et al. Benefit of surveillance for pancreatic cancer in high-risk individuals: outcome of long-term prospective follow-up studies from three European expert centers. J Clin Oncol 2016;34(17):2010–9.
4. Ryan DP, Hong TS, Bardeesy N. Pancreatic adenocarcinoma. N Engl J Med 2014;371(11):1039–49.
5. Regine WF, Winter KA, Abrams R, et al. Fluorouracil-based chemoradiation with either gemcitabine or fluorouracil chemotherapy after resection of pancreatic adenocarcinoma: 5-year analysis of the U.S. Intergroup/RTOG 9704 phase III trial. Ann Surg Oncol 2011;18(5):1319–26.
6. Oettle H, Neuhaus P, Hochhaus A, et al. Adjuvant chemotherapy with gemcitabine and long-term outcomes among patients with resected pancreatic cancer: the CONKO-001 randomized trial. JAMA 2013;310(14):1473–81.
7. Iacobuzio-Donahue CA, Fu B, Yachida S, et al. DPC4 gene status of the primary carcinoma correlates with patterns of failure in patients with pancreatic cancer. J Clin Oncol 2009;27(11):1806–13.
8. Liu RC, Traverso LW. Diagnostic laparoscopy improves staging of pancreatic cancer deemed locally unresectable by computed tomography. Surg Endosc 2005;19(5):638–42.
9. National Comprehensive Cancer Network. Pancreatic adenocarcinoma (version 2.2016). Available at: www.nccn.org/professionals/physician_gls/pdf/pancreatic.pdf. Accessed November 12, 2016.
10. Katz MH, Pisters PW, Evans DB, et al. Borderline resectable pancreatic cancer: the importance of this emerging stage of disease. J Am Coll Surg 2008;206(5):833–46 [discussion: 846–8].
11. Callery MP, Chang KJ, Fishman EK, et al. Pretreatment assessment of resectable and borderline resectable pancreatic cancer: expert consensus statement. Ann Surg Oncol 2009;16(7):1727–33.
12. Katz MH, Marsh R, Herman JM, et al. Borderline resectable pancreatic cancer: need for standardization and methods for optimal clinical trial design. Ann Surg Oncol 2013;20(8):2787–95.

13. Kalser MH, Ellenberg SS. Pancreatic cancer. Adjuvant combined radiation and chemotherapy following curative resection. Arch Surg 1985;120(8):899–903.
14. Klinkenbijl JH, Jeekel J, Sahmoud T, et al. Adjuvant radiotherapy and 5-fluorouracil after curative resection of cancer of the pancreas and periampullary region: phase III trial of the EORTC Gastrointestinal Tract Cancer Cooperative Group. Ann Surg 1999;230(6):776–82 [discussion: 782–4].
15. Smeenk HG, Erdmann J, van Dekken H, et al. Long-term survival after radical resection for pancreatic head and ampullary cancer: a potential role for the EGF-R. Dig Surg 2007;24(1):38–45.
16. Garofalo MC, Regine WF, Tan MT. On statistical reanalysis, the EORTC trial is a positive trial for adjuvant chemoradiation in pancreatic cancer. Ann Surg 2006;244(2):332–3 [author reply: 333].
17. Neoptolemos JP, Stocken DD, Friess H, et al. A randomized trial of chemoradiotherapy and chemotherapy after resection of pancreatic cancer. N Engl J Med 2004;350(12):1200–10.
18. Choti MA. Adjuvant therapy for pancreatic cancer–the debate continues. N Engl J Med 2004;350(12):1249–51.
19. Crane CH, Ben-Josef E, Small W Jr. Chemotherapy for pancreatic cancer. N Engl J Med 2004;350(26):2713–5 [author reply: 2713-5].
20. Corsini MM, Miller RC, Haddock MG, et al. Adjuvant radiotherapy and chemotherapy for pancreatic carcinoma: the Mayo Clinic experience (1975-2005). J Clin Oncol 2008;26(21):3511–6.
21. Herman JM, Chang DT, Goodman KA, et al. Phase 2 multi-institutional trial evaluating gemcitabine and stereotactic body radiotherapy for patients with locally advanced unresectable pancreatic adenocarcinoma. Cancer 2015;121(7):1128–37.
22. Kinsella TJ, Seo Y, Willis J, et al. The impact of resection margin status and postoperative CA19-9 levels on survival and patterns of recurrence after postoperative high-dose radiotherapy with 5-FU-based concurrent chemotherapy for resectable pancreatic cancer. Am J Clin Oncol 2008;31(5):446–53.
23. Hsu CC, Herman JM, Corsini MM, et al. Adjuvant chemoradiation for pancreatic adenocarcinoma: the Johns Hopkins Hospital–Mayo Clinic collaborative study. Ann Surg Oncol 2010;17(4):981–90.
24. Abrams RA, Winter KA, Regine WF, et al. Failure to adhere to protocol specified radiation therapy guidelines was associated with decreased survival in RTOG 9704–a phase III trial of adjuvant chemotherapy and chemoradiotherapy for patients with resected adenocarcinoma of the pancreas. Int J Radiat Oncol Biol Phys 2012;82(2):809–16.
25. Hammel P, Huguet F, van Laethem JL, et al. Effect of chemoradiotherapy vs chemotherapy on survival in patients with locally advanced pancreatic cancer controlled after 4 months of gemcitabine with or without erlotinib: the LAP07 Randomized Clinical Trial. JAMA 2016;315(17):1844–53.
26. Cheng TY, Sheth K, White RR, et al. Effect of neoadjuvant chemoradiation on operative mortality and morbidity for pancreaticoduodenectomy. Ann Surg Oncol 2006;13(1):66–74.
27. Chang DK, Johns AL, Merrett ND, et al. Margin clearance and outcome in resected pancreatic cancer. J Clin Oncol 2009;27(17):2855–62.
28. Raut CP, Tseng JF, Sun CC, et al. Impact of resection status on pattern of failure and survival after pancreaticoduodenectomy for pancreatic adenocarcinoma. Ann Surg 2007;246(1):52–60.

29. Burris HA 3rd, Moore MJ, Andersen J, et al. Improvements in survival and clinical benefit with gemcitabine as first-line therapy for patients with advanced pancreas cancer: a randomized trial. J Clin Oncol 1997;15(6):2403–13.
30. Conroy T, Desseigne F, Ychou M, et al. FOLFIRINOX versus gemcitabine for metastatic pancreatic cancer. N Engl J Med 2011;364(19):1817–25.
31. Evans DB, Rich TA, Byrd DR, et al. Preoperative chemoradiation and pancreaticoduodenectomy for adenocarcinoma of the pancreas. Arch Surg 1992; 127(11):1335–9.
32. Pisters PW, Abbruzzese JL, Janjan NA, et al. Rapid-fractionation preoperative chemoradiation, pancreaticoduodenectomy, and intraoperative radiation therapy for resectable pancreatic adenocarcinoma. J Clin Oncol 1998;16(12): 3843–50.
33. Pisters PW, Wolff RA, Janjan NA, et al. Preoperative paclitaxel and concurrent rapid-fractionation radiation for resectable pancreatic adenocarcinoma: toxicities, histologic response rates, and event-free outcome. J Clin Oncol 2002; 20(10):2537–44.
34. Hoffman JP, Lipsitz S, Pisansky T, et al. Phase II trial of preoperative radiation therapy and chemotherapy for patients with localized, resectable adenocarcinoma of the pancreas: an Eastern Cooperative Oncology Group Study. J Clin Oncol 1998;16(1):317–23.
35. Talamonti MS, Small W Jr, Mulcahy MF, et al. A multi-institutional phase II trial of preoperative full-dose gemcitabine and concurrent radiation for patients with potentially resectable pancreatic carcinoma. Ann Surg Oncol 2006;13(2):150–8.
36. Evans DB, Varadhachary GR, Crane CH, et al. Preoperative gemcitabine-based chemoradiation for patients with resectable adenocarcinoma of the pancreatic head. J Clin Oncol 2008;26(21):3496–502.
37. Varadhachary GR, Wolff RA, Crane CH, et al. Preoperative gemcitabine and cisplatin followed by gemcitabine-based chemoradiation for resectable adenocarcinoma of the pancreatic head. J Clin Oncol 2008;26(21):3487–95.
38. Kozak KR, Kachnic LA, Adams J, et al. Dosimetric feasibility of hypofractionated proton radiotherapy for neoadjuvant pancreatic cancer treatment. Int J Radiat Oncol Biol Phys 2007;68(5):1557–66.
39. Hong TS, Ryan DP, Borger DR, et al. A phase 1/2 and biomarker study of preoperative short course chemoradiation with proton beam therapy and capecitabine followed by early surgery for resectable pancreatic ductal adenocarcinoma. Int J Radiat Oncol Biol Phys 2014;89(4):830–8.
40. Mehta VK, Fisher G, Ford JA, et al. Preoperative chemoradiation for marginally resectable adenocarcinoma of the pancreas. J Gastrointest Surg 2001;5(1): 27–35.
41. Van Buren G 2nd, Ramanathan RK, Krasinskas AM, et al. Phase II study of induction fixed-dose rate gemcitabine and bevacizumab followed by 30 Gy radiotherapy as preoperative treatment for potentially resectable pancreatic adenocarcinoma. Ann Surg Oncol 2013;20(12):3787–93.
42. Shroff RT, Varadhachary GR, Crane CH, et al. Updated survival analysis of preoperative gemcitabine (gem) plus bevacizumab (bev)-based chemoradiation for resectable pancreatic adenocarcinoma. J Clin Oncol 2012;30(Suppl) [abstract: 4051].
43. Kim EJ, Ben-Josef E, Herman JM, et al. A multi-institutional phase 2 study of neoadjuvant gemcitabine and oxaliplatin with radiation therapy in patients with pancreatic cancer. Cancer 2013;119(15):2692–700.

44. Pipas JM, Zaki BI, McGowan MM, et al. Neoadjuvant cetuximab, twice-weekly gemcitabine, and intensity-modulated radiotherapy (IMRT) in patients with pancreatic adenocarcinoma. Ann Oncol 2012;23(11):2820–7.
45. Landry J, Catalano PJ, Staley C, et al. Randomized phase II study of gemcitabine plus radiotherapy versus gemcitabine, 5-fluorouracil, and cisplatin followed by radiotherapy and 5-fluorouracil for patients with locally advanced, potentially resectable pancreatic adenocarcinoma. J Surg Oncol 2010;101(7):587–92.
46. Shaib WL, Hawk N, Cassidy RJ, et al. A phase 1 study of stereotactic body radiation therapy dose escalation for borderline resectable pancreatic cancer after modified FOLFIRINOX (NCT01446458). Int J Radiat Oncol Biol Phys 2016; 96(2):296–303.
47. Ten Haken RK, Lawrence TS, McShan DL, et al. Technical considerations in the use of 3-D beam arrangements in the abdomen. Radiother Oncol 1991;22(1): 19–28.
48. Regine WF, Winter KA, Abrams RA, et al. Fluorouracil vs gemcitabine chemotherapy before and after fluorouracil-based chemoradiation following resection of pancreatic adenocarcinoma: a randomized controlled trial. JAMA 2008; 299(9):1019–26.
49. van der Geld YG, van Triest B, Verbakel WF, et al. Evaluation of four-dimensional computed tomography-based intensity-modulated and respiratory-gated radiotherapy techniques for pancreatic carcinoma. Int J Radiat Oncol Biol Phys 2008; 72(4):1215–20.
50. Kataria T, Rawat S, Sinha SN, et al. Intensity modulated radiotherapy in abdominal malignancies: our experience in reducing the dose to normal structures as compared to the gross tumor. J Cancer Res Ther 2006;2(4):161–5.
51. Brown MW, Ning H, Arora B, et al. A dosimetric analysis of dose escalation using two intensity-modulated radiation therapy techniques in locally advanced pancreatic carcinoma. Int J Radiat Oncol Biol Phys 2006;65(1):274–83.
52. Taylor R, Opfermann K, Jones BD, et al. Comparison of radiation treatment delivery for pancreatic cancer: Linac intensity-modulated radiotherapy versus helical tomotherapy. J Med Imaging Radiat Oncol 2012;56(3):332–7.
53. Chang DS, Bartlett GK, Das IJ, et al. Beam angle selection for intensity-modulated radiotherapy (IMRT) treatment of unresectable pancreatic cancer: are noncoplanar beam angles necessary? Clin Transl Oncol 2013;15(9):720–4.
54. Chang JS, Wang ML, Koom WS, et al. High-dose helical tomotherapy with concurrent full-dose chemotherapy for locally advanced pancreatic cancer. Int J Radiat Oncol Biol Phys 2012;83(5):1448–54.
55. Tunceroglu A, Park JH, Balasubramanian S, et al. Dose-painted intensity modulated radiation therapy improves local control for locally advanced pancreas cancer. ISRN Oncol 2012;2012:572342.
56. Yovino S, Poppe M, Jabbour S, et al. Intensity-modulated radiation therapy significantly improves acute gastrointestinal toxicity in pancreatic and ampullary cancers. Int J Radiat Oncol Biol Phys 2011;79(1):158–62.
57. Ling TC, Slater JM, Mifflin R, et al. Evaluation of normal tissue exposure in patients receiving radiotherapy for pancreatic cancer based on RTOG 0848. J Gastrointest Oncol 2015;6(2):108–14.
58. Chauffert B, Mornex F, Bonnetain F, et al. Phase III trial comparing intensive induction chemoradiotherapy (60 Gy, infusional 5-FU and intermittent cisplatin) followed by maintenance gemcitabine with gemcitabine alone for locally advanced unresectable pancreatic cancer. Definitive results of the 2000-01 FFCD/SFRO study. Ann Oncol 2008;19(9):1592–9.

59. Brown JM, Koong AC. High-dose single-fraction radiotherapy: exploiting a new biology? Int J Radiat Oncol Biol Phys 2008;71(2):324–5.
60. Chhabra A, Kaiser A, Regine WF, et al. The expanding role of stereotactic body radiation therapy for pancreatic cancer: a review of the literature. Transl Cancer Res 2015;4(6):659–70.
61. Chang DT, Schellenberg D, Shen J, et al. Stereotactic radiotherapy for unresectable adenocarcinoma of the pancreas. Cancer 2009;115(3):665–72.
62. Mahadevan A, Miksad R, Goldstein M, et al. Induction gemcitabine and stereotactic body radiotherapy for locally advanced nonmetastatic pancreas cancer. Int J Radiat Oncol Biol Phys 2011;81(4):e615–22.
63. Chuong MD, Springett GM, Freilich JM, et al. Stereotactic body radiation therapy for locally advanced and borderline resectable pancreatic cancer is effective and well tolerated. Int J Radiat Oncol Biol Phys 2013;86(3):516–22.
64. Rwigema JC, Heron DE, Parikh SD, et al. Adjuvant stereotactic body radiotherapy for resected pancreatic adenocarcinoma with close or positive margins. J Gastrointest Cancer 2012;43(1):70–6.
65. Nichols RC, Huh S, Li Z, et al. Proton therapy for pancreatic cancer. World J Gastrointest Oncol 2015;7(9):141–7.
66. Thompson RF, Mayekar SU, Zhai H, et al. A dosimetric comparison of proton and photon therapy in unresectable cancers of the head of pancreas. Med Phys 2014;41(8):081711.
67. Ding X, Dionisi F, Tang S, et al. A comprehensive dosimetric study of pancreatic cancer treatment using three-dimensional conformal radiation therapy (3DCRT), intensity-modulated radiation therapy (IMRT), volumetric-modulated radiation therapy (VMAT), and passive-scattering and modulated-scanning proton therapy (PT). Med Dosim 2014;39(2):139–45.
68. Nichols RC Jr, Huh SN, Prado KL, et al. Protons offer reduced normal-tissue exposure for patients receiving postoperative radiotherapy for resected pancreatic head cancer. Int J Radiat Oncol Biol Phys 2012;83(1):158–63.
69. Radiation-induced emesis: a prospective observational multicenter Italian trial. The Italian Group for Antiemetic Research in Radiotherapy. Int J Radiat Oncol Biol Phys 1999;44(3):619–25.
70. Nichols RC Jr, George TJ, Zaiden RA Jr, et al. Proton therapy with concomitant capecitabine for pancreatic and ampullary cancers is associated with a low incidence of gastrointestinal toxicity. Acta Oncol 2013;52(3):498–505.
71. Jones S, Zhang X, Parsons DW, et al. Core signaling pathways in human pancreatic cancers revealed by global genomic analyses. Science 2008; 321(5897):1801–6.
72. Biankin AV, Waddell N, Kassahn KS, et al. Pancreatic cancer genomes reveal aberrations in axon guidance pathway genes. Nature 2012;491(7424):399–405.
73. Collisson EA, Sadanandam A, Olson P, et al. Subtypes of pancreatic ductal adenocarcinoma and their differing responses to therapy. Nat Med 2011; 17(4):500–3.
74. Crane CH, Varadhachary GR, Yordy JS, et al. Phase II trial of cetuximab, gemcitabine, and oxaliplatin followed by chemoradiation with cetuximab for locally advanced (T4) pancreatic adenocarcinoma: correlation of Smad4(Dpc4) immunostaining with pattern of disease progression. J Clin Oncol 2011;29(22): 3037–43.
75. Han W, Cao F, Chen MB, et al. Prognostic value of SPARC in patients with pancreatic cancer: a systematic review and meta-analysis. PLoS One 2016; 11(1):e0145803.

76. Von Hoff DD, Ervin T, Arena FP, et al. Increased survival in pancreatic cancer with nab-paclitaxel plus gemcitabine. N Engl J Med 2013;369(18):1691–703.
77. Bryant HE, Schultz N, Thomas HD, et al. Specific killing of BRCA2-deficient tumours with inhibitors of poly(ADP-ribose) polymerase. Nature 2005;434(7035): 913–7.
78. Kaufman B, Shapira-Frommer R, Schmutzler RK, et al. Olaparib monotherapy in patients with advanced cancer and a germline BRCA1/2 mutation. J Clin Oncol 2015;33(3):244–50.
79. Huang Z, Liu F. Diagnostic value of serum carbohydrate antigen 19-9 in pancreatic cancer: a meta-analysis. Tumour Biol 2014;35(8):7459–65.
80. Ballehaninna UK, Chamberlain RS. The clinical utility of serum CA 19-9 in the diagnosis, prognosis and management of pancreatic adenocarcinoma: an evidence based appraisal. J Gastrointest Oncol 2012;3(2):105–19.
81. Hartwig W, Strobel O, Hinz U, et al. CA19-9 in potentially resectable pancreatic cancer: perspective to adjust surgical and perioperative therapy. Ann Surg Oncol 2013;20(7):2188–96.
82. Berger AC, Garcia M Jr, Hoffman JP, et al. Postresection CA 19-9 predicts overall survival in patients with pancreatic cancer treated with adjuvant chemoradiation: a prospective validation by RTOG 9704. J Clin Oncol 2008;26(36):5918–22.
83. Humphris JL, Chang DK, Johns AL, et al. The prognostic and predictive value of serum CA19.9 in pancreatic cancer. Ann Oncol 2012;23(7):1713–22.
84. Regine WF, Winter K, Kessel IL, et al. Prospective and concurrent analysis of postresection CA19-9 level and surgical margin status (SMS) as predictors of pattern of disease recurrence following adjuvant treatment for pancreatic carcinoma: NRG oncology/RTOG 9704 secondary analysis. Int J Radiat Oncol Biol Phys 2015;93(3):s153.
85. Tzeng CW, Balachandran A, Ahmad M, et al. Serum carbohydrate antigen 19-9 represents a marker of response to neoadjuvant therapy in patients with borderline resectable pancreatic cancer. HPB (Oxford) 2014;16(5):430–8.
86. Kimbara S, Kondo S. Immune checkpoint and inflammation as therapeutic targets in pancreatic carcinoma. World J Gastroenterol 2016;22(33):7440–52.
87. Dewan MZ, Galloway AE, Kawashima N, et al. Fractionated but not single-dose radiotherapy induces an immune-mediated abscopal effect when combined with anti-CTLA-4 antibody. Clin Cancer Res 2009;15(17):5379–88.
88. Van Laethem JL, Demols A, Gay F, et al. Postoperative adjuvant gemcitabine and concurrent radiation after curative resection of pancreatic head carcinoma: a phase II study. Int J Radiat Oncol Biol Phys 2003;56(4):974–80.
89. Wilkowski R, Thoma M, Duhmke E, et al. Concurrent chemoradiotherapy with gemcitabine and cisplatin after incomplete (R1) resection of locally advanced pancreatic carcinoma. Int J Radiat Oncol Biol Phys 2004;58(3):768–72.
90. Allen AM, Zalupski MM, Robertson JM, et al. Adjuvant therapy in pancreatic cancer: phase I trial of radiation dose escalation with concurrent full-dose gemcitabine. Int J Radiat Oncol Biol Phys 2004;59(5):1461–7.
91. Demols A, Peeters M, Polus M, et al. Adjuvant gemcitabine and concurrent continuous radiation (45 Gy) for resected pancreatic head carcinoma: a multicenter Belgian phase II study. Int J Radiat Oncol Biol Phys 2005;62(5):1351–6.
92. Blackstock AW, Mornex F, Partensky C, et al. Adjuvant gemcitabine and concurrent radiation for patients with resected pancreatic cancer: a phase II study. Br J Cancer 2006;95(3):260–5.
93. Brade A, Brierley J, Oza A, et al. Concurrent gemcitabine and radiotherapy with and without neoadjuvant gemcitabine for locally advanced unresectable or

resected pancreatic cancer: a phase I-II study. Int J Radiat Oncol Biol Phys 2007;67(4):1027–36.
94. Linehan DC, Tan MC, Strasberg SM, et al. Adjuvant interferon-based chemoradiation followed by gemcitabine for resected pancreatic adenocarcinoma: a single-institution phase II study. Ann Surg 2008;248(2):145–51.
95. Van Laethem JL, Hammel P, Mornex F, et al. Adjuvant gemcitabine alone versus gemcitabine-based chemoradiotherapy after curative resection for pancreatic cancer: a randomized EORTC-40013-22012/FFCD-9203/GERCOR phase II study. J Clin Oncol 2010;28(29):4450–6.
96. Morganti AG, Picardi V, Ippolito E, et al. Capecitabine based postoperative accelerated chemoradiation of pancreatic carcinoma. A dose-escalation study. Acta Oncol 2010;49(4):418–22.
97. Katz MH, Wolff R, Crane CH, et al. Survival and quality of life of patients with resected pancreatic adenocarcinoma treated with adjuvant interferon-based chemoradiation: a phase II trial. Ann Surg Oncol 2011;18(13):3615–22.
98. Picozzi VJ, Abrams RA, Decker PA, et al. Multicenter phase II trial of adjuvant therapy for resected pancreatic cancer using cisplatin, 5-fluorouracil, and interferon-alfa-2b-based chemoradiation: ACOSOG Trial Z05031. Ann Oncol 2011;22(2):348–54.
99. Schmidt J, Abel U, Debus J, et al. Open-label, multicenter, randomized phase III trial of adjuvant chemoradiation plus interferon alfa-2b versus fluorouracil and folinic acid for patients with resected pancreatic adenocarcinoma. J Clin Oncol 2012;30(33):4077–83.
100. Herman JM, Wild AT, Wang H, et al. Randomized phase III multi-institutional study of TNFerade biologic with fluorouracil and radiotherapy for locally advanced pancreatic cancer: final results. J Clin Oncol 2013;31(7):886–94.
101. Cho M, Wang-Gillam A, Myerson R, et al. A phase II study of adjuvant gemcitabine plus docetaxel followed by concurrent chemoradation in resected pancreaticobiliary carcinoma. HPB (Oxford) 2015;17(7):587–93.
102. Yeung RS, Weese JL, Hoffman JP, et al. Neoadjuvant chemoradiation in pancreatic and duodenal carcinoma. A phase II study. Cancer 1993;72(7):2124–33.
103. Joensuu TK, Kiviluoto T, Karkkainen P, et al. Phase I-II trial of twice-weekly gemcitabine and concomitant irradiation in patients undergoing pancreaticoduodenectomy with extended lymphadenectomy for locally advanced pancreatic cancer. Int J Radiat Oncol Biol Phys 2004;60(2):444–52.
104. Pipas JM, Barth RJ Jr, Zaki B, et al. Docetaxel/gemcitabine followed by gemcitabine and external beam radiotherapy in patients with pancreatic adenocarcinoma. Ann Surg Oncol 2005;12(12):995–1004.
105. Mornex F, Girard N, Scoazec JY, et al. Feasibility of preoperative combined radiation therapy and chemotherapy with 5-fluorouracil and cisplatin in potentially resectable pancreatic adenocarcinoma: the French SFRO-FFCD 97-04 phase II trial. Int J Radiat Oncol Biol Phys 2006;65(5):1471–8.
106. Desai SP, Ben-Josef E, Normolle DP, et al. Phase I study of oxaliplatin, full-dose gemcitabine, and concurrent radiation therapy in pancreatic cancer. J Clin Oncol 2007;25(29):4587–92.
107. Macchia G, Valentini V, Mattiucci GC, et al. Preoperative chemoradiation and intra-operative radiotherapy for pancreatic carcinoma. Tumori 2007;93(1):53–60.
108. Small W Jr, Berlin J, Freedman GM, et al. Full-dose gemcitabine with concurrent radiation therapy in patients with nonmetastatic pancreatic cancer: a multicenter phase II trial. J Clin Oncol 2008;26(6):942–7.

109. Turrini O, Ychou M, Moureau-Zabotto L, et al. Neoadjuvant docetaxel-based chemoradiation for resectable adenocarcinoma of the pancreas: new neoadjuvant regimen was safe and provided an interesting pathologic response. Eur J Surg Oncol 2010;36(10):987–92.
110. Small W Jr, Mulcahy MF, Rademaker A, et al. Phase II trial of full-dose gemcitabine and bevacizumab in combination with attenuated three-dimensional conformal radiotherapy in patients with localized pancreatic cancer. Int J Radiat Oncol Biol Phys 2011;80(2):476–82.
111. Leone F, Gatti M, Massucco P, et al. Induction gemcitabine and oxaliplatin therapy followed by a twice-weekly infusion of gemcitabine and concurrent external-beam radiation for neoadjuvant treatment of locally advanced pancreatic cancer: a single institutional experience. Cancer 2013;119(2):277–84.
112. Satoi S, Toyokawa H, Yanagimoto H, et al. Neo-adjuvant chemoradiation therapy using S-1 followed by surgical resection in patients with pancreatic cancer. J Gastrointest Surg 2012;16(4):784–92.
113. Jensen EH, Armstrong L, Lee C, et al. Neoadjuvant interferon-based chemoradiation for borderline resectable and locally advanced pancreas cancer: a Phase II pilot study. HPB (Oxford) 2014;16(2):131–9.
114. Wo JY, Mamon HJ, Ferrone CR, et al. Phase I study of neoadjuvant accelerated short course radiation therapy with photons and capecitabine for resectable pancreatic cancer. Radiother Oncol 2014;110(1):160–4.
115. Esnaola NF, Chaudhary UB, O'Brien P, et al. Phase 2 trial of induction gemcitabine, oxaliplatin, and cetuximab followed by selective capecitabine-based chemoradiation in patients with borderline resectable or unresectable locally advanced pancreatic cancer. Int J Radiat Oncol Biol Phys 2014;88(4):837–44.

Evolving Role of Radiotherapy in the Management of Rectal Carcinoma

Clayton A. Smith, MD, PhD[a,*], Lisa A. Kachnic, MD[b]

KEYWORDS

- Rectal • Cancer • Radiotherapy • Radiation • Neoadjuvant
- Intensity-modulated radiation therapy

KEY POINTS

- Neoadjuvant radiation improves local control of rectal cancer and reduces acute and late toxicity compared with adjuvant treatment.
- Neoadjuvant radiation combined with chemotherapy improves pathologic complete response rates.
- Alternative treatment strategies either omitting radiotherapy or omitting surgery may be feasible in select populations and are under evaluation in prospective trials.
- Intensity-modulated radiation therapy may reduce toxicity and treatment delays compared with traditional 3-dimensional conformal radiation therapy.

INTRODUCTION

The incidence of rectal cancer is estimated to be 39,220 in the United States in 2016, with an estimated 49,190 deaths from combined colon and rectal cancer.[1] Although surgery remains the primary definitive treatment of colorectal cancers, additional local treatment with radiotherapy is indicated in many patients because of the anatomy of the rectum and pelvis. The limited space within the pelvis can make complete surgical resection more difficult for rectal tumors while at the same time providing a fixed target for radiation treatments. The role of radiotherapy as adjunct to surgery has evolved over the decades with changes in the timing (preoperative vs postoperative), length (short course vs long course), intent (neoadjuvant vs definitive), and delivery (3-dimensional conformal radiation therapy [3D-CRT] vs intensity-modulated radiation therapy

Disclosure Statement: The authors have nothing to disclose.
[a] Division of Radiation Oncology, University of South Alabama Mitchell Cancer Institute, 1660 Spring Hill Avenue, Mobile, AL 36604, USA; [b] Department of Radiation Oncology, Vanderbilt University Medical Center, 2220 Pierce Avenue, Preston Research Building B-1003, Nashville, TN 37232, USA
* Corresponding author.
E-mail address: Claytonsmith@health.southalabama.edu

Surg Oncol Clin N Am 26 (2017) 455–466
http://dx.doi.org/10.1016/j.soc.2017.01.011 surgonc.theclinics.com
1055-3207/17/

[IMRT]), significantly improving the outcomes of patients. This review summarizes the evolution in radiation therapy (RT) for the management of rectal cancer and addresses some of the current questions regarding its role in the future.

FROM SURGERY ALONE TO COMBINED MODALITY THERAPY

Historically, the primary management of rectal carcinoma was surgical resection, with rates of local failure of 25% or higher with older surgical techniques.[2] It was also observed that positive resection margin resulted in significantly worse local failure rates.[3] The advent of total mesorectal excision (TME), which uses sharp dissection of mesorectal contents, further reduced the rate of local recurrence to as low as 8%.[4] For patients with higher risk disease (such as T3/T4 disease and node positivity), the risk of local and distant failure remained elevated, so adjuvant therapies including radiation and chemotherapy were administered in an attempt to reduce rates of local and distant failure. Multiple studies examined this adjuvant role of pelvic radiation and collectively found that adjuvant radiation alone decreased the risk of local recurrence but did not significantly improve overall survival.[5] The addition of adjuvant chemotherapy was noted to reduce the rates of distant metastases while improving disease-free survival.[6,7] Since that time, more modern trials have examined the appropriate sequencing of therapies (surgery, radiation, chemotherapy) and assessed which patients may be candidates for omission of certain modalities to reduce the late effects of treatment.

PREOPERATIVE RADIATION THERAPY REGIMENS

In the 1980s and 1990s, the standard management of rectal cancer was surgical resection with low anterior resection (LAR) or abdomino-perineal resection for proximal and distal tumors, respectively, followed by adjuvant radiation (with or without chemotherapy) and further chemotherapy. For some patients, it was difficult to complete the entire postoperative course of adjuvant treatment, which led to the emergence of several trials to address the question of whether neoadjuvant radiation therapy (RT) with or without chemotherapy could be safely administered without sacrificing disease control. The German Rectal Cancer Study CAO/ARO/AIO-94 randomly assigned more than 800 patients to treatment with either neoadjuvant RT to 5040 cGy with continuous infusion 5-fluorouracil (5-FU) or adjuvant RT to 5580 cGy with 5-FU.[8] Both groups underwent TME resection and 4 cycles of adjuvant 5-FU. With the long-term update, neoadjuvant chemoradiation (chemo-RT) was found to decrease local recurrence (7.1% vs 10.1%; $P = .048$); however, there were no differences in overall survival [OS] rate (59.6% vs 59.9%; $P = .85$) or distant metastases (29.8% vs 29.6%; $P = .9$).[9] Pathologic complete response (pCR) rate in the preoperative group was 9% as of the long-term update. In the initial publication, acute grade 3 or higher toxicity, an important endpoint, was significantly less in the preoperative group (27% vs 40%; $P = .001$), and late grade 3 or higher toxicity was also decreased with preoperative therapy (14% vs 24%; $P = .01$).

Two additional trials, the European Organisation for Research and Treatment of Cancer (EORTC) 22,921 and the Federation Francophone de Cancerologie (FFCD) 9203, examined the effect of neoadjuvant chemo-RT over RT alone (with or without adjuvant chemotherapy) on outcomes for patients with cT3-4 resectable disease.[10–12] Pooled analysis of the data found that chemo-RT significantly improved 3-year local control (92.3% vs 84.7%; $P<.0001$) and pCR rates (11.2% vs 3.7%; $P<.0001$).[13] However, there were no differences in 5-year OS (66.3% vs 65.9%; $P = .66$) or 3-year distant progression-free rates (71.3% vs 70.7%; $P = .5$). Based on the totality of the above data, neoadjuvant chemo-RT has become the current standard of care in the United States and many regions of Europe.

In contrast to the neoadjuvant chemo-RT approach with 5 to 6 weeks of daily RT (long course), other countries have assessed whether preoperative short-course RT alone is sufficient to reduce the local recurrence risk in stage II and III rectal cancers. The Swedish Rectal Cancer Trial investigated whether preoperative short-course RT of 25 Gy in 5 fractions followed by surgery 1 week later improved outcomes over surgery alone.[14] TME was not mandated in this trial. On long-term follow-up, short-course RT improved OS (38% vs 30%; *P* = .008) and reduced local recurrence (9% vs 26%; *P*<.001). One of the criticisms of this trial is that TME was not mandated, which may have resulted in worse outcomes in the control group as demonstrated by the high rate of local recurrence. The Dutch TME trial therefore sought to address the benefit of short-course RT in patients undergoing TME by comparing preoperative RT, 25 Gy/5 fractions, with surgery alone (although patients with positive margins received mandatory adjuvant RT).[15] Long-term follow-up found that short-course RT reduced the 10-year local recurrence rate (5% vs 11%; *P*<.0001) but had no effect on 10-year OS (48% vs 49%; *P* = .86).[16] However, nearly two-thirds of patients on this study had stage I/II disease for which radiation may not provide a benefit, so subset analysis was performed and discovered that patients with stage III and negative circumferential margins had increased OS with short-course RT (50% vs 40%; *P* = .032).

Two additional trials addressed whether preoperative short-course RT results in inferior outcomes to those of standard long-course chemo-RT.[17,18] Bujko and colleagues[17] randomly assigned more than 300 patients with cT3/T4 disease to preoperative short-course RT, 25 Gy/5 fractions, followed by surgery within 7 days or to preoperative long-course chemo-RT, 50.4 Gy/28 fractions, with 5-FU/leucovorin followed by surgery 4 to 6 weeks later. No differences were detected in 4-year local recurrence rates (9% vs 14.2%; *P* = .17), OS (67.2% vs 66.2%; *P* = .96), disease-free survival (58.4% vs 55.6%; *P* = .82), or late toxicity (10.1% vs 7.1%; *P* = .36) for short- versus long-course RT, respectively.[19] Notably, short-course RT showed lower rates of pCR (0.7% vs 16.1%; *P*<.001) and increased rates of positive circumferential margins (12.9% vs 4.4%; *P* = .017) but no difference in sphincter preservation (61.2% vs 58%; *P* = .57).[17] In a similar trial design, the Trans-Tasman Radiation Oncology Group (TROG) 01.04 randomly assigned more than 300 patients with cT3N0-2 disease less than 12 cm from anal verge to short-course RT, 25 Gy/5 fractions, followed by surgery and 6 cycles of adjuvant chemotherapy versus long-course RT, 50.4 Gy/28 fractions, with 5-FU and 4 additional cycles of adjuvant chemotherapy.[18] Although patients were randomly assigned, there were more patients with distal tumors (<5 cm from anal verge) in the short-course RT arm (30% vs 19%) and fewer patients with proximal tumors (10–12 cm) in the short-course arm (16% vs 26%). No differences were detected in 3-year local recurrence (7.5% vs 4.4%; *P* = .24), 5-year OS (74% vs 70%; *P* = .62), 5-year distant recurrence (27% vs 30%; *P* = .92), or late toxicity (5.8% vs 8.2%; *P* = .53). Similar to the Polish trial, pCR rates were lower in the short-course group (1% vs 15%; *P* value not reported), and there were no differences in sphincter preservation rates (63% vs 69%; *P* = .22). Although not statistically significant, the actuarial rates of local failure were higher in patients with distal tumors who received short-course RT (12.5% vs 0.3%; *P* = .21), which the authors concluded may favor long course in patients with distal tumors.

Short-course RT has not been routinely adopted in the United States because of concern over the late gastrointestinal (GI) morbidity from hypofractionated RT. Although neither the Polish nor Australian trials observed a difference in late GI toxicity between short-course and long-course arms, there is concern that a median follow-up of 4 and 6 years, respectively, may not be sufficient time to observe the late effects of the hypofractionated treatment. Current National Comprehensive Cancer Network guidelines (v2.2016), however, do allow for the use of short-course RT in cT3 or cN1-2 patients but recommends against its use in T4 tumors or in patients for whom down-staging is desired.[20]

ALTERNATIVE NEOADJUVANT TREATMENT STRATEGIES

Although the current standard of care for locally advanced rectal cancer is neoadjuvant RT (with or without chemotherapy) and surgical resection followed by adjuvant chemotherapy, several recent and ongoing clinical trials have addressed the sequencing of the adjuvant therapies. These studies were conducted with the intent to ensure completion of all therapy, improve pCR rates, and potentially reduce the late effects of treatment. Because it has been observed that pCR rates are associated with superior survival and outcomes, it is important to define treatment strategies that best accomplish this goal (**Table 1**).[21,22]

In the Spanish GCR-3 phase II randomized trial, patients with locally advanced cT3-T4 or cN+ disease were randomly assigned to chemo-RT using 5040 cGy with capecitabine/oxaliplatin (CAPOX) followed by TME and 4 additional adjuvant cycles of CAPOX or to the experimental arm of induction CAPOX followed by chemo-RT and then TME.[23] There were no differences in 5-year local recurrence (2% vs 5%; $P = .61$), distant metastases (21% vs 23%; $P = .79$), OS (78% vs 75%; $P = .64$), or pCR rates (13% vs 14%; $P = .94$). This finding shows that induction chemotherapy (with a delay in chemo-RT and surgery) may be safely administered in lieu of postoperative adjuvant chemotherapy treatment.

Garcia-Aguilar and colleagues[24] conducted a multi-institutional, nonrandomized phase II trial examining the effect of increasing preoperative chemotherapy cycles on pCR rates in patients with locally advanced rectal cancer. Patients in all arms

Table 1
Table of pathologic complete response rates from select randomized trials

Trial	Neoadjuvant Regimens	Pathologic Complete Response Rates
German CAO/ARO/AIO-94[8]	RT–5-FU	9%
EORTC 22921/FFCD9203[13]	RT	3.7%
	RT–5-FU	11.2%
Bujko et al,[19] 2006	SC-RT	0.7%
	LC-RT 5-FU	16.1%
TROG 01.04[18]	SC-RT	1%
	LC-RT 5-FU	15%
Spanish GCR-3[23]	RT-CAPOX	13%
	CAPOX- > RT-CAPOX	14%
Garcia-Aguilar et al,[24] 2015	RT–5-FU	18%
	RT–5-FU - > mFOLFOX x2	25%
	RT–5-FU - > mFOLFOX x4	30%
	RT–5-FU - > mFOLFOX x6	38%
Chinese FOWARC[25]	RT–5-FU	14%
	RT-mFOLFOX	27.5%
	mFOLFOX	6.6%

Abbreviations: SC, short course; LC, long course.

received chemo-RT to 5040 to 5400 cGy with 5-FU followed by either (1) TME; (2) 2 cycles of modified leucovorin, 5-FU, and oxaliplatin (mFOLFOX6) then TME; (3) 4 cycles mFOLFOX6 then TME; or (4) 6 cycles mFOLFOX6 and TME. They observed that increasing cycles of neoadjuvant mFOLFOX6 resulted in higher pCR rates (groups 1–4: 18% vs 25% vs 30% vs 38%; P = .0036). Although lengthening the interval between completion of chemo-RT and TME did result in increased pelvic fibrosis at the time of TME, it did not adversely affect the ability to achieved R0 resections. Long-term follow-up with recurrence rates and survival outcomes have not been published at this time.

Preliminary results from the Chinese Neoadjuvant FOLFOX6 Chemotherapy with or without Radiation in Rectal Cancer (FOWARC) study have recently been published providing information on the role of neoadjuvant radiation in achieving pCR.[25] Nearly 500 patients were randomly assigned to (1) standard chemo-RT with 5-FU and postoperative 5-FU, (2) chemo-RT with mFOLFOX6 and postoperative mFOLFOX6, or (3) neoadjuvant mFOLFOX6 alone (RT is omitted) and postoperative mFOLFOX6. pCR rates varied significantly between arms (groups 1–3: 14% vs 27.5% vs 6.6%; P = .005 for group 1 vs group 2). This trial concluded that radiotherapy provides a clear improvement in pCR rates that is further enhanced by intensified preoperative chemotherapy. There were no differences in R0 resection or sphincter preservation rates between groups. The addition of mFOLFOX6 to RT over 5-FU resulted in worse acute grade 3 to 4 GI toxicity (14.5% vs 7.7% diarrhea; P value not reported), but it did not impair the ability of patients to receive the full course of radiation (86.4% vs 90.5%; P value not reported). Recurrence and survival outcomes are pending.

The ongoing Alliance PROSPECT trial is investigating whether RT may be safely omitted in select LAR candidates with good response to induction FOLFOX6. Patients are randomly assigned to induction FOLFOX6 and assessed for response to the primary tumor; those with regression greater than 20% will undergo LAR, while those with poor response or regression will receive standard neoadjuvant chemo-RT with 5-FU followed by resection. The outcomes of this arm will be compared against the standard of care chemo-RT with 5-FU arm; both arms will receive adjuvant chemotherapy. This study population has more favorable disease than those in the Chinese FOWARC trial in that only T2N1 and T3N0-1 who will undergo LAR are eligible, so it will be interesting to determine whether the omission of neoadjuvant RT significantly decreases the ability to achieve pCR in this population.

Movement toward a total neoadjuvant therapy approach allows for novel clinical trial designs that may incorporate targeted systemic agents or radiation sensitizers with focus on improving pCR rates and reducing distant metastatic disease. NRG Oncology GI-002 (clinicaltrials.gov ID 02921256) is a randomized phase II trial opened in October 2016 that compares a standard arm (mFOLFOX6 x 8 cycles followed by preoperative RT plus capecitabine and surgery) versus additional experimental arms that incorporate new systemic agents. The first planned experimental arm will add the polyADP-ribose inhibitor, veliparib, to RT plus capecitabine. The study populations are patients with locally advanced rectal cancer at high risk for distant disease meeting one of the following criteria: (1) cT3-4 and distal location (< 5 cm from anal verge), (2) bulky cT4 tumor within 3 mm of the mesorectal fascia, (3) cN2 disease, or (4) not a candidate for sphincter preservation before preoperative therapy. The primary endpoint is an improvement in pathologic Neoadjuvant Rectal Cancer score (total downstaging) compared with the control arm. Other agents under investigation for addition to neoadjuvant therapy include COX-2 inhibitors and statins after early preclinical and clinical work demonstrated poorer outcomes in tumors overexpressing COX-2 and improved outcomes in patients being treated with statins, respectively.[26–28] Strategies such as this may allow further refinement of neoadjuvant therapies to improve the outcomes of patients with more aggressive disease.

NONOPERATIVE MANAGEMENT

As refinements in neoadjuvant therapy are resulting in improving pCR rates, it may now be reasonable to assess whether a planned local surgery may be safely omitted in select patients to reduce the associated long-term morbidity and allow for sphincter preservation. This has been termed *nonoperative management, watch and wait*, or *watchful waiting*. In one of the earliest descriptions of this approach, Habr-Gama and colleagues[29] reported their series of 265 patients with distal (< 7 cm), nonmetastatic rectal cancers treated with chemo-RT to 5040 cGy in combination with 5-FU/leucovorin.[29] Eight weeks after completion of treatment, restaging was performed with physical (digital) examination, procto/colonoscopy with biopsy, and CT imaging. Patients without abnormality at the time of re-evaluation underwent nonoperative management with monthly surveillance (physical examination, scope, biopsy) and biannual CT imaging. All other patients went on to TME. The outcomes of patients found to have pCR at the time of surgery were then compared with those patients with clinical CR (cCR). Roughly 27% of patients were found to have cCR, whereas about 8% did not have a cCR but showed pCR at resection. The observational cCR group had slightly increased 5-year OS (100% vs 88%; $P = .01$) but was not different from the pCR group in disease-free survival (92% vs 83%; $P = .09$). There was no difference between overall recurrence rates between groups (7% vs 13.6%; $P = .2$). The cCR rate of 27% in this study was higher than the pCR rates of approximately 15% reported by many trials (see **Table 1**) despite having similar local control outcomes, suggesting that time between completion of chemo-RT and surgery has a significant effect on pathologic tumor response. These encouraging retrospective findings suggested that nonoperative management in carefully selected patients may allow for organ preservation without increased risk of recurrence or death.

Martens and colleagues[30] recently published patient outcomes from a prospective cohort of patients offered nonoperative management or transanal excision for complete or near complete clinical response. One hundred patients made up the cohort, of which, 61 had initial cCR at 8-week postneoadjuvant therapy assessment. An additional 24 patients were found to have cCR at second assessment 3 months later, and the remaining 15 patients underwent transanal excision. Locoregional recurrences developed in 15% of patients (12 luminal, 3 nodal), and those patients survived. Three-year OS was 96.6%, distant metastasis-free survival was 96.8%, and colostomy-free survival was 94.8%. In addition to these findings, multiple retrospective and prospective cohort studies have been published that show favorable outcomes in patients undergoing nonoperative management with chemo-RT.[30–35] Local recurrence rates have ranged from 15% to 38% but in all series, salvage therapies have been successful in most (90+%) patients with local recurrences. This results in excellent overall survival rates ranging from 96% to 100% up to 5 years out from treatment.

One of the inherent difficulties in the nonsurgical approach is appropriate patient selection after chemo-RT. A meta-analysis of the ability of MRI to adequately restage disease after chemo-RT found the sensitivity to detect yT0 was 19.1% but with a specificity of 94.6%.[36] This number improved to a sensitivity of 55.3% when differentiating yT0-2 from yT3-4. A more recent multicenter prospective validation study has tried to define MR values that predict for complete tumor response to neoadjuvant therapy, with magnetic resonance volumetry providing accuracy up to 80%.[37] This area remains an active area of investigation particularly with the use of newer multiparametric MRI technology. Additionally, investigators have also searched for potential biomarkers that may predict for complete response, including low serum carcinoembryonic antigen and gene expression and protein translation profiles, but no marker has shown sufficient predictive value to prospectively guide treatment recommendation.[28,38] At this time, the centers that have reported outcomes of a nonoperative management approach carefully select patients based on favorable response assessed by multiple methods: digital rectal examination, direct visualization with endoscopy, MRI/CT, and biopsies. Such encouraging results warrant further assessment in large multicenter prospective trials.

REDUCING TOXICITY WITH ADVANCED RADIATION TREATMENT PLANNING

Advances in immobilization and technology have allowed for refinements in radiation treatment planning and delivery to reduce dose to adjacent organs at risk within the pelvis. With regard to immobilization, prone positioning of the patient on a bowel displacement or "belly board" device allows for anatomic displacement of the small bowel away from the pelvis. Using conventional 3D-CRT delivery, the pelvis may then be treated with a 3-field (posterioranterior and 2 laterals) technique to further reduce dose to the anterior small bowel. For patients with adjacent organ involvement (T4), a 4-field (anteroposterior /posterioranterior and 2 laterals) beam arrangement is often used to adequately treat the nodal regions at risk. The development of IMRT has allowed for more conformal shaping of the delivered dose around the tumor while minimizing dose to adjacent nontarget organs (**Fig. 1**). It also allows for variable dose prescriptions to gross disease and prophylactic areas with dose painting, or simultaneous integrated boost, technique. RTOG 0529 was a phase II trial that investigated whether IMRT with concurrent chemotherapy could reduce the treatment-related toxicity of anal cancer relative to historical trial outcomes.[39] It was observed that the use of IMRT reduced grade 3+ acute GI toxicity (21% vs 36%; $P = .0082$) and grade 3+ acute skin toxicity (23% vs 49%; $P<.0001$). Thus, a reasonable question is whether patients treated with radiotherapy for rectal cancer might also receive a similar benefit from IMRT.

Multiple retrospective series have attempted to determine whether IMRT reduces acute toxicity from rectal cancer treatment. Samuelian and colleagues[40] reviewed outcomes from 31 patients treated with IMRT and 61 patients treated with 3D-CRT. They observed a significant decrease in overall grade 2+ GI toxicity with IMRT (32% vs 62%; $P = .006$), which was accounted for by significant reductions in diarrhea and enteritis. There was not a significant difference in grade 3 GI toxicity between groups (3% vs 10%; $P = .42$). Jabbour and colleagues[41] compared 30 patients treated with IMRT with 56 patients treated with 3D-CRT. They observed a significant reduction in all grade 3+ toxicities with IMRT ($P = .016$) but did not find a difference in rates of grade 3 diarrhea (9% vs 3%; $P = .31$). They also examined the effect of treatment on treatment breaks and hospitalizations/emergency department visits. IMRT resulted in significantly fewer treatment breaks (0% vs 20%; $P = .0002$) and fewer hospitalizations (2% vs 14%; $P = .005$). Similarly, Parekh and colleagues[42] examined the records of 48 patients treated with either IMRT or 3D-CRT and bowel displacement and found that IMRT resulted in significant decreased rates of grade 2+ acute GI toxicity (30% vs 60.7%; $P = .036$) and had significantly shorter treatment duration (35 days vs 39 days; $P<.0001$).[42] More recently, Hong and colleagues[43] reported the outcomes of 144 patients treated with either preoperative helical tomotherapy IMRT or 3D-CRT. They also observed a decrease in grade 3+ acute GI toxicity with IMRT (6.7% vs 15.1%;

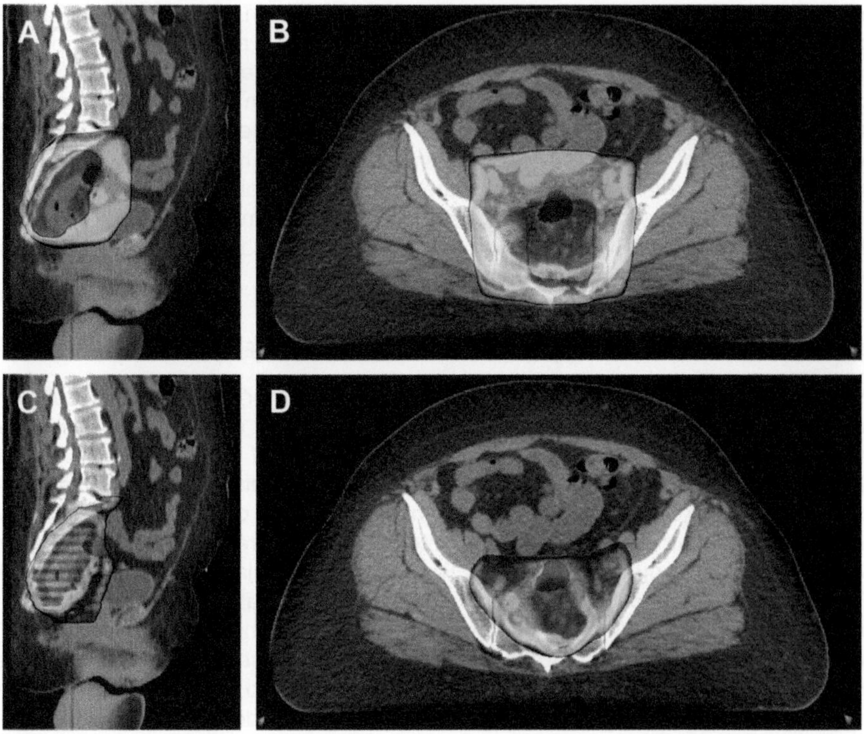

Fig. 1. High-dose distribution of 3D-CRT versus IMRT planning. This is a patient for whom prone positioning on a belly board device did not displace bowel. Sagittal (*A*, *C*) and axial (*B*, *D*) views of 3D-CRT (*A*, *B*) and IMRT (*C*, *D*) plans are presented. The IMRT plan shows reduction in high-dose region to bowel and bladder. Dose color wash reflects 4500 cGy in blue and 5000 cGy in red.

P = .039) in line with prior reports. Collectively, these retrospective series show the potential for IMRT to reduce GI toxicity and prevent treatment breaks and costly hospitalizations in patients with locally advanced rectal cancer.

RTOG 0822 was a phase II trial determining the toxicity of preoperative IMRT delivered with concurrent CAPOX in patients with locally advanced rectal cancer.[43] The results of this treatment regimen were compared with the RT-CAPOX arm of RTOG 0247, which was delivered with 3D-CRT. With 68 evaluable patients, rates of grade 2+ acute GI toxicity did not significantly differ between patients treated with IMRT in 0822 and those treated with 3D-CRT in 0247 (51.5% vs 40%; *P* = .93). A primary criticism of this trial is the use of concurrent oxaliplatin, which multiple phase III trials have found does not improve surgical or survival outcomes but does increase rates of grade 3+ toxicity.[44–46]

Based on the equivocal results between the retrospective and prospective data, the benefit of IMRT in patients with locally advanced rectal cancer treated concurrently with single-agent 5-FU or capecitabine remains to be determined. It may be considered in cases in which prone positioning on a belly board device does not allow sufficient repositioning of bowel outside of the pelvis, with T4 primary tumors in which the external iliac nodal chain is covered prophylactically, and with distal tumors that approach the anal canal in which prophylactic coverage of the inguinal nodal chain is planned.

SUMMARY

Management of locally advanced rectal cancer has evolved over time from surgical resection alone to multimodality therapy with preoperative radiation, chemotherapy, and TME resulting in excellent local control rates. Refinements in neoadjuvant therapies and their sequencing have improved pathologic complete response rates such that consideration of selective radiation and nonoperative management are now active clinical trial questions in select patients. Advances in radiation treatment planning and delivery techniques such as IMRT may allow for further reduction in acute treatment-related toxicity in select patient populations. Collectively, therapeutic strategies remain focused on improving outcomes for patients with higher-risk disease and reducing the morbidity of treatment.

REFERENCES

1. Colorectum Statistics | American Cancer Society - Cancer Facts & Statistics. Available at: https://cancerstatisticscenter.cancer.org/?_ga=1.8691186.615191375.1476052195#/cancer-site/Colorectum. Accessed October 8, 2016.
2. McCall JL, Cox MR, Wattchow DA. Analysis of local recurrence rates after surgery alone for rectal cancer. Int J Colorectal Dis 1995;10(3):126–32. Available at: http://www.ncbi.nlm.nih.gov/pubmed/7561427. Accessed October 8, 2016.
3. Quirke P, Durdey P, Dixon MF, et al. Local recurrence of rectal adenocarcinoma due to inadequate surgical resection. Histopathological study of lateral tumour spread and surgical excision. Lancet 1986;2(8514):996–9. Available at: http://www.ncbi.nlm.nih.gov/pubmed/2430152. Accessed October 8, 2016.
4. Heald RJ, Moran BJ, Ryall RD, et al. Rectal cancer: the Basingstoke experience of total mesorectal excision, 1978-1997. Arch Surg 1998;133(8):894–9. Available at: http://www.ncbi.nlm.nih.gov/pubmed/9711965. Accessed October 9, 2016.
5. Colorectal Cancer Collaborative Group. Adjuvant radiotherapy for rectal cancer: a systematic overview of 8,507 patients from 22 randomised trials. Lancet 2001;358(9290):1291–304.
6. Thomas PR, Lindblad AS. Adjuvant postoperative radiotherapy and chemotherapy in rectal carcinoma: a review of the Gastrointestinal Tumor Study Group experience. Radiother Oncol 1988;13(4):245–52. Available at: http://www.ncbi.nlm.nih.gov/pubmed/3064191. Accessed October 9, 2016.
7. Krook JE, Moertel CG, Gunderson LL, et al. Effective surgical adjuvant therapy for high-risk rectal carcinoma. N Engl J Med 1991;324(11):709–15.
8. Sauer R, Becker H, Hohenberger W, et al. Preoperative versus postoperative chemoradiotherapy for rectal cancer. N Engl J Med 2004;351(17):1731–40.
9. Sauer R, Liersch T, Merkel S, et al. Preoperative versus postoperative chemoradiotherapy for locally advanced rectal cancer: results of the German CAO/ARO/AIO-94 randomized phase III trial after a median follow-up of 11 years. J Clin Oncol 2012;30(16):1926–33.
10. Gérard J-P, Conroy T, Bonnetain F, et al. Preoperative radiotherapy with or without concurrent fluorouracil and leucovorin in T3-4 rectal cancers: results of FFCD 9203. J Clin Oncol 2006;24(28):4620–5.
11. Bosset J-F, Collette L, Calais G, et al. Chemotherapy with preoperative radiotherapy in rectal cancer. N Engl J Med 2006;355(11):1114–23.
12. Bosset J-F, Calais G, Mineur L, et al. Fluorouracil-based adjuvant chemotherapy after preoperative chemoradiotherapy in rectal cancer: long-term results of the EORTC 22921 randomised study. Lancet Oncol 2014;15:184–90.

13. Bonnetain F, Bosset JF, Gerard JP, et al. What is the clinical benefit of preoperative chemoradiotherapy with 5FU/leucovorin for T3-4 rectal cancer in a pooled analysis of EORTC 22921 and FFCD 9203 trials: surrogacy in question? Eur J Cancer 2012;48(12):1781–90.
14. Folkesson J, Birgisson H, Pahlman L, et al. Swedish rectal cancer trial: long lasting benefits from radiotherapy on survival and local recurrence rate. J Clin Oncol 2005;23(24):5644–50.
15. Kapiteijn E, Marijnen CA, Nagtegaal ID, et al. Preoperative radiotherapy combined with total mesorectal excision for resectable rectal cancer. N Engl J Med 2001;345(9):638–46.
16. van Gijn W, Marijnen CAM, Nagtegaal ID, et al. Preoperative radiotherapy combined with total mesorectal excision for resectable rectal cancer: 12-year follow-up of the multicentre, randomised controlled TME trial. Lancet Oncol 2011;12(6):575–82.
17. Bujko K, Nowacki MP, Nasierowska-Guttmejer A, et al. Sphincter preservation following preoperative radiotherapy for rectal cancer: report of a randomised trial comparing short-term radiotherapy vs. conventionally fractionated radiochemotherapy. Radiother Oncol 2004;72(1):15–24.
18. Ngan SY, Burmeister B, Fisher RJ, et al. Randomized trial of short-course radiotherapy versus long-course chemoradiation comparing rates of local recurrence in patients with T3 rectal cancer: Trans-Tasman Radiation Oncology Group trial 01.04. J Clin Oncol 2012;30(31):3827–33.
19. Bujko K, Nowacki MP, Nasierowska-Guttmejer A, et al. Long-term results of a randomized trial comparing preoperative short-course radiotherapy with preoperative conventionally fractionated chemoradiation for rectal cancer. Br J Surg 2006;93(10):1215–23.
20. Deborah Freedman-Cass N, Gregory KM, Bekaii-Saab T, et al. NCCN guidelines rectal version 2.2015. J Natl Compr Canc Netw 2015;13(6):719–28.
21. Zorcolo L, Rosman AS, Restivo A, et al. Complete pathologic response after combined modality treatment for rectal cancer and long-term survival: a meta-analysis. Ann Surg Oncol 2012;19(9):2822–32.
22. Martin ST, Heneghan HM, Winter DC. Systematic review and meta-analysis of outcomes following pathological complete response to neoadjuvant chemoradiotherapy for rectal cancer. Br J Surg 2012;99(7):918–28.
23. Fernandez-Martos C, Garcia-Albeniz X, Pericay C, et al. Chemoradiation, surgery and adjuvant chemotherapy versus induction chemotherapy followed by chemoradiation and surgery: long-term results of the Spanish GCR-3 phase II randomized trial†. Ann Oncol 2015;26(8):1722–8.
24. Garcia-Aguilar J, Chow OS, Smith DD, et al. Effect of adding mFOLFOX6 after neoadjuvant chemoradiation in locally advanced rectal cancer: a multicentre, phase 2 trial. Lancet Oncol 2015;16(8):957–66.
25. Deng Y, Chi P, Lan P, et al. Modified FOLFOX6 with or without radiation versus fluorouracil and leucovorin with radiation in neoadjuvant treatment of locally advanced rectal cancer: initial results of the Chinese FOWARC multicenter, open-label, randomized three-arm phase III trial. J Clin Oncol 2016;34(27):3300–7.
26. Wang LW, Hsiao CF, Chen WT, et al. Celecoxib plus chemoradiotherapy for locally advanced rectal cancer: a phase II TCOG study. J Surg Oncol 2014;109(6):580–5.

27. Smith FM, Reynolds JV, Kay EW, et al. COX-2 overexpression in pretreatment biopsies predicts response of rectal cancers to neoadjuvant radiochemotherapy. Int J Radiat Oncol Biol Phys 2006;64(2):466–72.
28. Armstrong D, Raissouni S, Price Hiller J, et al. Predictors of pathologic complete response after neoadjuvant treatment for rectal cancer: a multicenter study. Clin Colorectal Cancer 2015;14(4):291–5.
29. Habr-Gama A, Perez RO, Nadalin W, et al. Operative versus nonoperative treatment for stage 0 distal rectal cancer following chemoradiation therapy: long-term results. Ann Surg 2004;240(4):717–8. Available at: http://www.ncbi.nlm.nih.gov/pubmed/15383798. Accessed October 14, 2016.
30. Martens MH, Maas M, Heijnen LA, et al. Long-term outcome of an organ preservation program after neoadjuvant treatment for rectal cancer. J Natl Cancer Inst 2016;108(12) [pii:djw171].
31. Appelt AL, Pløen J, Harling H, et al. High-dose chemoradiotherapy and watchful waiting for distal rectal cancer: a prospective observational study. Lancet Oncol 2015;16(8):919–27.
32. Smith JD, Ruby JA, Goodman KA, et al. Nonoperative management of rectal cancer with complete clinical response after neoadjuvant therapy. Ann Surg 2012;256(6):965–72.
33. Habr-Gama A, Gama-Rodrigues J, São Julião GP, et al. Local recurrence after complete clinical response and watch and wait in rectal cancer after neoadjuvant chemoradiation: impact of salvage therapy on local disease control. Int J Radiat Oncol Biol Phys 2014;88(4):822–8.
34. Renehan AG, Malcomson L, Emsley R, et al. Watch-and-wait approach versus surgical resection after chemoradiotherapy for patients with rectal cancer (the OnCoRe project): a propensity-score matched cohort analysis. Lancet Oncol 2016;17(2):174–83.
35. Maas M, Beets-Tan RG, Lambregts DM, et al. Wait-and-see policy for clinical complete responders after chemoradiation for rectal cancer. J Clin Oncol 2011;29(35):4633–40.
36. van der Paardt MP, Zagers MB, Beets-Tan RG, et al. Patients who undergo preoperative chemoradiotherapy for locally advanced rectal cancer restaged by using diagnostic MR imaging: a systematic review and meta-analysis. Radiology 2013;269(1):101–12.
37. Martens MH, van Heeswijk MM, van den Broek JJ, et al. Prospective, multicenter validation study of magnetic resonance volumetry for response assessment after preoperative chemoradiation in rectal cancer: can the results in the literature be reproduced? Int J Radiat Oncol Biol Phys 2015;93(5):1005–14.
38. Ryan JE, Warrier SK, Lynch AC, et al. Predicting pathological complete response to neoadjuvant chemoradiotherapy in locally advanced rectal cancer: a systematic review. Colorectal Dis 2016;18(3):234–46.
39. Kachnic LA, Winter K, Myerson RJ, et al. RTOG 0529: a phase 2 evaluation of dose-painted intensity modulated radiation therapy in combination with 5-fluorouracil and mitomycin-C for the reduction of acute morbidity in carcinoma of the anal canal. Int J Radiat Oncol Biol Phys 2013;86(1):27–33.
40. Samuelian JM, Callister MD, Ashman JB, et al. Reduced acute bowel toxicity in patients treated with intensity-modulated radiotherapy for rectal cancer. Int J Radiat Oncol Biol Phys 2012;82(5):1981–7.
41. Jabbour SK, Patel S, Herman JM, et al. Intensity-modulated radiation therapy for rectal carcinoma can reduce treatment breaks and emergency department visits. Int J Surg Oncol 2012;2012:891067.

42. Parekh A, Truong MT, Pashtan I, et al. Acute gastrointestinal toxicity and tumor response with preoperative intensity modulated radiation therapy for rectal cancer. Gastrointest Cancer Res 2013;6(5–6):137–43. Available at: http://www.ncbi.nlm.nih.gov/pubmed/24312687. Accessed October 16, 2016.
43. Hong TS, Moughan J, Garofalo MC, et al. NRG oncology radiation therapy oncology group 0822: a phase 2 study of preoperative chemoradiation therapy using intensity modulated radiation therapy in combination with capecitabine and oxaliplatin for patients with locally advanced rectal cancer. Int J Radiat Oncol Biol Phys 2015;93(1):29–36.
44. Gérard JP, Azria D, Gourgou-Bourgade S, et al. Comparison of two neoadjuvant chemoradiotherapy regimens for locally advanced rectal cancer: results of the phase III trial ACCORD 12/0405-Prodige 2. J Clin Oncol 2010;28(10):1638–44.
45. O'Connell MJ, Colangelo LH, Beart RW, et al. Capecitabine and oxaliplatin in the preoperative multimodality treatment of rectal cancer: surgical end points from National Surgical Adjuvant Breast and Bowel Project trial R-04. J Clin Oncol 2014;32(18):1927–34.
46. Allegra CJ, Yothers G, O'Connell MJ, et al. Neoadjuvant 5-FU or capecitabine plus radiation with or without oxaliplatin in rectal cancer patients: a phase III randomized clinical trial. J Natl Cancer Inst 2015;107(11) [pii:djv248].

Radiotherapy for Anal Cancer

Intensity-Modulated Radiotherapy and Future Directions

Serguei A. Castaneda, MD[a,b], Lindsay B. Romak, MD[a,*]

KEYWORDS

- Anal cancer • Anus neoplasms • Radiotherapy • Intensity-modulated radiotherapy
- Volumetric-modulated arc therapy • Chemoradiotherapy • Antineoplastic agents
- Toxicity

KEY POINTS

- Chemoradiotherapy is the standard of care for most patients with anal cancer; surgery is largely reserved for salvage.
- Intensity-modulated radiotherapy is a radiation delivery technique that allows conformal dose distribution, limiting unnecessary dose to nearby normal tissues.
- Prospective data have demonstrated improvement in treatment toxicity with use of intensity-modulated radiotherapy.

INTRODUCTION

Although anal squamous-cell carcinoma (ASCC) is a rare disease, its incidence is rising. Definitive chemoradiotherapy is widely accepted as the standard of care for most patients diagnosed with this disease. Intensity-modulated radiotherapy (IMRT) is a sophisticated treatment delivery modality that uses multiple dynamically modified beams to create a highly conformal dose distribution. This allows for improvement in sparing of normal tissues, thereby decreasing the toxicity associated with treatment. Ongoing studies aim to optimize and improve treatments to maximize efficacy of treatment and further reduce side effects.

The authors have nothing to disclose.
[a] Department of Radiation Oncology, Helen F. Graham Cancer Center & Research Institute, Christiana Care Health System, 4701 Ogletown-Stanton RR, S-1110, Newark, DE 19713, USA; [b] Department of Radiation Oncology, Drexel University College of Medicine, 245 North 15th Street, MS #200, Philadelphia, PA 19102, USA
* Corresponding author.
E-mail address: Lindsay.B.Romak@christianacare.org

Surg Oncol Clin N Am 26 (2017) 467–475
http://dx.doi.org/10.1016/j.soc.2017.01.004

EPIDEMIOLOGY

ASCC diagnoses have increased by an average of 2.2% per year over the past decade. It is estimated that 8080 cases will be diagnosed in the United States in 2016, representing 0.5% of new cancer diagnoses. Crude incidence rates of anal cancer in the United States are 1.8 per 100,000.[1] Approximately 88% to 91% of ASCC is human papilloma virus–driven.[2,3] That given, the immunosuppressed, including HIV-infected patients and solid organ transplant recipients, are at higher risk than the general public.

HISTORICAL CONTEXT

Before the 1980s, surgical resection was the mainstay of treatment of ASCC. In 1983, Nigro and colleagues[4] published a landmark report detailing treatment of ASCC with chemoradiotherapy. They delivered 30 Gy in 15 fractions to the tumor and draining pelvic and inguinal lymph nodes, with concurrent 5-fluorouracil (5-FU) and mitomycin-C (mitomycin). Half of treated patients had complete clinical regression of disease and no microscopic residual; an additional 25% underwent abdominoperineal resection and were found to have no residual disease in the specimen.

This finding prompted future research regarding nonoperative management of ASCC. Two randomized trials have addressed the value of the addition of chemotherapy to radiation.[5,6] Both used a combination of 5-FU, administered as a continuous infusion on Days 1 to 5 and 29 to 33, and a single dose of mitomycin, administered on Day 1. A study conducted by the EORTC[5] randomized patients with T3-4N0 or T1-2N1-3 ASCC to radiation with or without concomitant chemotherapy. Patients receiving chemoradiotherapy experienced more frequent complete remission (80% vs 54%; $P = .02$) and improved locoregional control and event-free survival. A similar study performed by the UK Coordinating Committee on Cancer Research[6] randomized 585 patients with ASCC of any stage to receive radiotherapy alone or combination chemoradiotherapy. Local control was improved with the addition of chemotherapy (local failure 59% vs 36%; $P<.0001$). Cause-specific survival was superior in the combined modality arm ($P = .02$).

Subsequent studies aimed to define the optimal chemotherapy regimen. Flam and colleagues[7] evaluated the possibility of omitting mitomycin. Their study demonstrated that inclusion of mitomycin improved colostomy-free survival (71 vs 59%; $P = .014$) and disease-free survival (73 vs 51%; $P = .0003$). Unfortunately, improvement in oncologic outcomes with mitomycin came at the price of increased toxicity (23 vs 7% grade 4–5 toxicity; $P\leq.001$). Radiation Therapy Oncology Group (RTOG) 98-11[8] aimed to compare 5-FU and cisplatin with 5-FU and mitomycin. The study showed that the cumulative rate of colostomy was better for mitomycin than cisplatin (10 vs 19%; $P = .02$) and, with mature follow-up,[9] the cisplatin arm was associated with poorer disease-free survival and overall survival; however, the findings of the study were somewhat difficult to interpret, because patients on the cisplatin arm received 56 days of induction chemotherapy before radiotherapy initiation.

More recently, the ACT II trial[10] was designed with two randomizations: to receive mitomycin versus cisplatin with 5-FU and radiotherapy; and to receive versus not receive maintenance chemotherapy. Improvement in outcomes was noted neither with cisplatin versus mitomycin, nor with additional maintenance therapy. Toxicity was similar between the two chemotherapy regimens. Based on the sum of these data, radiotherapy with mitomycin and 5-FU remains the standard of care for most patients with anal cancer. **Table 1** summarizes the outcomes of patients treated with radiotherapy, 5-FU, and mitomycin on prospective trials.

Table 1
Clinical outcomes of definitive chemoradiotherapy with 5-FU/MMC in selected prospective trials

Study and Reference	Sample Size, n	Treatment Arm	Median Follow-up, mo	Time Point, y	LC, %	CFS, %	OS, %
UKCCR ACT I[7,8]	585	3DCRT + 5-FU/MMC	157	10	66	36	42
EORTC[9]	103	3DCRT + 5-FU/MMC	42	5	69	—	69
RTOG 87-04/ ECOG 1289[10]	310	3DCRT + 5-FU/MMC	36	4	—	59	—
RTOG 98-11[11,12]	644	3DCRT + 5-FU/MMC	156	5	80	72	78
ACCORD-03[13]	307	3DCRT + 5-FU/MMC	50	5	—	77	—
ACT II[14]	940	3DCRT + 5-FU/MMC	1	3	89	—	—
RTOG 0529[30]	52	IMRT + 5-FU/MMC	23	2	—	86	88

Abbreviations: 3DCRT, three-dimensional conformal radiotherapy; 5-FU, fluorouracil; CFS, colostomy-free survival rates; ECOG, Eastern Cooperative Oncology Group; IMRT, intensity-modulated radiotherapy; LC, local control rates; MMC, mitomycin; OS, overall survival rates.

TOXICITY OF DEFINITIVE CHEMORADIOTHERAPY

The toxicity, however, of concurrent chemoradiotherapy with 5-FU and mitomycin for ASCC is significant. Flam and colleagues[7] reported grade 4 + acute toxicity in 23% of patients and James and colleagues[10] demonstrated grade 3 + acute dermatologic toxicity in 48% of their population. Ajani and colleagues[8] reported that 34% of patients had acute grade 4 toxicity (26% hematologic and 13% nonhematologic) and 36% of patients had late grade 3 to 4 toxicity. Toxicity statistics from major trials of chemoradiotherapy are summarized in **Table 2**.

Table 2
Acute toxicity of definitive chemoradiotherapy with 5-FU/MMC in prospective trials

Study and Reference	Sample Size, n	Treatment Arm	G3+ GI Toxicity, %	G3+ Skin Toxicity, %
RTOG 87-04/ECOG 1289[10]	310	3DCRT + 5-FU/MMC	—	55
EORTC[9]	103	3DCRT + 5-FU/MMC	19.6	54.9
RTOG 98-11[11]	644	3DCRT + 5-FU/MMC	36	49
EORTC 22011-40014[16]	88	3DCRT + 5-FU/MMC	17.9	43.6
ACT II[14]	940	3DCRT + 5-FU/MMC	16	48
RTOG 0529[15]	52	IMRT + 5-FU/MMC	21	23

Abbreviations: 3DCRT, three-dimensional conformal radiotherapy; 5-FU, fluorouracil; ECOG, Eastern Cooperative Oncology Group; GI, gastrointestinal; IMRT, intensity-modulated radiotherapy; MMC, mitomycin.

This significant treatment-related toxicity raises concern regarding the impact of treatment on patient's well-being and functional capacity. Furthermore, it has been demonstrated previously that treatment breaks for squamous-cell carcinomas lead to poorer outcomes.[11,12] This phenomenon was demonstrated in ASCC in an RTOG pilot study of dose escalation.[13] RTOG 92-08 mandated that patients receive dose-escalated chemoradiotherapy to 59.4 Gy with concurrent 5-FU and mitomycin, with a required 2-week break. The 2-year colostomy rate was 30%, compared with only 7% in a historical RTOG 87-04 cohort treated to 45 Gy to 50.4 Gy in a continuous fashion. Thus, when toxicity is severe enough to necessitate treatment breaks, it may have a negative impact on tumor control.

INTENSITY-MODULATED RADIATION THERAPY AND TOXICITY REDUCTION

The previously discussed trials used two-dimensional and three-dimensional treatment techniques, in which four static photon beams and matched electron beams are used to treat the pelvis, resulting in a "box" of high-dose radiation that exposes nearby normal tissues, including the small bowel, bladder, and uninvolved skin to unnecessary radiation. IMRT is a modern, more sophisticated radiation delivery technique, in which beams are dynamically modulated to allow for sculpting of dose around uninvolved structures (**Fig. 1**). Following a simulation computed tomography scan, the treating physician delineates target tissues and uninvolved organs at risk, and determines goals for target coverage and normal tissue avoidance. These goals are given to a team of dosimetrists and physicists, who in turn work with complex treatment algorithms to develop an inverse treatment plan that aims to achieve the requested constraints via dynamic collimation (shaping) and varying intensity of radiation delivery from multiple beam angles. Early dosimetric studies demonstrated a theoretic advantage with use of IMRT versus three-dimensional treatment planning, with reduced dose to the genitalia, skin, bladder, bowel, bone marrow, and femoral heads while maintaining comparable target coverage,[14–16] generating great interest in the possible use of IMRT in routine treatment of ASCC.

The RTOG thus conducted a phase 2 trial evaluating IMRT in the treatment of anal cancer.[17] RTOG 0529 treated patients with stage T2-4 N0-3 ASCC with 5-FU and mitomycin and dose-painted IMRT, in which elective regions at risk were treated to a lower dose while gross disease was simultaneously treated with a higher dose. Total dose ranged from 50.4 Gy to 54 Gy, depending on the tumor stage and nodal size. The primary end point was reduction of grade 2 + combined acute gastrointestinal and genitourinary adverse events by at least 15% compared with the standard arm of RTOG 9811.[8] This primary end point was not met; however, with 52 evaluable patients, the authors were able to demonstrate a significant reduction in acute grade 3 + gastrointestinal (21% vs 36%; $P = .01$), grade 3 + dermatologic (23% vs 49%; $P<.0001$), and grade 2 + hematologic (73% vs 85%; $P = .03$) toxicities with IMRT compared with the historical cohort. Treatment breaks were necessary in 49% versus 62% of patients ($P = .09$) and the median duration of treatment interruption was 0 versus 3 days ($P = .005$). This has important implications for treatment efficacy, as previously discussed.

The growing adoption of IMRT by the radiation oncology community, aided greatly by published atlases and treatment guidelines,[18–20] seems to be associated with improved toxicity, as demonstrated in recent report from the United Kingdom.[21] Emerging technologies, such as volumetric modulated arc therapy and proton therapy, may allow even greater conformality of treatment and reduction in toxicity.

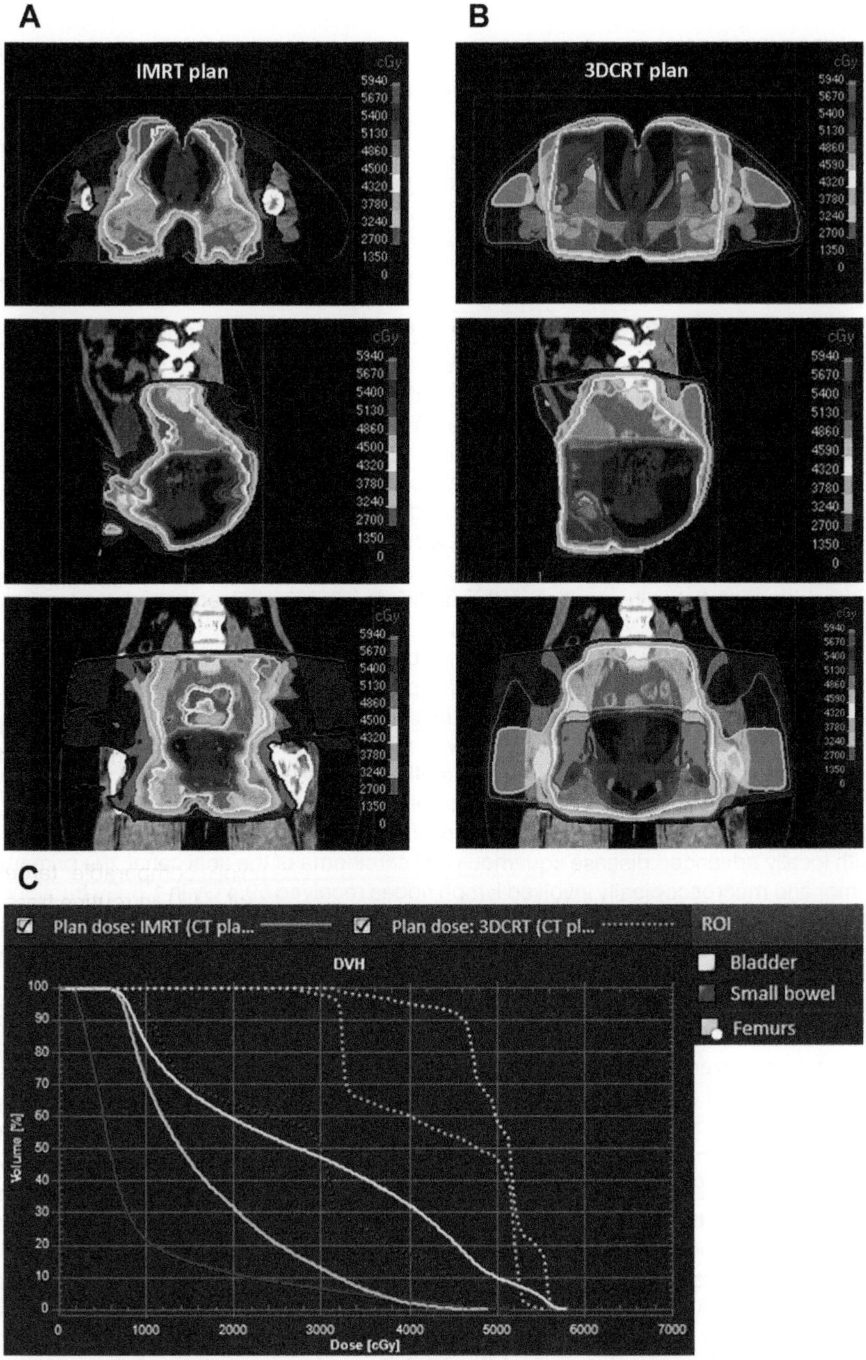

Fig. 1. (*A*) An IMRT plan showing a more conformal distribution of radiation doses compared with (*B*) a three-dimensional conformal radiotherapy (3DCRT) plan from the same patient. (*C*) Comparison of the dose-volume histogram (DVH) analyses of these two radiotherapy plans with attention to three normal structures (bladder, small bowel, and femurs); the IMRT plan in solid lines compared with the 3DCRT plan in dotted lines represented lower mean doses of radiation to normal structures with the use of an IMRT technique. ROI, region of interest.

FUTURE DIRECTIONS

Despite the gains afforded by the adoption of IMRT, there remains great potential for improvement in the treatment of ASCC. Clinicians and researchers are striving to appropriately risk-stratify patients to identify those who may be adequately treated with lower doses and less likelihood of toxicity, and to identify those at risk for locoregional failure, for whom treatment intensification may be of benefit. There is also great interest in the potential use of biologic and immunotherapeutic agents in the treatment of ASCC.

Dose Escalation for Locally Advanced Disease

Dose escalation was investigated in the ACCORD 03 trial,[22] in which patients with tumors greater than 4 cm or less than 4 cm and node positive were assigned to receive or not receive induction chemotherapy and to receive a standard-dose (15 Gy) or high-dose (20–25 Gy) boost following an initial 45 Gy in 25 fractions. Chemotherapy consisted of 5-FU and cisplatin. Radiation used a simple four-field box or anteroposterior/posteroanterior beam arrangement and there was a 3-week break between delivery of the initial 45 Gy and the boost dose. 5-year colostomy-free survival was 73.7% versus 77.8% in the standard boost versus high boost arms (P = .067). Although not statistically significant, this finding is intriguing, given the relatively small difference in dose between the two arms.

Prior attempts at dose escalation have reported significant toxicity, including RTOG 92-08, in which 78% and 28% of patients experienced grade 3 to 4 dermatologic and gastrointestinal toxicities, respectively. However, with modern treatment techniques, there is renewed interest in the possibility of treatment escalation for patients at high risk of local failure. In a phase 1 trial of radiotherapy dose-intensification,[23] a simultaneous integrated boost using IMRT concurrently with capecitabine and mitomycin for locally advanced anal cancer showed promising safety and effectiveness. In this study with locally advanced disease squamous cell carcinoma of the anal canal, the primary tumor and macroscopically involved lymph nodes received 59.4 Gy in 1.8-Gy fractions while the electively treated lymph nodes received 49.5 Gy in 1.5-Gy per fraction, using a dose-painted or simultaneous integrated boost technique. For residual disease in the fifth week of treatment, a boost dose of 5.4 Gy using 1.8-Gy per fraction was given. Fifteen out of 18 patients (83%) had a complete response with an acceptable toxicity profile. The PLATO (PersonaLising Anal cancer radioTherapy dOse) trial in the United Kingdom is currently investigating dose escalation for patients with locally advanced disease, defined as T2 N1-3 or T3-4 Nx.[24] Patients are randomized to 53.2 Gy in 28 fractions versus 58.8 Gy or 61.6 Gy in 28 fractions with concurrent chemotherapy.

Dose De-escalation for Early Stage Disease

Simultaneously, there is also great interest in selecting patients for whom dose de-escalation may be appropriate and feasible, knowing that many people experienced complete response and durable tumor control with the initially reported Nigro regimen of 30 Gy. The PLATO trial is also addressing this critical question, randomizing patients with intermediate risk disease to concurrent capecitabine and mitomycin with either 50.4 Gy at 1.8 Gy per fraction or 41.4 Gy at 1.8 Gy per fraction, in the definitive setting. The target patient population includes patients with T1-2 (up to 4 cm) N0 or NX anal canal or anal margin tumor.[24] Patients with T1N0 or NX anal margin tumors that have been completed excised are also eligible for the trial, and will be observed if margins are greater than 1 mm or treated with low-dose chemoradiation (41.4 Gy) for margins less than or equal to 1 mm.

Biologic and Immunotherapy

After success with cetuximab in the treatment of head and neck squamous cell carcinoma,[25] there was enthusiasm for possible similar benefit for ASCC. The Eastern Cooperative Oncology Group phase 2 trial E3205[26] showed promising early results with combination cetuximab and chemoradiotherapy for ASCC, generating further interest in this approach. Unfortunately, more recent reports have shown significant rates of acute toxicities, prolonged treatment time, and no clear improvement in outcomes, leading to a dampening of enthusiasm about the role of cetuximab in treatment of ASCC.[27,28]

In past years, interest in the possibility of integrating immunotherapy in the treatment of ASCC has increased significantly. The immune checkpoint inhibitor nivolumab (anti-PD-1 monoclonal antibody) has shown activity in treatment of metastatic ASCC. In a phase 2 trial with 37 patients, 24% had treatment response and 46% had stable disease, and overexpression of PD-1 and PD-L1 was shown to correlate with treatment responses. Acute toxicities were acceptable.[29] The combination of nivolumab with ipilimumab (anti-CTLA-4 monoclonal antibody) is currently being investigated in patients with HIV and solid tumors including anal cancer (ClinicalTrials.gov identifiers: NCT02408861). A similar trial is underway for patients with rare forms of anal cancer, including anal canal undifferentiated and neuroendocrine carcinomas (NCT02834013). Pembrolizumab (anti-PD-1 monoclonal antibody) is also currently being evaluated in metastatic anal cancer. The potential additive efficacy of immune checkpoint inhibitors with concurrent with radiotherapy with or without conventional chemotherapy is an area of great interest.

SUMMARY

Definitive chemoradiotherapy is the standard of care for patients with ASCC, allowing organ preservation and maintenance of continence for most patients. Recent advances in radiotherapy planning and delivery have resulted in clinically meaningful improvements in treatment-related toxicity. Most notably, the advent and wide adoption of IMRT provides a superior toxicity profile compared with older techniques, while maintaining similar oncologic outcomes. However, there remains great potential for improvement. Current areas of active research include optimizing and individualizing treatment intensity and possible integration of biologic and immunotherapies in the treatment of ASCC.

ACKNOWLEDGMENTS

The authors thank Dr Poli and the superb dosimetry teams from our institutions for their contribution creating the plans illustrated in **Fig. 1**, especially Ngoc Thai and Bryan Streitfeld.

REFERENCES

1. National Institutes of Health, National Cancer Institute, Surveillance, Epidemiology, and End Results Program. SEER stat fact sheets: anal cancer. Available at: http://seer.cancer.gov/statfacts/html/anus.html/. Accessed September 30, 2016.
2. De Martel C, Ferlay J, Franceschi S, et al. Global burden of cancers attributable to infections in 2008: A review and synthetic analysis. Lancet Oncol 2012;13:607–15.

3. Centers for Disease Control and Prevention. HPV-associated anal cancer rates by race and ethnicity. Available at: http://www.cdc.gov/cancer/hpv/statistics/anal.htm/. Accessed September 30, 2016.
4. Nigro ND, Seydel HG, Considine B, et al. Combined preoperative radiation and chemotherapy for squamous cell carcinoma of the anal canal. Cancer 1983; 51(10):1826–9.
5. Bartelink H, Roelofsen F, Eschwege F, et al. Concomitant radiotherapy and chemotherapy is superior to radiotherapy alone in the treatment of locally advanced anal cancer-phase III EORTC. J Clin Oncol 1997;15:2040–9.
6. Northover JMA, Arnott SJ, Cunningham D, et al. Epidermoid anal cancer: results from the UKCCCR randomised trial of radiotherapy alone versus radiotherapy, 5-fluorouracil, and mitomycin. Lancet 1996;348:1049–54.
7. Flam M, John M, Paajk TF, et al. Role of mitomycin in combination with fluorouracil and radiotherapy, and of salvage chemoradiation in the definitive nonsurgical treatment of epidermoid carcinoma of the anal canal: results of a phase III randomized intergroup study. J Clin Oncol 1996;14:2527–39.
8. Ajani JA, Winter KA, Gunderson LL, et al. Fluorouracil, mitomycin, and radiotherapy vs fluorouracil, cisplatin, and radiotherapy for carcinoma of the anal canal: a randomized controlled trial. JAMA 2008;299(16):1914–21.
9. Gunderson LL, Winter KA, Ajani JA, et al. Long-term update of US GI intergroup RTOG 98-11 phase III trial for anal carcinoma: survival, relapse, and colostomy failure with concurrent chemoradiation involving fluorouracil/mitomycin versus fluorouracil/cisplatin. J Clin Oncol 2012;30(35):4344–51.
10. James RD, Glynne-Jones R, Meadows HM, et al. Mitomycin or cisplatin chemoradiation with or without maintenance chemotherapy for treatment of squamous-cell carcinoma of the anus (ACT II): a randomised, phase 3, open-label, 2×2 factorial trial. Lancet Oncol 2013;14:516–24.
11. Gonzalez Ferreira JA, Jaen Olasolo J, Azinovic I, et al. Effect of radiotherapy delay in overall treatment time on local control and survival in head and neck cancer: review of the literature. Rep Pract Oncol Radiother 2015;20:328–39.
12. Choan E, Dahrouge S, Samant R, et al. Radical radiotherapy for cervix cancer: the effect of waiting time on outcome. Int J Radiat Oncol Biol Phys 2005;61(4): 1071–7.
13. Konski A, Garcia M, John M, et al. Evaluation of planned treatment breaks during radiation therapy for anal cancer: update of RTOG 92-08. Int J Radiat Oncol Biol Phys 2008;72:114–8.
14. Chen YJ, Liu A, Tsai PT, et al. Organ sparing by conformal avoidance intensity-modulated radiation therapy for anal cancer: dosimetric evaluation of coverage of pelvis and inguinal/femoral nodes. Int J Radiat Oncol Biol Phys 2005;63(1): 274–81.
15. Milano MT, Jani AB, Farrey KJ, et al. Intensity-modulated radiation therapy (IMRT) in the treatment of anal cancer: toxicity and clinical outcome. Int J Radiat Oncol Biol Phys 2005;63(2):354–61.
16. Mell LK, Schomas DA, Salama JK, et al. Association between bone marrow dosimetric parameters and acute hematologic toxicity in anal cancer patients treated with concurrent chemotherapy and intensity-modulated radiotherapy. Int J Radiat Oncol Biol Phys 2008;70(5):1431–7.
17. Kachnic LA, Winter K, Myerson RJ, et al. RTOG 0529: A phase 2 evaluation of dose-painted intensity modulated radiation therapy in combination with 5-fluorouracil and mitomycin-C for the reduction of acute morbidity in carcinoma of the anal canal. Int J Radiat Oncol Biol Phys 2013;86(1):27–33.

18. Muirhead R, Adams RA, Gilbert DC, et al. Anal cancer: developing an intensity-modulated radiotherapy solution for ACT2 fractionation. Clin Oncol 2014;26(11): 720–1.
19. Myerson RJ, Garofalo MC, El Naqa I, et al. Elective clinical target volumes for conformal therapy in anorectal cancer: a radiation therapy oncology group consensus panel contouring atlas. Int J Radiat Oncol Biol Phys 2009;74(3): 824–30.
20. Myerson RJ, Garofalo MC, El Naqa I, et al. Elective clinical target volumes in anorectal cancer: an RTOG consensus panel contouring atlas. Available at: https://www.rtog.org/LinkClick.aspx?fileticket=DgflROvKQ6w=&tabid=231.
21. Gilbert DC, Drinkwater K, O'Cathail SM, et al. Stepwise multicenter introduction of intensity modulated radiation therapy for anal cancer in the United Kingdom: from consensus guidance to large-scale prospective audit, prior to future clinical trials. Int J Radiat Oncol Biol Phys 2016;96(2S):S105–6.
22. Peiffert D, Tournier-Rangeard L, Gérard JP, et al. Induction chemotherapy and dose intensification of the radiation boost in locally advanced anal canal carcinoma: final analysis of the randomized UNICANCER ACCORD 03 trial. J Clin Oncol 2012;30(16):1941–8.
23. Deenen MJ, Dewit L, Boot H, et al. Simultaneous integrated boost-intensity modulated radiation therapy with concomitant capecitabine and mitomycin C for locally advanced anal carcinoma: a phase 1 study. Int J Radiat Oncol Biol Phys 2013; 85(5):e201–7.
24. ISRCTN registry. PLATO - Personalising anal cancer radiotherapy dose. ISRCTN88455282. Available at: http://www.isrctn.com/. Accessed September 27, 2016.
25. Bonner JA, Harari PM, Giralt J, et al. Radiotherapy plus cetuximab for squamous-cell carcinoma of the head and neck. N Engl J Med 2006;354:567–78.
26. Garg M, Lee JY, Kachnic LA, et al. Phase II trials of cetuximab (CX) plus cisplatin (CDDP), 5-fluorouracil (5-FU) and radiation (RT) in immunocompetent (ECOG 3205) and HIV-positive (AMC045) patients with squamous cell carcinoma of the anal canal (SCAC): safety and preliminary efficacy result. J Clin Oncol 2012;30:S15.
27. Olivatto LO, Vieira FM, Pereira BV, et al. Phase 1 study of cetuximab in combination with 5-fluorouracil, cisplatin, and radiotherapy in patients with locally advanced anal canal carcinoma. Cancer 2013;119(16):2973–80.
28. Deutsch E, Lemanski C, Pignon JP, et al. Unexpected toxicity of cetuximab combined with conventional chemoradiotherapy in patients with locally advanced anal cancer: results of the UNICANCER ACCORD 16 phase II trial. Ann Oncol 2013;24(11):2834–8.
29. Morris VK, Ciombor KK, Salem ME, et al. NCI9673: a multi-institutional eETCTN phase II study of nivolumab in refractory metastatic squamous cell carcinoma of the anal canal (SCCA). J Clin Oncol 2016;34 [abstract: 3503].
30. Kachnic L, Winter K, Myerson R, et al. Two-year outcomes of RTOG 0529: a phase II evaluation of dose-painted IMRT in combination with 5-fluorouracil and mitomycin-C for the reduction of acute morbidity in carcinoma of the anal canal. J Clin Oncol 2011;29(Suppl 4) [abstract: 368].

Radiation Oncology Management of Stage I–III Cervix Cancer

Lana de Souza Lawrence, MD

KEYWORDS

• Cervix • Cancer • Radiation • Brachytherapy

KEY POINTS

- Postoperative radiotherapy (with or without concurrent chemotherapy) is indicated for patients with intermediate or high-risk pathologic features, whereas up-front definitive radiotherapy with concurrent sensitizing chemotherapy is indicated for locoregionally advanced disease.
- Definitive radiotherapy typically consists of a combination of external beam treatment and central pelvic brachytherapy boost.
- Commonly used external beam techniques include 3-D conformal radiotherapy, and intensity-modulated radiotherapy (IMRT).
- Selection of brachytherapy boost technique depends on the geometry of the primary tumor and adjacent pattern of spread.
- External beam techniques should not be routinely used in lieu of brachytherapy for pelvic boost outside of clinical trial.

INTRODUCTION

Cervical cancer is the third most common cancer in women around the world and in the developing world is the second leading cause of cancer death among women.[1] Largely due to use of cytologic screening, however, cervical cancer death rate declined by 74% between 1955 and 1992 in developed countries,[2] with a sustained trend to decline thereafter.[3]

Multidisciplinary evaluation for the management of newly diagnosed cervical cancer is strongly encouraged. The treatment of choice depends on the presenting stage, availability of resources, and the general health of a patient. Cervical cancer is clinically staged according to the International Federation of Gynecology and Obstetrics (FIGO) guidelines, and, in terms of treatment, patients can be grouped into 3

Disclosure Statement: The author has nothing to disclose.

Department of Radiation Oncology, Christiana Care Health Services, 4701 Ogletown Stanton Road, Suite 1109, Newark, DE 19713, USA
E-mail address: ldesouzalawrence@christianacare.org

Surg Oncol Clin N Am 26 (2017) 477–489
http://dx.doi.org/10.1016/j.soc.2017.01.002
surgonc.theclinics.com

categories: early-stage disease, locally advanced disease, and metastatic disease. To minimize morbidity, primary therapy should avoid the planned use of both radical surgery and radiation. Therefore, in general, early-stage cervix cancers (FIGO stages 1A, IB1, and IIA1) are managed surgically, whereas locoregionally advanced nonmetastatic cases (stage IB2 or greater) are managed with definitive chemoradiotherapy.

POSTOPERATIVE RADIOTHERAPY

Postoperative radiotherapy is offered to women who have undergone surgical resection and have been found on pathology to have intermediate-risk or high-risk features suggestive of increased risk for disease recurrence.

Gynecologic Oncology Group (GOG) 92 was a trial conducted to evaluate the benefits and risks of adjuvant pelvic radiotherapy in women with stage IB cervical cancer treated by radical hysterectomy and pelvic lymphadenectomy. Inclusion criteria specified at least 2 of the following intermediate-risk factors (Sedlis criteria): greater than one-third stromal invasion, capillary lymphatic space involvement, and large clinical tumor diameter. The findings of the trial were that adjuvant pelvic radiotherapy after radical surgery significantly reduces the risk of recurrences in women with stage IB cervical cancer by 47% (relative risk = 0.53; $P = .008$, 1-tail) compared with no further treatment, with recurrence-free rates at 2 years of 88% versus 79% for the radiation and observation groups, respectively. The benefit from radiotherapy came at the cost of 6% grade 3 to grade 4 adverse events versus 2.1% in the observation group.[4] With longer follow-up, there was trend toward overall survival with the addition of radiation (hazard ratio [HR] 0.70), but it did not reach statistical significance.[5] There is some debate as to whether concurrent chemotherapy should be added for patients with the intermediate-risk factors (discussed previously), and an ongoing study is comparing adjuvant radiation versus adjuvant chemoradiation in these patients (ClinicalTrials Gov NCT01101451).

Postoperative chemoradiotherapy is standardly used for patients with high-risk features of positive lymph nodes or positive parametria discovered on final pathology. Peters and colleagues[6] reported outcomes for postoperative radiotherapy with or without concurrent chemotherapy in this population and found significant improvements in both disease recurrence (HR 2.01, $P = .003$) and overall survival (HR 1.96, $P = .007$) in favor of the addition of concurrent chemotherapy. Both pelvic and extrapelvic recurrences were less frequent in those patients receiving chemoradiotherapy compared with radiotherapy alone, but there was no statistically significant difference in the pattern of recurrence between the 2 treatment arms. Ideally, an adequate staging work-up should prevent this situation from occurring frequently.

DEFINITIVE RADIOTHERAPY

Definitive radiotherapy with concurrent chemotherapy is standard of care for the management of locoregionally advanced cervix cancer. Definitive radiotherapy consists of a combination of external beam treatment to the pelvis and brachytherapy.

There seems to be no added benefit to routinely adding surgery after completion of chemoradiotherapy with definitive intent. GOG 71 was a randomized clinical trial that evaluated the role of adjuvant hysterectomy after standardized radiation for bulky stage IB cervical cancer. The results demonstrated no statistical differences in outcomes between regimens and, overall, there was no clinically important benefit with the use of extrafascial hysterectomy after definitive radiotherapy.[7] Pelvic exenteration remains an option, however, in the uncommon event of isolated local pelvic recurrence or persistent disease.

EXTERNAL BEAM TECHNIQUES

Radiotherapy to the pelvis is typically delivered using a 3-D conformal approach to target the gross disease in the cervix and the parametria as well as elective coverage to the surrounding nodal regions at risk, including the common iliac nodes and internal and external iliac nodes. Standard technique involves a 4-field approach (anteroposterior, posteroanterior, and opposed laterals) with customized blocks to shield the femoral heads, bladder, and rectum. Patients may be instructed on a daily bladder-filling protocol to displace small bowel out of the pelvis.

IMRT, however, is increasingly used and accepted. IMRT allows for more conformal shaping of radiotherapy dose to a specified target, with the intention of reducing high-dose exposure to surrounding organs at risk, including the small bowel, sigmoid bowel, bladder, rectum, femoral heads, and pelvic bone marrow. IMRT is particularly useful in situations in which dose escalation is required, such as in the case of gross nodal positivity,[8] or in candidates who are ineligible for brachytherapy boost due to comorbid conditions.[9]

IMRT is now also considered standard in postoperative settings where removal of the uterus results in displacement of small bowel into the pelvis. Several retrospective studies have suggested that IMRT in the postoperative setting for gynecologic malignancies achieves excellent rates of local control with low rates of toxicity.[10,11] A phase III randomized controlled trial has also recently been completed, directly comparing 3-D conformal radiotherapy to IMRT in the postoperative setting for gynecologic malignancies.[12] Preliminary results demonstrate that patients who received IMRT had better bowel and bladder functions scores and required fewer antidiarrheal medications, with less significant decline in quality-of-life measures. Continued follow-up is ongoing to determine if differences in acute toxicity result in lower rates of long-term toxicity. A comparison of dose distribution between IMRT and 3-D conformal planning is illustrated in **Fig. 1**.

IMRT has not been yet similarly well validated in the setting of definitive treatment to the intact cervix. One potential disadvantage of IMRT in the case of the intact cervix is potential for marginal miss of the primary target, because the cervix is a highly mobile structure that can demonstrate significant variability in position between radiotherapy treatment sessions as well as during radiotherapy treatment with variations in bladder and rectal filling. For example, Beadle and colleagues[13] demonstrated a mean maximum change in cervix center of mass position of 2.1 cm in the superior-inferior dimension, 1.6 cm in the anterior-posterior direction, and 0.82 cm in the right-left lateral dimension when comparing CT scans performed before, weekly during, and after 5 weeks of radiation to the pelvis. In addition, the tumor changes geometry as it regresses, thereby potentially making a highly conformal technique less accurate. Fiducial marker placement in combination with daily image guidance can accommodate for these changes to some degree; however, shifts in treatment positioning must be limited to prevent marginal miss to the pelvic nodal volumes, which are fixed in geometry compared with a patient's bony anatomy. It is the author's institutional practice to obtain CT scans with a full bladder as well as an empty bladder at the time of treatment planning to account for motion of the cervix, using a so-called internal target volume approach in which additional planning margin is allowed to the cervix primary compared with the other relatively fixed targets, such as the pelvic nodes.

BRACHYTHERAPY BOOST TECHNIQUES

Brachytherapy is internal radiotherapy that is delivered using an applicator that is in direct proximity to the target. It is an essential component of treatment to the cervix to achieve the biologically equivalent dose necessary to sterilize disease, which

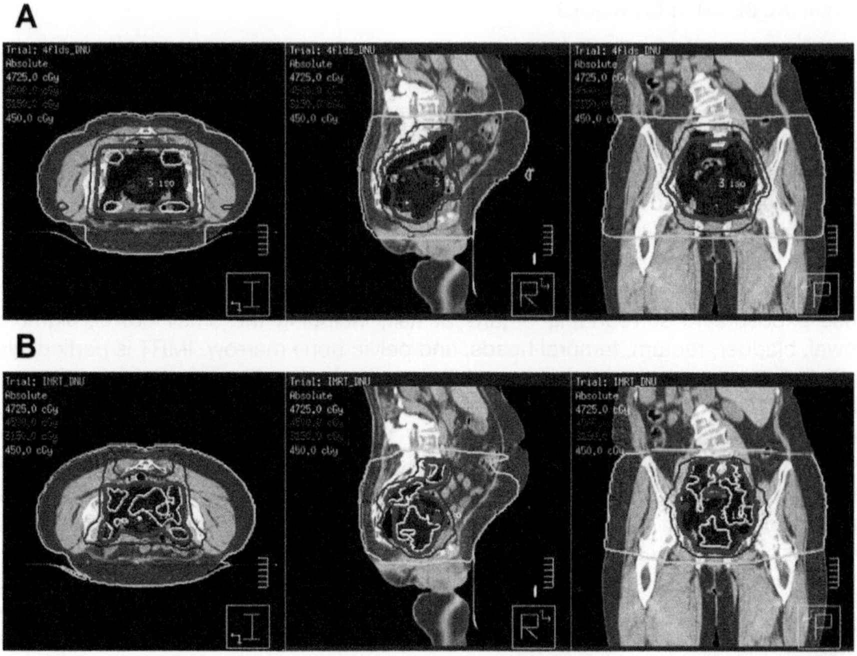

Fig. 1. (*A*) A 3 D conformal plan. Left panel: axial view. Middle panel: saggital view. Right panel: coronal view. The target volume is shaded blue, the prescription dose is the thick red line, the 105% isodose line is yellow, and the surrounding other lines represent lower dose fall-off. Note that the surrounding organs near the target (such as the bowel and parts of the femoral heads) are included within the full prescription dose region. (*B*) An IMRT plan. Left panel: axial view. Middle panel: saggital view. Right panel: coronal view. The target volume is shaded blue, the prescription dose is the thick red line, the 105% isodose line is yellow, and the surrounding other lines represent dose fall-off. The IMRT plan is more conformal to the shape of the target and is useful to keep high dose out of surrounding organs, such as the bowel.

reduces radiotherapy exposure to surrounding organs. The skill and expertise of the radiation oncologist performing the brachytherapy have a significant impact on the placement of the applicator devices, which in turn affects dosimetry and ultimate disease outcome.[14] Centers with no or limited experience with brachytherapy should refer patients to institutions with more expertise for optimal treatment outcomes.[15]

Brachytherapy is able to spare normal surrounding structures due to disproportionate rapid fall-off in the dose with increasing distance from the radioactive source. The applicator for the radioactive source is typically located in the center of the target, which results in a high dose to the middle of the tumor and a lower dose at the periphery (**Fig. 2**).

Also, brachytherapy is able to overcome one major limitation of external beam treatments, previously discussed, which is variability in the intrapelvic position of the cervix, because the brachytherapy applicator moves along with the target. By eliminating the source of positioning uncertainty, there is no need to add additional margin for the area intended to receive high dose, which would otherwise likely extend into to the adjacent bowel, bladder, or rectum.

Timing of Brachytherapy

The entire treatment course, including external beam and brachytherapy, should be completed within 8 weeks, because better disease control and outcomes can be

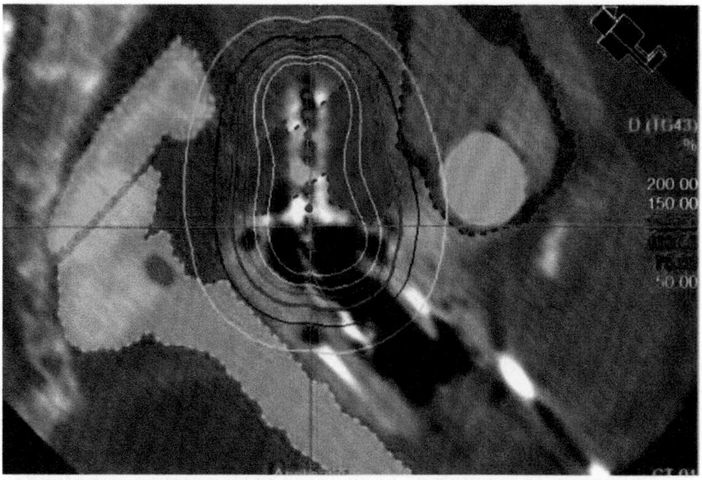

Fig. 2. Brachytherapy allows for higher dose at the center of the target with rapid dose fall-off at the periphery, which allows sparing of surrounding normal structures. This is a lateral view of a ring and tandem brachytherapy treatment. The target is shaded red, the bladder is shaded blue, the rectum is shaded yellow, and the sigmoid bowel is shaded green. The 100% prescription dose level is the red line covering the target, and the surrounding lines represent the 75% and 50% dose fall-off.

expected with a shorter time frame.[16,17] Brachytherapy may be interdigitated with the external beam or may follow sequentially. When treatment is interdigitated with external beam, the duration of the treatment course is likely to be shorter, but this means that brachytherapy may be performed when tumor is still bulky. If a tumor undergoing brachytherapy is still too bulky, there is the potential that the peripheral aspect of the tumor may be underdosed and lead to poor disease control. Many institutions opt to wait until a minimum of 5 weeks of chemoradiotherapy is complete for tumor shrinkage, which improves the geometry of the tumor for optimal dose coverage at time of brachytherapy. In the United States, the most common treatment scheme prescribes 2 intracavitary brachytherapy fractions per week for a total of 5 fractions, but several different treatment fractionation schemes have been performed.[18]

Concurrent weekly cisplatin chemotherapy may be ongoing when a patient is ready to start brachytherapy. The American Brachytherapy Society recommends that chemotherapy not be delivered on the same day that a patient is to receive brachytherapy, due to the potential for radiosensitization of the high radiotherapy doses used per fraction, which can translate to increased risk of toxicity.[19]

High-Dose Rate Brachytherapy Versus Low-Dose Rate Brachytherapy

Historically, brachytherapy treatment exclusively uses low-dose rate brachytherapy sources, such as cesium 137, in which treatments were delivered in 1 to 2 fractions each over 1 to 3 days. This technique has largely fallen out of favor in the United States due to requirements for prolonged patient immobilization, long treatment times, and wariness of radiation exposure to staff caring for patients receiving treatment.

High-dose rate brachytherapy uses a treatment source (typically iridium 192), which has the ability to deliver treatment over a matter of minutes rather than days in an outpatient setting. High-dose rate brachytherapy is now the predominant technique for delivery of brachytherapy in the United States.[20]

Applicator Selection

Brachytherapy may be performed using intracavitary techniques, interstitial techniques, or a combination of both. Applicator selection is based on the geometry of the target at the time of brachytherapy boost. The dose distribution can further be shaped by varying the dwell times of the radioactive source at specific positions within the applicator devices; the longer the source sits in a position, the higher the dose that is delivered at that location.

Ring/ovoid and tandem

The most common applicator used for management of the intact cervix is an intracavitary device using an intrauterine tube called a tandem, which is used in conjunction with a ring or ovoids that sit in the region of the lateral vaginal fornices. There is a classic pear-shaped dose distribution achieved with this approach (**Fig. 3**).

The tandem traverses the cervix os to enter the uterine cavity and, therefore, the cervix os must be dilated to accommodate the device. A hollow plastic tube called a smit sleeve is often placed into the dilated cervix os at the time of examination under anesthesia prior to start of brachytherapy to maintain an open passage for insertion of the tandem device. To prevent uterine perforation, a uterine sound is also used at the time of examination under anesthesia to determine the length of the uterine canal, which in turn used to select the tandem length. A longer tandem is preferable because it allows better coverage to the entire cervix as well as the lower uterine segment of the uterus, which is often involved due to direct extension of tumor. Applicator sets include tandems of varying curvature, and the curvature best suiting a patient's anatomy should be selected.

Ovoids have been classically used in conjunction with tandem, with the purpose of better encompassing the lateral spread of tumor. It is most helpful for a barrel-shaped cervix. Size of the applicator should not be so large that it slips out of the vaginal fornices, which would result in underdosing to the tumor. Careful vaginal packing,

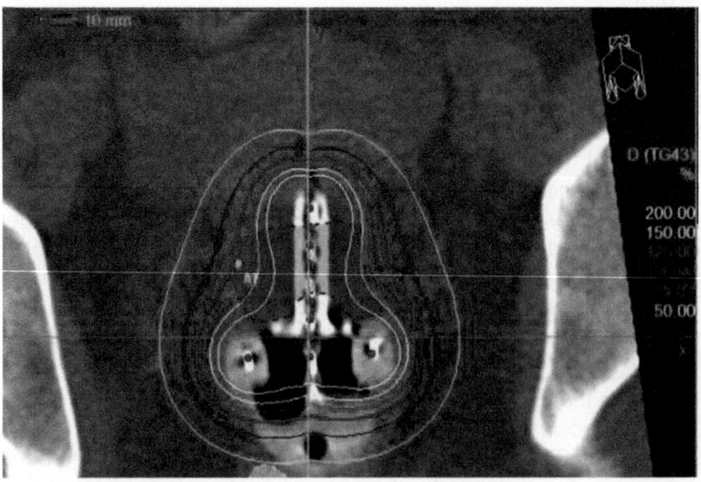

Fig. 3. Coronal view of the typical dose distribution achieved with an intracavitary brachytherapy approach, in this circumstance, with a ring and tandem. The tandem is traversing a smit sleeve, which was placed in the cervix os prior to the treatment. The cervix target is shaded red, and the 100% prescription dose line is the solid red line encompassing the target volume. The surrounding lines represent dose fall-off (Dark blue=75% of prescribed dose, Light blue=50% of prescribed dose).

often with gauze, is crucial to maintain the correct position of the ovoids and to push the bladder and rectal structures away from the applicator surface.

A ring applicator allows for a fixed geometry setup because it is rigidly attached to the tandem device and, therefore, is convenient and easier to reliably place compared with ovoids, especially in cases of women with shallow vaginal fornices. In addition, the ring device has dwell positions available around the entire periphery of the cervix. The anterior and posterior dwell positions are often not used to spare the bladder and rectum; however, this does allow for more flexibility in dosimetry in the event the device is slightly rotated if the disease is extending asymmetrically anterolaterally or posterolaterally. The potential disadvantages of the ring device compared with the ovoids are that it may produce a narrower dose distribution with underdosing to lateral structures, and it may have a higher surface dose to the vagina.

Vaginal cylinder

A vaginal cylinder is an intracavitary device used for brachytherapy boost in the postoperative setting (in the absence of an intact cervix) or may be used in combination with a tandem for patients with a narrow vagina that would not accommodate a ring or ovoids or in cases of minimal vaginal extension (<5 mm thick). In general, the largest diameter applicator that a patient's anatomy allows is selected to achieve the most homogenous dose distribution to the target of the deeper vaginal tissues, and to limit overdose to the vaginal mucosa, which may result in late toxicities, such as telangiectasia formation and vaginal fibrosis and or/closure. Vaginal cylinders usually have a single central channel through which the radioactive source traverses. Multichannel vaginal cylinders are also available, however, which can allow further optimization of dose. An example of a single-channel vaginal cylinder plan is shown in **Fig. 4**.

Interstitial brachytherapy

Interstitial brachytherapy involves insertion of catheters directly into the soft tissues of the target to facilitate placement of radioactive sources. Indications for interstitial boost include the following:

- Inability to locate the cervix os
- Vaginal disease thicker than 5 mm
- Persistent palpable disease on pelvic sidewall

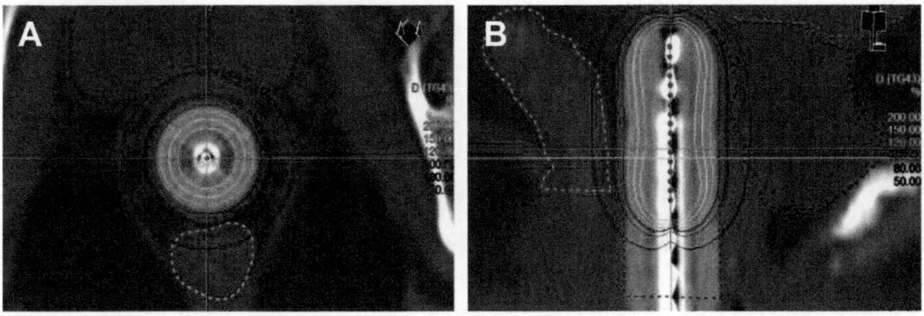

Fig. 4. (*A*) Axial and (*B*) sagittal views of a vaginal cylinder treatment plan in the postoperative setting. The bladder is outlined by a dotted blue line, the rectum by a dotted yellow line, and the bowel by a dotted orange line. The 100% prescription isodose is solid red. In this patient's case, the dose was prescribed to the vaginal surface of the upper vaginal cuff. The surrounding lines represent dose fall-off (Purple line=80% of prescribed dose. Dark blue line=50% of prescribed dose).

- Bulky lesions
- Lower vaginal extension
- A narrow vagina that does not accommodate intracavitary device placement

Interstitial brachytherapy catheters may be guided using templates placed in the region of the perineum, such as a modified Syed-Neblett template[21] (Best Medical International Inc., Springfield, VA) or Martinez Universal Perineal Interstitial Template (MUPIT) (Elekta AB, Stockholm, Sweden) applicator.[22] Whenever possible, a tandem should be placed in the case of an intact cervix to avoid cold spots in the central tissue. An example of an interstitial plan using a modified Syed-Neblett template is shown in **Fig. 5**. Modified ring and ovoid applicators have also recently become available that have the ability to deliver a combined intracavitary and interstitial approach.

Imaging for Brachytherapy Treatment Planning

In the past, 2-D imaging was used for brachytherapy planning, with doses prescribed to clinical point landmarks; however, plain film imaging does not give an accurate assessment of the tumor size, extent of disease, or organs at risk. When available, MRI should be performed because it is more sensitive than pelvic examination or for detecting parametrial involvement and estimating tumor size.[23] The RetroEMBRACE trial was a multi-institutional European trial that prospectively evaluated 3-D volume-based planning using MRI for brachytherapy. Results demonstrated improved pelvic control and survival compared with historical 2-D treatment approaches as well as limited severe morbidity.[24]

Although less sensitive than MRI, CT imaging is more widely available in the United States within radiation oncology departments and is, therefore, most commonly used for the purposes of brachytherapy planning. Many institutions use a hybrid imaging approach for brachytherapy planning, where a prebrachytherapy MRI is obtained for assistance with tumor delineation and CT imaging is used for planning once the device is in place. The hybrid approach may be comparable to MRI only–based planning with regard to local control rates and toxicity and is reasonable to consider when MRI is not readily available.[25]

A B

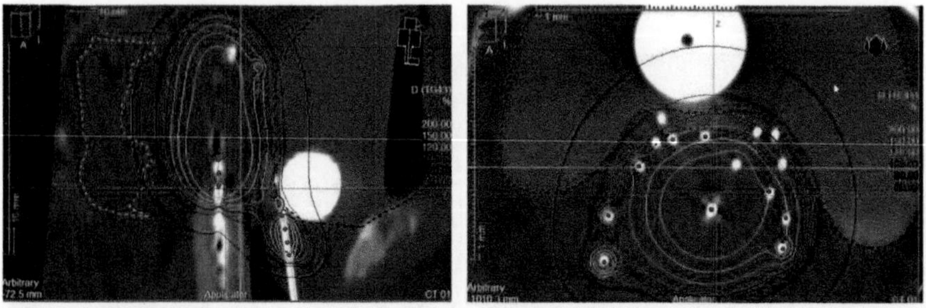

Fig. 5. (*A*) Sagittal and (*B*) axial views, respectively, of an interstitial brachytherapy plan using a modified Syed-Neblett template. This patient presented with bulky extension to the anterior vagina and right parametrial invasion. A central tandem was used and peripheral catheter placement was determined by distribution on residual disease at the time of brachytherapy planning. The target is represented by the red dotted line, the rectum by the dotted yellow line, and the bladder by the dotted blue line. The solid red line is the 100% prescription dose line. The surrounding lines represent dose fall-off (Purple line=80% prescribed dose. Dark Blue line=50% prescribed dose).

FUTURE DIRECTIONS

As discussed previously, brachytherapy is an essential component for radiotherapy management of cervix cancer. Unfortunately, brachytherapy is resource intensive, technically challenging, and not universally available. In addition, brachytherapy is relatively invasive and ideally should be performed in patients with a good performance status. For these reasons, and with emergence of new technologies, brachytherapy use seems to be on the decline. Han and colleagues[26] noted a decline in the use of brachytherapy for cervix cancer from 83% in 1988 to 58% in 2009, with a significant decline in 2003, which coincided with the introduction of a health care rebate for IMRT in the United Sates. Higher rates of cause-specific survival and overall survival rates, however, were noted in patients treated with brachytherapy, signifying that brachytherapy cannot reasonably be replaced by currently available external beam approaches in patients who are candidates for brachytherapy treatment. Alternative techniques for cervix cancer treatment currently under exploration include stereotactic body radiotherapy (SBRT) and proton therapy.

Stereotactic Body Radiotherapy

SBRT is an external beam radiotherapy technique, which delivers high doses of radiotherapy in fewer fractions compared with standard external beam radiotherapy (usually 5 or fewer fractions) and often uses advanced imaging techniques for tumor localization and/or tumor motion management strategies. The goal behind utilization of SBRT for a central pelvic boost is to noninvasively mimic the dose distribution of brachytherapy.

Dosimetric studies have been reported showing that SBRT may provide adequate target coverage with similar doses to organs at risk compared with brachytherapy.[27–30] Clinical outcome data is limited, however, to small single-institutional experiences at this point and, therefore, SBRT cannot be recommended for routine replacement of brachytherapy outside of a clinical trial.

Proton Therapy

Proton therapy is an external beam technology that relies on the acceleration of protons to deposit dose in the region of disease rather than using photons as in conventional radiotherapy techniques. The physical characteristics of protons allow narrow beams with minimal side scatter and minimal deposition of dose past the particle range, which is determined by the beam energy. These physical characteristics may make proton therapy a better alternative to IMRT or SBRT in patients who are not candidates for brachytherapy, assuming that adequate tumor localization can be achieved. Single-institution dosimetric data suggest that proton therapy provides good target coverage and conformity and sparing of normal tissues within guidelines suggested for MRI-guided brachytherapy and also seem to provide superior dosimetry compared with IMRT approaches.[31] Proton therapy is resource intensive, however, and not yet widely available. Sufficient prospective data in the management of cervix cancers are lacking and proton therapy should only be used in the context of a clinical trial at this point in time.

Ongoing National Trials

There are 2 active national protocols addressing whether there may be benefit to the addition of chemotherapy after completion of concurrent chemoradiotherapy for high-risk patients.

The Radiation Therapy Oncology Group (RTOG) 0724/GOG 0724 is a phase III randomized study of concurrent chemotherapy and pelvic radiotherapy with or without adjuvant chemotherapy after radical hysterectomy for high-risk cervix cancer patients, defined as patients with any of the following risk features: positive pelvic nodes, positive parametria, and/or PET/CT-negative para-aortic nodes that are found at time of surgery and completely resected. The primary endpoint is to determine if there will be benefit to progression-free survival with the addition of adjuvant systemic chemotherapy composed of carboplatin and paclitaxel compared with cisplatin-based chemoradiotherapy alone. In the previously discussed trial by Peters and colleauges,[6] the investigators found that high-risk patients who received less than or equal to 2 courses of concurrent cisplatin and 5-fluorouracil–based chemotherapy had a 31% recurrence rate compared with 13% for patients who received 2 cycles of concurrent chemotherapy and another 1 to 2 cycles postradiation, suggesting that additional chemotherapy may be beneficial. There is some concern of toxicity, however, with continued cisplatin, particularly with regard to potential neurotoxicity, and, therefore, there has been increased interest in carboplatin-based regimens. Carboplatin-paclitaxel was selected for this study based on mounting evidence that it is an effective regimen and less toxic compared with cisplatin-paclitaxel in advanced-stage or recurrent cervix cancer. For instance, in a multi-institutional retrospective study, Moore and colleagues[32] demonstrated objective responses of 53% with carboplatin-paclitaxel compared with 29% with cisplatin-paclitaxel.

The OUTBACK trial (Australia New Zealand Gynaecological Oncology Group [ANZGOG] 0902/GOG 0274/RTOG 1174) is a sister protocol to the RTOG 0724/GOG 0724 and was developed on the same basis as discussed previously but for patients undergoing chemoradiotherapy with definitive intent. It is a phase III randomized trial of cisplatin-based chemoradiotherapy with or without adjuvant carboplatin-paclitaxel chemotherapy for locally advanced cervix cancer (node-positive FIGO stage IB1 and FIGO stage IB2-IVA). After definitive chemoradiotherapy, most failures are distant, and only a small percent fail in the pelvis. Therefore, there is interest in trying to decrease the rate of distant failures, thereby improving disease-free survival and hopefully overall survival.

Another ongoing study is the National Research Group (NRG)-GY006, which is a randomized phase II trial of cisplatin-based chemoradiotherapy with or without intravenous triapine in women with bulky stage IB2–IVA cervix cancer as well as those with stage II–IVA vaginal cancer. Triapine is a more potent inhibitor of ribonucleotide reductase than hydroxyurea, which has activity in cervix cancer, and earlier preclinical and phase I–II studies using triapene have demonstrated promising results.[33] This protocol is also noteworthy because it is a randomized trial allowing the use of either IMRT or 3-D conformal radiotherapy, and one of the secondary endpoints of the study is to assess quality of life, progression-free survival, and overall survival of IMRT compared with 3-D conformal external beam techniques.

SUMMARY

Cervix cancer requires multidisciplinary input for selection of an appropriate treatment strategy. Radiotherapy is used in the postoperative management of patients with early-stage cervix cancer with intermediate-risk or high-risk features and also with definitive intent in patients presenting with locoregionally advanced disease. Radiotherapy with definitive intent is composed of a combination of external beam treatment and brachytherapy. Although brachytherapy use seems to be on the decline for several reasons, it remains the gold standard for treatment in patients who are candidates for definitive treatment. Emerging technologies for cervix cancer boost, such as SBRT and proton therapy, warrant further investigation before they can be clinically adopted.

REFERENCES

1. Parkin DM, Bray F, Ferlay J, et al. Global cancer statistics, 2002. CA Cancer J Clin 2005;55(2):74–108.
2. Gustafsson L, Ponten J, Zack M, et al. International incidence rates of invasive cervical cancer after introduction of cytological screening. Cancer Causes Control 1997;8(5):755–63.
3. Ferlay J, Soerjomataram I, Ervik M, et al. GLOBOCAN 2012: estimated cancer incidence, mortality, and prevalence worldwide in 2012. Lyon (France): International Agency for Research on Cancer; 2013. Available at: http://globocan.iarc.fr.
4. Sedlis A, Bundy BN, Rotman MZ, et al. A randomized trial of pelvic radiation therapy versus no further therapy in selected patients with stage IB carcinoma of the cervix after radical hysterectomy and pelvic lymphadenectomy: a Gynecologic Oncology Group Study. Gynecol Oncol 1999;73(2):177–83.
5. Rotman M, Sedlis A, Piedmonte MR, et al. A phase III randomized trial of postoperative pelvic irradiation in Stage IB cervical carcinoma with poor prognostic features: follow-up of a gynecologic oncology group study. Int J Radiat Oncol Biol Phys 2006;65(1):169–76.
6. Peters WA 3rd, Liu PY, Barrett RJ 2nd, et al. Concurrent chemotherapy and pelvic radiation therapy compared with pelvic radiation therapy alone as adjuvant therapy after radical surgery in high-risk early-stage cancer of the cervix. J Clin Oncol 2000;18(8):1606–13.
7. Keys HM, Bundy BN, Stehman FB, et al, Gynecologic Oncology Group. Radiation therapy with and without extrafascial hysterectomy for bulky stage IB cervical carcinoma: a randomized trial of the Gynecologic Oncology Group. Gynecol Oncol 2003;89(3):343–53.
8. Schefter TE, Kavanagh BD, Wu Q, et al. Technical considerations in the application of intensity-modulated radiotherapy as a concomitant integrated boost for locally-advanced cervix cancer. Med Dosim 2002;27(2):177–84.
9. Chan P, Yeo I, Perkins G, et al. Dosimetric comparison of intensity-modulated, conformal, and four-field pelvic radiotherapy boost plans for gynecologic cancer: a retrospective planning study. Radiat Oncol 2006;1:13.
10. Beriwal S, Jain SK, Heron DE, et al. Clinical outcome with adjuvant treatment of endometrial carcinoma using intensity-modulated radiation therapy. Gynecol Oncol 2006;102(2):195–9.
11. Chen MF, Tseng CJ, Tseng CC, et al. Adjuvant concurrent chemoradiotherapy with intensity-modulated pelvic radiotherapy after surgery for high-risk, early stage cervical cancer patients. Cancer J 2008;14(3):200–6.
12. Klopp AH, Yeung AR, Deshmukh S, et al. NRG RTOG-1203: a phase III randomized trial comparing patient reported toxicity and quality of life (QOL) during pelvic IMRT as compared to conventional RT. NRG Oncology Press Release: Embargoed Until September 28, 2016, 7:45 AM Eastern Time. Available at: https://www.rtog.org/News/tabid/72/articleType/ArticleView/articleId/109/Intensity-Modulated-Pelvic-Radiation-Therapy-Reduces-Patient-Reported-Toxicities.aspx.
13. Beadle BM, Jhingran A, Salehpour M, et al. Cervix regression and motion during the course of external beam chemoradiation for cervical cancer. Int J Radiat Oncol Biol Phys 2009;73(1):235–41.

14. Viswanathan A, Moughan JW, Small J, et al. The quality of cervical-cancer brachytherapy implantation and the impact on local recurrence and disease-free survival in RTOG Prospective Trials 0116and 0128. Int J Radiat Oncol Biol Phys 2010;75:S86.
15. Erickson B, Eifel P, Moughan J, Eifel PJ. Patterns of brachytherapy practice for patients with carcinoma of the cervix (1996-1999): a Patterns of Care study. Int J Radiat Oncol Biol Phys 2005;63:1083–92.
16. Petereit DG, Sarkaria JN, Chappell R, et al. The adverse effect of treatment prolongation in cervical carcinoma. Int J Radiat Oncol Biol Phys 1995;32:1301–7.
17. Lanciano RM, Pajak TF, Martz K, et al. The influence of treatment time on outcome for squamous cell cancer of the uterine cervixtreated with radiation: a Patterns-of-care study. Int J Radiat Oncol Biol Phys 1993;25:391–7.
18. Viswanathan AN, Creutzberg C, Craighead P, et al. International brachytherapy practice patterns: a survey of the Gynecologic Cancer Intergroup. Int J Radiat Oncol Biol Phys 2010;82(1):250–5.
19. Viswanathan AN, Beriwal S, De Los Santos JF, et al, American Brachytherapy Society. American Brachytherapy Society consensus guidelines for locally advanced carcinoma of the cervix. Part II: high-dose-rate brachytherapy. Brachytherapy 2012;11(1):47–52.
20. Viswanathan AN, Erickson BA. Three-dimensional imaging in gynecologic brachytherapy: a survey of the American Brachytherapy Society. Int J Radiat Oncol Biol Phys 2010;76(1):104–9.
21. Beriwal S, Bhatnagar A, Heron DE, et al. High-dose-rate interstitial brachytherapy for gynecologic malignancies. Brachytherapy 2006;5(4):218–22.
22. Martinez A, Cox RS, Edmundson GK. A multiple-site perineal applicator (MUPIT) for treatment of prostatic, anorectal, and gynecologic malignancies. Int J Radiat Oncol Biol Phys 1984;10(2):297–305.
23. Hricak H, Gatsonis C, Coakley FV, et al. Early invasive cervicalcancer: CTand MR imaging in preoperative evaluationdACRIN/-GOG comparative study of diagnostic performance and interobservervariability. Radiology 2007;245:491–8.
24. Sturdza A, Pötter R, Fokdal LU, et al. Image guided brachytherapy in locally advanced cervical cancer: Improved pelvic control and survival in RetroEMBRACE, a multicenter cohort study. Radiother Oncol 2016;120(3):428–33.
25. Choong ES, Bownes P, Musunuru HB, et al. Hybrid (CT/MRI based) vs. MRI only based image-guided brachytherapy in cervical cancer: dosimetry comparisons and clinical outcome. Brachytherapy 2016;15(1):40–8.
26. Han K, Milosevic M, Fyles A, et al. Trends in the utilization of brachytherapy in cervical cancer in the United States. Int J Radiat Oncol Biol Phys 2013;87(1):111–9.
27. Sethi RA, Jozsef G, Grew D, et al. Is there a role for an external beam boost in cervical cancer radiotherapy? Front Oncol 2013;3:3.
28. Hsieh CH, Wei MC, Hsu YP, et al. Should helical tomotherapy replace brachytherapy for cervical cancer? Case Report. BMC Cancer 2010;10:637.
29. Marnitz S, Kohler C, Budach V, et al. Robotic radiosurgery: emulating brachytherapy in patients with locally advanced cervical carcinoma. Technique, feasibility and acute toxicity. Radiat Oncol 2013;8(1):109.
30. Haas JA, Witten MR, Clancey O, et al. CyberKnife boost for patients with cervical cancer unable to undergo brachytherapy. Front Oncol 2012;2:25.
31. Clivio A, Kluge A, Cozzi L, et al. Intensity modulated proton beam radiation for brachytherapy in patients with cervical carcinoma. Int J Radiat Oncol Biol Phys 2013;87(5):897–903.

32. Moore KN, Herzog TJ, Lewin SL, et al. A comparison of cisplatin/paclitaxel and carboplatin/paclitaxel in stage IVB, recurrent or persistent cervical cancer. Gynecol Oncol 2007;105:299–303.
33. Kunos C, Radivoyevitch T, Waggoner S, et al. Radiochemotherapy plus 3-aminopyridine-2-carboxaldehyde thiosemicarbazone (3-AP, NSC #663249) in advanced-stage cervical and vaginal cancers. Gynecol Oncol 2013;130(1): 75–80.

Brachytherapy in the Management of Prostate Cancer

Bradley J. Stish, MD[a,*], Brian J. Davis, MD, PhD[a], Lance A. Mynderse, MD[b], Christopher L. Deufel, PhD[a], Richard Choo, MD[a]

KEYWORDS

- Prostate cancer • High dose rate brachytherapy • Low dose rate brachytherapy
- Radiation therapy • Image guidance • Dose escalation

KEY POINTS

- Brachytherapy is an important tool for radiation oncologists in the curative management of men with all risk categories of localized prostate cancer.
- By delivering radiation directly to the prostate gland via implantation, brachytherapy allows clinicians to deliver significant radiation dose escalation while minimizing doses to nearby normal tissues.
- Both low dose rate and high dose rate brachytherapy have published long-term data supporting their use for the treatment of prostate cancer.
- The long-term safety and tolerability of brachytherapy has been reported in multiple trials and series.
- Outcomes with brachytherapy compare favorably with other definitive treatment modalities.

INTRODUCTION

In 2016, there will be an estimated 180,890 men with a new diagnosis of prostate cancer, of whom approximately 80% will have localized disease, with an estimated 26,120 prostate-cancer specific deaths. Prostate cancer is the second leading cause of

Disclosure State: Dr B.J. Stish, L.A. Mynderse, C.L. Deufel, and R. Choo have nothing to disclose. Dr B.J. Davis: Speaking honoraria from the American Brachytherapy Society, American College of Radiation Oncology, American Society Radiation Oncology, Prospect Medical Inc; Stock ownership; Pfizer Inc, Research grants from Takeda UK Inc, and a grant Augmenix; Travel expenses from American Board of Radiology.

[a] Department of Radiation Oncology, Mayo Clinic, 200 First Street Southwest, Rochester, MN 55905, USA; [b] Department of Urology, Mayo Clinic, 200 First Street Southwest, Rochester, MN 55905, USA

* Corresponding author.

E-mail address: stish.bradley@mayo.edu

Surg Oncol Clin N Am 26 (2017) 491–513
http://dx.doi.org/10.1016/j.soc.2017.01.008 surgonc.theclinics.com

cancer-related death among men in the United States.[1] For men diagnosed with nonmetastatic prostate cancer who pursue an active treatment approach, the National Comprehensive Cancer Network (NCCN) guidelines currently recommend radical prostatectomy and radiation therapy as appropriate definitive local therapy modalities.[2] Both treatments have long been considered equivalent in cancer outcomes for the treatment of prostate cancer, an assertion that has been confirmed in a recently published randomized trial for low-risk patients.[3] Among radiation therapy strategies, brachytherapy is an important treatment option with compelling data supporting its use for appropriately selected men with any NCCN risk category of nonmetastatic prostate cancer.

The term brachytherapy is derived from the Greek term "brachy," which means "short," and generally is used to describe a variety of therapeutic techniques using radioactive sources placed into or near tissues. The French physicians Pasteau and Degrais published the first description of prostate brachytherapy in 1914, which was performed using radium inserted through a catheter placed in the urethra.[4] The first use of interstitial radioactive needle implantation, a technique more akin to modern methods, was published in 1917 by Benjamin Barringer, who was Chief of Urology at Memorial Hospital in New York.[5] During the ensuing century, the technique and use of prostate brachytherapy has evolved to make it a safe and highly effective treatment modality for prostate cancer.

THE RATIONALE FOR BRACHYTHERAPY IN THE MANAGEMENT OF PROSTATE CANCER

Prostate cancer represents a favorable clinical scenario for the use of brachytherapy. The anatomic location of the prostate gland renders it relatively accessible for percutaneous placement of brachytherapy catheters. Incorporation of transrectal ultrasound imaging at the time of the brachytherapy procedure for visualization of the prostate gland and nearby anatomy allows accurate needle or catheter placement, which is vital for optimal radioactive source localization.

Brachytherapy allows a number of potential advantages over external beam radiation therapy (EBRT) delivered using either high-energy photons or protons. The most commonly used radioactive sources for modern prostate brachytherapy emit relatively low-energy (20–400 keV) photons that are typically absorbed by the surrounding tissues within a few centimeters.[6] Megavoltage photons, which are standard for modern EBRT, have significantly greater energy than those used in brachytherapy applications. As such, photons from EBRT sources deposit energy over greater distances beyond their target before being attenuated fully. This physical property, along with the fact that EBRT inherently requires an entrance dose (ie, dose delivered on the pathway to the radiation target), results in a greater integral dose exposure to the normal tissue in proximity to the prostate. Although modern radiation techniques, such as intensity modulated radiation therapy (IMRT), have improved EBRT dose delivery, the dose concentration in the target allowed by brachytherapy is superior.[7] **Fig. 1** shows a comparison of the relative dose distribution achieved treating the prostate with high dose rate (HDR) brachytherapy (see **Fig. 1**A) and IMRT (see **Fig. 1**B). This image clearly demonstrates the ability of brachytherapy to limit both higher dose exposure to the rectum and low dose level exposure to the surrounding soft tissues. Proton beam therapy has physical characteristics that can decrease deposition of low to medium dose radiation compared with photon-based treatments. However, even a state-of-the art proton beam treatment plan (see **Fig. 1**C) does not achieve the conformity provided by brachytherapy. Detailed dosimetric analyses have confirmed the superiority of brachytherapy treatments for decreasing radiation dose to the

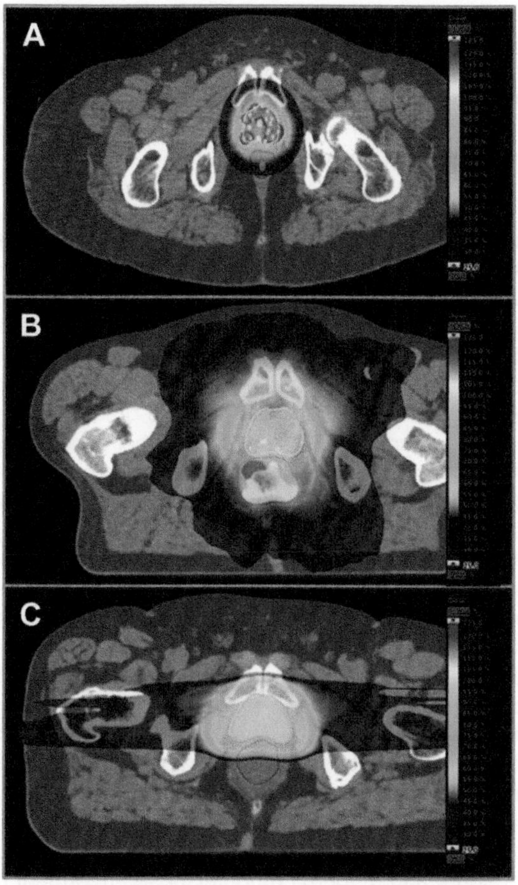

Fig. 1. Dosimetric comparison of radiation techniques for prostate cancer. Calculated radiation dose distributions are shown on a representative axial computed tomography image of 3 separate patients treated with (*A*) high dose rate brachytherapy (*B*) intensity modulated radiation therapy with photons, or (*C*) intensity modulated proton therapy with proton beam therapy. Radiation dose (relative to prescription dose) is represented as a color dose wash according the legend shown on the right side of each panel.

bladder and rectum compared with either IMRT or proton beam therapy with modern treatment regimens and technologies.[8]

An additional point to consider is the ability of brachytherapy to provide dose-escalated treatment. Randomized studies have shown that improved clinical outcomes are associated with increased EBRT dose delivery to the prostate.[9–12] With its favorable dosimetric conformality, brachytherapy allows clinicians to deliver radiation doses to the prostate far exceeding those able to be safely administered with external beam techniques. Most patients treated with modern EBRT receive a dose of approximately 74 to 80 Gy to the prostate, whereas commonly used brachytherapy prescription doses deliver a biological effective dose that is 1.5 to 3.0 times greater.[13] Large brachytherapy treatment series have demonstrated the treatment with an increased biological effective dose is associated with improved disease control outcomes.[14] Furthermore, by placing radioactive sources directly within the target tissue, brachytherapy creates focal "hot spots" or regions of dose more than 2-fold greater than the prescription level (see **Fig. 1**A). Owing to their restricted location within the prostate, these areas of dose heterogeneity may confer improved cancer control rates without significantly affecting toxicity.[15]

PROSTATE BRACHYTHERAPY TECHNICAL FACTORS

Early applications of prostate brachytherapy were typically performed with placement of radioactive sources under visual guidance or by palpation, using a retropubic approach requiring open laparotomy for access.[16] However, widespread adoption of this technique was hindered by the need for an open surgical procedure, suboptimal radiation dose coverage, and concerns related to radiation safety.

Modern prostate brachytherapy is almost exclusively performed by insertion of radioactive sources by way of transperineally implanted hollow catheters or needles with real-time image guidance (**Fig. 2**). Most prostate brachytherapy procedures are performed as a same-day surgical procedure using either general anesthesia or spinal anesthesia with intravenous sedation. The number of needles required is variable and is influenced by prostate size, patient pelvic anatomy, and physics of the particular radioisotope used. Typically, 14 to 22 needles are used. The majority of implants are performed with transrectal ultrasound guidance, which allows excellent visualization of the prostate and brachytherapy needles. A Foley catheter is usually placed during the procedure to assist with identification of the urethra. A template with needle guidance holes at regular intervals is commonly placed on the perineum to assist with the identification, spacing, and securing of catheters. The positions of the template's needle holes are registered and projected onto the ultrasound electronic display screen to guide and coregister the needle localization. The location and pattern for the placement of the interstitial needles and radiation sources into the prostate can be determined before the actual procedure using existing transrectal ultrasound images to optimize radiation dose delivery in a method known as "preplanning." Conversely, needles can be inserted in a templated arrangement at the time of the procedure and modern computer-based treatment planning software

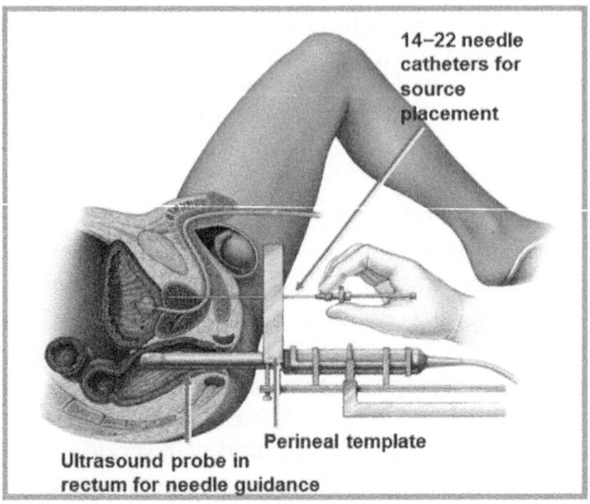

Fig. 2. Patient position and vital component of prostate brachytherapy with transrectal ultrasound guidance. (*From* Mayo Clinic. Radiation seed implants for prostate cancer [patient education brochure]. 2002. Used with permission of Mayo Foundation for Medical Education and Research, all rights reserved.)

can then be used to determine the optimal distribution of radiation sources to allow real-time planning.[17] Real-time planning allows clinicians to account for differences in prostate volume or position at the time of the procedure and may improve clinical outcomes compared with preplanning.[18] However, real-time planning typically prolongs the duration of the procedure compared with preplanning. After the implant is complete, the needles are removed and the patient is discharged after appropriate recovery from anesthesia. After the procedure, specific dosimetric parameters that quantify the dose to the prostate and nearby organs at risk (ie, urethra, bladder, and rectum) are recorded as a means to measure the quality of the implant and subsequent risk of toxicity.

CATEGORIES OF PROSTATE BRACHYTHERAPY

Low Dose Rate Brachytherapy

Prostate brachytherapy techniques are often broadly categorized according to the physical properties of the radiation sources being used.[19] Low dose rate (LDR) brachytherapy is used to describe treatments delivered by radioactive sources with dose rates of less than 2 Gy per hour. Modern transperineal implanted LDR brachytherapy, also known as permanent prostate brachytherapy, has been used for more than 30 years and is estimated to have been performed on more than 250,000 patients in the United States.[20,21] Although a number of different radioactive isotopes have been used for LDR brachytherapy, the 3 most commonly used and commercially available sources, their physical properties, and typical prescription doses are shown in **Table 1**. With an introduction year of 1965, ^{125}I has a longer clinical track record than either palladium-103 (^{103}Pd, 1986) or cesium-131 (^{131}Cs, 2004). Given the similar average energies of these 3 radionuclides, they possess comparable relative dose distributions and photon attenuation properties. The relatively shorter half-lives of ^{103}Pd and ^{131}Cs result in more rapid radiation dose rate delivery for these isotopes compared with ^{125}I. Both ^{103}Pd and ^{131}Cs offer a theoretic radiobiological advantage for improving tumor control, but do require lower prescription doses.[22,23] However, multiple studies, including 1 randomized trial, have demonstrated no significant difference in patient clinical outcomes when comparing implants performed with either ^{125}I or ^{103}Pd.[24–26] The current American Brachytherapy Society (ABS) and American Society for Radiation Oncology/American College of Radiology guidelines for permanent prostate brachytherapy provide recommendations relating to the use of either ^{125}I or ^{103}Pd for management of prostate cancer, with no preference given for either radionuclide.[21,27] Given the growing experience with ^{131}Cs, its routine use has also gained acceptance among brachytherapy clinicians.

Table 1
Common radionuclide used in low dose rate brachytherapy and their properties

Radionuclide	Half-Life (d)	Average Energy (keV)	Prescription Dose Range (Gy; Monotherapy)	Prescription Dose Range (Gy; Combined with EBRT)
Iodine-125 (^{125}I)	59.4	28.4	140–160	108–110
Palladium-103 (^{103}Pd)	17.0	20.7	110–125	90–100
Cesium-131 (^{131}Cs)	9.7	30.4	115	80–85

Abbreviation: EBRT, external beam radiation therapy.

Patient selection is an important consideration for delivery of LDR prostate brachytherapy. The ABS consensus guidelines provide a thorough overview of patient-specific factors that should be evaluated when determining candidacy for permanent prostate brachytherapy. As with any active treatment strategy being considered, all patients should have a recent biopsy (within <12 months from treatment) confirming prostate adenocarcinoma with Gleason score grading, a pretreatment serum prostate-specific antigen, physical examination including a digital rectal examination to determine tumor classification (T stage), and a thorough clinical history documenting pertinent past medical/surgical history.[21] **Table 2** lists both absolute and relative contraindications for LDR prostate brachytherapy according to the ABS consensus guidelines, which are similar to the recommendations published in other professional group guidelines for brachytherapy.[27,28] Both obstructive and irritative lower urinary symptoms before implantation are an important factor to evaluate before proceeding with LDR brachytherapy. A number of publications have shown that patients with elevated International Prostate Symptom Scores before treatment are at greater risk of developing urinary retention or increased toxicity after permanent prostate brachytherapy.[29–33] Patients who present with potentially prohibitive lower urinary tract symptoms at baseline can be treated with either medical (ie, alpha blockers) or surgical (transurethral resection of the prostate [TURP]) interventions with hopes to improve symptoms and render the risk of subsequent brachytherapy acceptable. However, medical treatments are generally preferred and TURP is generally reserved in the pre-implant setting for men with large median lobes. Furthermore, although large TURP defects are considered a contraindication to permanent prostate brachytherapy owing to concerns regarding limitations in seed placement resulting in inadequate dosimetry, there are number of reports detailing excellent outcomes when brachytherapy is used in patients with previous TURP.[34–36] Nevertheless, some studies still suggest an increased risk of urinary incontinence in the setting of prior TURP.[37] Thus, careful patient evaluation with a detailed urinary function evaluation, volumetric imaging, and cystoscopy can be helpful in determining whether a TURP defect is prohibitory. Adequate placement of brachytherapy needles can be limited further by pubic arch interference related to individual pelvic anatomy, patient positioning at the time of procedure and prostate size.[38] Generally, for men with prostate gland volumes of greater than 60 cm^3, prebrachytherapy androgen deprivation therapy (ADT) with both luteinizing hormone-releasing hormone agonists and antiandrogens is recommended to mitigate pubic arch interference. A 4-month course of ADT will result in an average prostate volume reduction of 30%.[39–41] Ultimately, the decision to proceed with

Table 2
Absolute and relative contraindications for low dose rate prostate brachytherapy According to the American Brachytherapy Society Consensus Guidelines

Absolute contraindications	Relative contraindications
Limited life expectancy	Inflammatory bowel disease
Unacceptable operative risks	History of prior pelvic radiation therapy
Ataxia telangiectasia	Large median lobe
Presence of distant metastasis	Prostate gland size >60 cm^3 at the time of implantation
Absence of a rectum which preclude transrectal ultrasound	Poor urinary function, typically defined by an International Prostate Symptom Score of >20
Large transurethral resection of the prostate defects that preclude seed placement and acceptable dosimetry	

LDR prostate brachytherapy should be undertaken after careful review of each patient and only after obtaining informed consent. The factors that determine brachytherapy candidacy often vary between individual physicians and are often guided by practitioner experience, skill, and training.

High Dose Rate Brachytherapy

Modern HDR prostate brachytherapy, defined as treatment using a radionuclide with a calculated delivery rate of 12 Gy or greater per hour, emerged in the early 1990s as a novel and promising tool for the treatment of prostate cancer.[19,42] Unlike LDR brachytherapy sources, which remain permanently implanted into the prostate, HDR sources are inserted temporarily into hollow needle catheters before being removed. Depending on the strength of the source being used and the dose prescribed, the radiation treatment is often delivered in 15 to 30 minutes. Nearly all modern prostate HDR brachytherapy treatments are performed using the radionuclide iridium-192 (^{192}Ir). ^{192}Ir has a half-life of 73.8 days and emits photons with an average energy of 380 keV, primarily via beta minus decay. Commercially available ^{192}Ir sources are typically small (eg, $\sim$5 mm in length and <1 mm in diameter) and are normally housed within a shielded robotic afterloader that also serves as the control mechanism for their deployment to and retrieval from catheters.[43] One advantage provided by HDR brachytherapy is that a single source can be used for multiple treatments, across multiple tumor types such as breast and gynecologic malignancies, during its 90- to 120-day practical lifetime. Whereas the use of a remotely controlled radionuclide source delivery afterloader results in essentially no radiation exposure to staff with HDR brachytherapy, the absolute advantage in exposure over manually loaded LDR brachytherapy is insignificant.[44] HDR brachytherapy does typically require more capital equipment costs upfront than LDR brachytherapy given the need to obtain an afterloader and remote control panel. Furthermore, the recurring costs of replacing the ^{192}Ir source multiple times per year must be justified by adequate clinical volume. An additional consideration for HDR brachytherapy is the need for significantly greater room and storage area shielding than is required for most LDR sources.[45]

Patient selection criteria for consideration of prostate HDR brachytherapy are very similar to those for LDR prostate brachytherapy. ABS consensus guidelines are available for HDR prostate brachytherapy and list absolute contraindications of preexisting rectal fistula, medically unsuited for anesthesia, and no proof of other major malignancy.[46] According to the European Society for Therapeutic Radiology and Oncology, additional factors that should be evaluated on an individual patient basis to determine candidacy for HDR prostate brachytherapy include prior pelvic radiation or surgery, inflammatory bowel disease, previous urethral procedures, urinary function, and prostate volume.[47]

Consideration of brachytherapy according to prostate cancer risk group stratification

Although the American Joint Commission Cancer staging guidelines have long been used to stage prostate cancer patients for prognostic and treatment considerations based on pathologic and radiographic findings, risk group stratification has emerged as a means to use clinically available data for classification of newly diagnosed patients.[48–50] A number of organizations, including the American Urologic Association, European Association of Urology, NCCN, and European Society for Medical Oncology have published risk group stratification parameters that divide patient into either low-, intermediate-, or high-risk categories based on clinical tumor classification (T stage), pretreatment prostate-specific antigen levels, and Gleason Score grade.[2,51–53] Both the ABS and European Society for Therapeutic Radiology and Oncology consensus guidelines for LDR and HDR brachytherapy provide guidance with regard to the appropriateness of brachytherapy for men with prostate cancer according to their clinical risk group.[21,28,46,47] However, these guidelines do also caution that recommendations are limited by a lack of level I evidence guiding patient selection. It should be emphasized that the existing literature reporting clinical outcomes for prostate brachytherapy are primarily institutional reports with heterogeneous inclusion criteria and methodologies.

In men with low-risk disease, there is universal consensus that brachytherapy alone is an excellent treatment modality for men undergoing LDR brachytherapy and those not pursuing active surveillance. In patients with intermediate risk factors, there remains differing perspectives whether brachytherapy is suitable as a stand-alone treatment, or should only be considered when used in combination with EBRT or ADT. This concern stems from the fact that certain patients with intermediate-risk prostate cancer will likely harbor clinically occult tumor extraprostatic disease, such as extraprostatic extension, seminal vesicle invasion, or lymph node metastases, which may be treated Inadequately with brachytherapy alone.[54,55] Detailed reviews of pathologic prostatectomy specimens has shown that radial extension of extraprostatic tumor rarely exceeds 5 mm, and thus should be adequately treated by brachytherapy treatments incorporating an appropriate planning margin.[21,56–59] Some studies have suggested that patients with more concerning intermediate risk factors, often termed "unfavorable intermediate risk," have a poorer prognosis when treated with brachytherapy alone.[60,61] However, the addition of supplemental EBRT in intermediate-risk prostate cancer has not yet been proven to improve outcomes. Further study is needed to elucidate if there are subsets of intermediate risk patients that derive benefit from the addition other treatment modalities to brachytherapy for definitive management. Men with high-risk prostate cancer have the poorest prognosis and seem to benefit from the use of multimodality therapy given their risk of non–organ-confined disease. Thus, brachytherapy is only recommended as a boost to EBRT for these patients. However, the importance of brachytherapy as a means to provide dose escalation and improve local control in high-risk prostate cancer should not be discounted, because its incorporation in multimodal therapy has been shown to improve outcomes compared with EBRT or surgery-based strategies.[62,63]

Clinical Outcomes of Prostate Cancer

Brachytherapy alone

Table 3 lists the pertinent details and clinical outcomes from selected published studies of both LDR and HDR monotherapy for the treatment of men with prostate cancer. These data clearly demonstrate that long-term prostate-specific antigen control exceeding 82% can be expected with the use of brachytherapy alone for men with low-risk prostate cancer, whereas biochemical control rates of 70% to 89% are typical in men with intermediate-risk disease. These outcomes compare very favorably to those seen in similar patients enrolled on contemporary studies assessing treatment with EBRT or radical prostatectomy.[62,64–66]

Outcomes for patients with high-risk disease treated with LDR monotherapy are expectedly less favorable, further supporting strong consideration for combination therapy (EBRT + brachytherapy) in this population. Although select institutional series shown in **Table 3** do show promising outcomes for HDR brachytherapy in high-risk patients, many did not meet the NCCN definition of high-risk disease and received prolonged ADT as a component of their treatment. ADT was used for a portion of men on the listed studies, either to induce prostate volume reduction or for oncologic benefit, and the results must be interpreted accordingly. Controversy currently exists

Table 3
Selected published studies of prostate brachytherapy

Study	Years of Treatment	Number of Patients	Risk Group (%)			Dose Prescription	Biochemical Control (%)		
			Low	Intermediate	High		Low	Intermediate	High
Low dose rate brachytherapy									
Kittel et al,[136] 2015	1996–2007	1989	61	30	5	144 Gy (^{125}I)	87 (10 y)	79 (10 y)	68 (5 y)
Funk et al,[137] 2015	1998–2013	966	71	29	—	145 Gy (^{125}I)	90 (10 y)	74 (10 y)	—
Tran et al,[138] 2013	2003–2007	615	—	100	—	145 Gy (^{125}I)	—	89 (5 y)	—
Sylvester et al,[139] 2011	1988–1992	215	74	21	5	144 Gy (^{125}I)	86 (15 y)	80 (15 y)	62 (15 y)
Henry et al,[140] 2010	1995–2004	1298	44	33	14	145 Gy (^{125}I)	86 (10 y)	77 (10 y)	61 (10 y)
Zelefsky et al,[141] 2007	1988–1998	2693	55	40	5	144 Gy (^{125}I), 130 Gy (^{103}Pd)	82 (8 y)	70 (8 y)	48 (8 y)
Guedea et al,[142] 2006	1998–2003	1050	64	28	6	145 Gy (^{125}I)	93 (3 y)	88 (3 y)	80 (3 y)
Grimm et al,[143] 2001	1988–1990	126	77	23	—	145 Gy (^{125}I)	87 (10 y)	79 (10 y)	—
Blasko et al,[144] 2000	1988–1995	230	45	46	9	115 Gy (^{103}Pd)	94 (5 y)	82 (5 y)	65 (5 y)
High dose rate brachytherapy									
Yoshioka et al,[145] 2016	1995–2012	190	—	42	58	45.5–54 Gy in 7–9 fractions	—	91 (8 y)	77 (8 y)
Jawad et al,[91] 2016	1999–2013	494	68	32	—	24–38 Gy in 2–4 fractions	97 (5 y)	88 (5 y)	—
Hauswald et al,[90] 2016	1996–2009	448	64	36	—	42–43.5 Gy in 6 fractions	99 (10 y)	95 (10 y)	—
Zamboglou et al,[93] 2013	2002–2009	718	55	25	20	34.5–38 Gy in 3–4 fractions	95 (5 y)	93 (5 y)	93 (5 y)
Rogers et al,[146] 2012	2001–2011	248	—	100	—	39 Gy in 6 fractions	—	94 (5 y)	—
Hoskin et al,[95] 2012	2003–2009	197	4	52	44	26–36 Gy in 2–4 fractions	—	99 (3 y)	91 (3 y)

regarding what role, if any, ADT plays in combination with brachytherapy for improving disease control in men with prostate cancer. Randomized studies are needed to clarify this question.[67,68] Although further controlled trials are needed, it is generally considered appropriate to incorporate ADT with brachytherapy and EBRT when they are used in concert for the management of high-risk prostate cancer.

Additionally, although these data show relative uniformity in the LDR prescription doses used, there is more variability in the HDR dose and fractionation schemes being delivered. The ABS consensus guidelines recognized the heterogeneity of reported treatment approaches and did not recommend any single dose fractionation schedule.[46] One negative aspect of HDR compared with LDR monotherapy is the requirement for 2 to 4 separate implants based on currently published dose fractionation schemes. Although many practitioners will deliver up to 4 fractions with a single implant by treating twice daily on consecutive days, the long-term safety and efficacy of a more convenient single implant fractionation scheme for monotherapy are currently limited.

Brachytherapy in combination with external beam radiation therapy

Treating prostate cancer patients with a combination of EBRT and brachytherapy is a strategy that has been used at many centers. Supplemental EBRT, typically given as a dose of 35 to 50 Gy over 3 to 5 weeks, in addition to brachytherapy, offers the ability to deliver an increased dose to the periprostatic regions, treat portions of the seminal vesicles outside of the implant volume, improve dose coverage in the setting of a technically inadequate implant, and radiate pelvic lymph nodes. Brachytherapy dose prescriptions used in combination with EBRT vary somewhat, but are typically 20% to 40% lower than those used for monotherapy. Retrospective studies have demonstrated that gastrointestinal (GI)/genitourinary (GU) toxicity rates and patient-reported quality of life are worsened in patients treated with both brachytherapy and EBRT compared with brachytherapy alone, although most of the observed increased toxicity is grade 2 or lower.[69–73] These results must be interpreted with some caution, because most patients did not receive modern EBRT or image guidance, both of which have been associated with a lower toxicity.[74,75]

As discussed, there remains controversy regarding the benefit of adding EBRT to high-quality brachytherapy in men with intermediate-risk prostate cancer. A large, retrospective study with detailed multivariable analyses showed that, when controlling for disease characteristics, supplemental EBRT did not improve biochemical control or cause-specific survival compared with brachytherapy alone.[76] This question was further assessed in a randomized trial of men with primarily intermediate risk disease and compared ^{103}Pd monotherapy (125 Gy) with ^{103}Pd (115 Gy) plus 20 Gy EBRT.[77] With 8 years of follow-up, there was no difference in biochemical failure (2.1% vs 3.6%), prostate cancer–specific mortality (0% vs 0%), or overall mortality (14.4% vs 16.1%) between the groups. Although the supplemental EBRT dose in this trial was lower than typically used, its use was justified by a preceding randomized trial that had shown no differences in outcomes when comparing supplemental doses of 20 Gy EBRT with 44 Gy EBRT.[78] The recently reported initial findings of RTOG 0232, a phase III randomized trial comparing brachytherapy alone to brachytherapy plus EBRT, provide the strongest evidence to date in this setting.[79] This study further demonstrated that in a population of patients with mostly favorable intermediate risk prostate cancer, supplemental EBRT did not improve progression-free survival with 5 years of follow-up, but did increase the risk of late grade 3 or higher toxicity. Thus, there are no data to date demonstrating clear clinical improvement for combination therapy in men with intermediate risk prostate cancer, although subgroup analyses from RTOG 0232 will provide insight regarding whether benefit is seen within any portion of this population.

In men with both intermediate- and high-risk prostate cancer, brachytherapy serves as a tool to provide dose escalation and overcome radiation insensitivity that may exist in some higher grade tumors.[80] Multiple, retrospective, institutional studies have demonstrated improved biochemical control outcomes when combining EBRT and brachytherapy compared with EBRT alone.[62,81–83] One published randomized clinical trial comparing EBRT with EBRT plus HDR boost has further supported improvements in biochemical control, without an impact on overall survival.[84] ASCENDE-RT (A multicenter, randomized trial of dose-escalated external beam radiation therapy [EBRT-B] versus low-dose-rate brachytherapy [LDR-B] for men with unfavorable-risk localized prostate cancer) recently reported in abstract form, is a phase III randomized, clinical trial of patients with intermediate and high-risk prostate treated with 12 months of ADT that compared EBRT (78 Gy) with EBRT (46 Gy) plus LDR boost (^{125}I, 115 Gy), with all patients receiving elective radiation to the pelvic lymph nodes.[85] Although biochemical control was improved significantly in the combination therapy arm (75% vs 86% at 7 years), no differences in prostate cancer–specific mortality or overall survival were noted. Longer term follow-up and further publications are needed to ascertain fully the benefits of a brachytherapy boost in select intermediate- and high-risk patients. Database analyses of larger patient populations powered to detect differences in relevant clinical endpoints have suggested that the addition of a brachytherapy boost may indeed translate into improved survival by reducing prostate cancer–related deaths, particularly in high-risk patients.[86,87] These results, although hypothesis generating, are limited by their observational nature. The optimal duration of ADT and the role of elective pelvic lymph radiation for patients receiving EBRT in combination with a brachytherapy boost remains uncertain. A currently accruing phase III trial (RTOG 0924 [Androgen Deprivation Therapy and High Dose Radiotherapy With or Without Whole-Pelvic Radiotherapy in Unfavorable Intermediate or Favorable High Risk Prostate Cancer: A Phase III Randomized Trial]) that randomizes men with intermediate and high-risk prostate to high-dose radiation therapy with or without pelvic lymph node radiation allows either HDR or LDR brachytherapy boost, as well as variable durations of ADT at the physician's discretion. Results from this study should provide additional data relating to these important questions.

Brachytherapy Toxicities and Quality of Life Impacts

As with any definitive treatment for prostate cancer, it is important for both the clinician and patient to consider the potential toxicities of brachytherapy before proceeding. In appropriately selected patients, periprocedural adverse effects are relatively uncommon (<5%), but can include infection, bleeding, anesthesia complications, and temporary postimplant bladder outlet obstruction requiring catheterization.[88,89] Owing to the proximity of the bladder and rectum, GU and GI toxicities are the primary adverse effects reported with any radiation treatment for prostate cancer, including brachytherapy. Irritative voiding symptoms, such as frequency, urgency, dysuria, and nocturia, represent the primary manifestation of acute GU toxicity from brachytherapy. Late GU effects are less common, but can include a higher prevalence of obstructive symptoms such as stricture and incomplete emptying. Large, retrospective series have shown that for both HDR and LDR brachytherapy rates of grades 2 and 3 toxicity range from 7% to 30% and 3% to 10%, respectively.[90–96] The time course for development and resolution of urinary symptoms after brachytherapy differs based on the dose delivery rate used. Expectedly, patients treated with HDR or ^{103}Pd brachytherapy tend to have an earlier peak in International Prostate Symptom Scores (3–6 weeks) than those treated with ^{125}I (2–5 months), followed by a more rapid return to baseline urinary function.[25,97–99] GI toxicities generally occur at a lower frequency after prostate brachytherapy than those reported in pre-IMRT EBRT series and primarily manifest themselves as increased bowel frequency in the acute phase. Grades 2 and 3 rectal toxicity rates range from 5% to 10% and 1% to 5%, respectively, in the literature.[100–104] Grade 4 GI or GU toxicities are rare after brachytherapy (0%–2%) and are typically limited to ulceration and/or hemorrhage of the bladder or rectum.

Although physician-reported toxicities represent an important tool for assessing the safety of interventions, including brachytherapy, patient-reported outcomes serve as a more reliable metric to document treatment effects. This information can be especially helpful when counseling men about treatment options for prostate cancer. Comparative studies of men with prostate cancer treated with brachytherapy, EBRT, or radical prostatectomy have been published to quantify differences in patient-reported outcomes between treatment modalities.[105,106] In general, these studies show that brachytherapy, like EBRT, provides superior preservation of continence and erectile function relative to radical prostatectomy, while being associated with more prominent irritative bladder and bowel symptoms. The favorable quality of life profile for brachytherapy is further supported by patient-reported outcomes from the Canadian SPIRIT trial (Surgical Prostatectomy versus Interstitial Radiation Intervention Trial). This randomized study was intended to assess prostate cancer outcomes for LDR brachytherapy compared with radical prostatectomy, but failed to meet accrual goals. However, 168 patients who were randomized to either treatment modality before trial closure completed quality of life assessments. Although no differences were noted in bowel and hormonal domains, brachytherapy was associated with significant improvements in the urinary domain, the sexual domain, and patient satisfaction scores.[107]

Although exposure to ionizing radiation can result in development of second malignancies (SM), the risk of carcinogenesis after prostate brachytherapy is uncertain. A recent metaanalysis found that exposure to therapeutic radiation for the treatment of prostate cancer was associated with a significantly increased risk of bladder, colon, and rectal cancer, although absolute rates of these malignancies were very low.[108] However, compared with EBRT, brachytherapy reduces integral radiation dose to nearby tissues at risk, and thus theoretically should result in lower rates of SM.[109] Large retrospective studies with long-term follow-up have shown no difference in SM rates when comparing patients treated with brachytherapy and radical prostatectomy.[110,111] Taken together, these data provide evidence that SM risk should not be a significant concern after brachytherapy for the treatment of prostate cancer.

When considering LDR brachytherapy, many patients and family members express concerns regarding radiation exposure risks to those who are in contact with the patient after implantation. Direct measurements with radiation monitors have shown that radiation exposure to family members after an ^{125}I or ^{103}Pd implant are below the limit for the general public established by the United State Nuclear Regulatory Commission (<0.5 mSv per year).[112,113] Despite these reassuring data, patients are typically given instructions to minimize prolonged contact with those most at risk from radiation exposure (children, pregnant women) as a further assurance that unnecessary exposure is avoided.

Brachytherapy as a Salvage Treatment

Both LDR and HDR brachytherapy have been used as a salvage treatment for local failure after primary definitive treatment for prostate cancer. Although the use of salvage brachytherapy is relatively uncommon, the largest experience with the longest follow-up exists for LDR brachytherapy after previous EBRT.[114–117] More recent studies have demonstrated HDR salvage brachytherapy is also a very viable alternative treatment strategy.[118,119] Although there is significant variation in the methods of these reports, most use a brachytherapy dose prescription that is similar to those used in the primary treatment setting (LDR = 90–145 Gy, HDR = 30–36 Gy in 3–6 fractions). Although most reports in the salvage setting have treated the entire prostate gland, some report partial gland treatments.[120,121] Biochemical control rates from these series are 34% to 89.5% at timeframes ranging from 3 to 10 years. Generally, toxicities in the salvage setting have been reasonable, although the risk of more severe (grade 3 or greater) GU or GI adverse effects seems to be significantly greater than that seen in the primary treatment setting.[122] Thus, careful patient selection and appropriate informed consent regarding the risks and benefits are important aspects when considering salvage brachytherapy.

There are some reports documenting the use of salvage brachytherapy for treating local recurrences after radical prostatectomy.[123–125] Although outcomes from these limited series are reasonable, it is unclear if brachytherapy as a postprostatectomy salvage therapy confers any advantages over salvage EBRT, which is considered the preferred treatment and has been endorsed in a prominent multidisciplinary consensus statement.[126]

Recent Developments and Future Directions

Current and future research will focus on methods designed to improve the safety and efficacy of brachytherapy for the treatment of prostate cancer. One recent development that is being adopted into clinical practice quickly is a commercially available absorbable retroprostatic spacer (SpaceOAR, Augmenix, Waltham, MA). This polyethylene glycol-based polymer is injected transperineally into the retroprostatic space anterior to Denonvilliers' fascia in an outpatient procedure and is resorbed by the body within 4 to 6 months. A prospective study of this product demonstrated a 99% placement success rate resulting in an average posterior displacement of the rectum of 1 cm from the prostate (**Fig. 3**).[127] Early experiences with the spacer in conjunction with LDR and HDR brachytherapy have yielded favorable clinical and dosimetric results that may lead to more widespread adoption of this tool.[128,129]

Multiparametric MRI (mpMRI) is being used increasingly for the diagnosis and assessment of disease burden in patients with prostate cancer.[130] The detailed image resolution afforded by mpMRI has been shown to be able to predict the presence of clinically occult extraprostatic extension, which may help aid in patient selection for

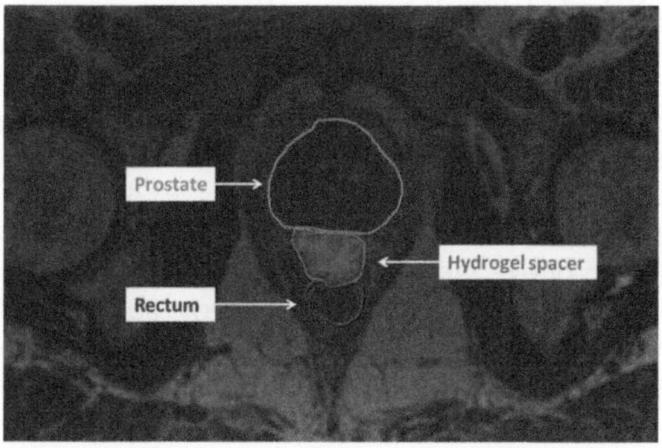

Fig. 3. T2-weighted axial MRI scan demonstrating retroprostatic spacer (SpaceOAR) placement. The image demonstrates that T2-hyperintense spacer (*blue*) displaces the rectum (*red*) approximately 1.5 cm posteriorly from the prostate (*orange*) allowing decreased radiation dosing the anterior wall of the rectum.

brachytherapy monotherapy or with supplement EBRT.[131] Further interest has emerged in using brachytherapy to provide a focal boost to mpMRI-detected dominant intraprostatic lesions. Both LDR and HDR brachytherapy possess the ability to deliver highly localized regions of dose escalation to areas of concern seen on mpMRI.[132,133] These approaches are considered typically with simultaneous treatment of the whole prostate with standard doses. However, there has also been some interest in focal treatments, directed only at the mpMRI-defined tumor and without concurrent whole gland dosing, as means to improve toxicity rates by decreasing the dose delivered to the bladder and rectum.[134] One prospective, non-randomized study has reported favorable early outcomes for patients receiving LDR brachytherapy to the peripheral zone of the prostate only.[135] However, at this time, partial gland treatments should be considered investigational and should only be pursued within the context of a clinical study.

SUMMARY

Brachytherapy represents an effective treatment option to be considered for many men with prostate cancer. Both LDR and HDR treatments have demonstrated excellent outcomes confirmed by up to 15 years of follow-up for treating men in all risk groups of localized prostate cancer. Ongoing research will continue to further define the best methods to integrate and optimize brachytherapy in the always evolving treatment of men with prostate cancer. It is important for clinicians to discuss the safety, efficacy, and convenience of brachytherapy with their patients when addressing treatment options for prostate cancer.

REFERENCES

1. Siegel RL, Miller KD, Jemal A. Cancer statistics, 2016. CA Cancer J Clin 2016; 66(1):7–30.
2. Network NCC. NCCN Clinical Practice Guidelines-Prostate Cancer (Version 3.2016). 2016. Available at: https://www.nccn.org/professionals/physician_gls/pdf/prostate.pdf. Accessed August 8, 2016.
3. Hamdy FC, Donovan JL, Lane JA, et al. 10-year outcomes after monitoring, surgery, or radiotherapy for localized prostate cancer. N Engl J Med 2016;375(15): 1415–24.
4. Holm HH. The history of interstitial brachytherapy of prostatic cancer. Semin Surg Oncol 1997;13(6):431–7.
5. Barringer BS. Radium in the treatment of carcinoma of the bladder and prostate. JAMA 1916;67:1442–5.
6. Rivard MJ, Coursey BM, DeWerd LA, et al. Update of AAPM task group no. 43 report: a revised AAPM protocol for brachytherapy dose calculations. Med Phys 2004;31(3):633–74.
7. Spratt DE, Scala LM, Folkert M, et al. A comparative dosimetric analysis of virtual stereotactic body radiotherapy to high-dose-rate monotherapy for intermediate-risk prostate cancer. Brachytherapy. 2013;12(5):428–33.
8. Georg D, Hopfgartner J, Gora J, et al. Dosimetric considerations to determine the optimal technique for localized prostate cancer among external photon, proton, or carbon-ion therapy and high-dose-rate or low-dose-rate brachytherapy. Int J Radiat Oncol Biol Phys 2014;88(3):715–22.
9. Pollack A, Zagars GK, Starkschall G, et al. Prostate cancer radiation dose response: results of the M. D. Anderson phase III randomized trial. Int J Radiat Oncol Biol Phys 2002;53(5):1097–105.

10. Dearnaley DP, Sydes MR, Graham JD, et al. Escalated-dose versus standard-dose conformal radiotherapy in prostate cancer: first results from the MRC RT01 randomised controlled trial. Lancet Oncol 2007;8(6):475–87.
11. Zietman AL, Bae K, Slater JD, et al. Randomized trial comparing conventional-dose with high-dose conformal radiation therapy in early-stage adenocarcinoma of the prostate: long-term results from Proton Radiation Oncology Group/American College of Radiology 95-09. J Clin Oncol 2010;28(7):1106–11.
12. Peeters ST, Heemsbergen WD, Koper PC, et al. Dose-response in radiotherapy for localized prostate cancer: results of the Dutch multicenter randomized phase III trial comparing 68 Gy of radiotherapy with 78 Gy. J Clin Oncol 2006;24(13):1990–6.
13. Jani AB, Hand CM, Lujan AE, et al. Biological effective dose for comparison and combination of external beam and low-dose rate interstitial brachytherapy prostate cancer treatment plans. Med Dosim 2004;29(1):42–8.
14. Marshall RA, Buckstein M, Stone NN, et al. Treatment outcomes and morbidity following definitive brachytherapy with or without external beam radiation for the treatment of localized prostate cancer: 20-year experience at Mount Sinai Medical Center. Urol Oncol 2014;32(1):38.e1-7.
15. Herstein A, Wallner K, Merrick G, et al. There is a wide range of predictive dosimetric factors for I-125 and Pd-103 prostate brachytherapy. Am J Clin Oncol 2008;31(1):6–10.
16. Whitmore WF Jr, Hilaris B, Grabstald H. Retropubic implantation to iodine 125 in the treatment of prostatic cancer. J Urol 1972;108(6):918–20.
17. Nag S, Ciezki JP, Cormack R, et al. Intraoperative planning and evaluation of permanent prostate brachytherapy: report of the American Brachytherapy Society. Int J Radiat Oncol Biol Phys 2001;51(5):1422–30.
18. Shah JN, Wuu CS, Katz AE, et al. Improved biochemical control and clinical disease-free survival with intraoperative versus preoperative preplanning for transperineal interstitial permanent prostate brachytherapy. Cancer J 2006;12(4):289–97.
19. International Commission on Radiological Units and Measurements. Dose and volume specification for reporting intracavitary therapy in gynecology. Bethesda (MD): ICRU; 1985.
20. Charyulu KK. Transperineal interstitial implantation of prostate cancer: a new method. Int J Radiat Oncol Biol Phys 1980;6(9):1261–6.
21. Davis BJ, Horwitz EM, Lee WR, et al. American Brachytherapy Society consensus guidelines for transrectal ultrasound-guided permanent prostate brachytherapy. Brachytherapy 2012;11(1):6–19.
22. King CR. LDR vs. HDR brachytherapy for localized prostate cancer: the view from radiobiological models. Brachytherapy 2002;1(4):219–26.
23. Ghilezan M. Role of high dose rate brachytherapy in the treatment of prostate cancer. Cancer Radiother 2012;16(5–6):418–22.
24. Wallner K, Merrick G, True L, et al. 125I versus 103Pd for low-risk prostate cancer: preliminary PSA outcomes from a prospective randomized multicenter trial. Int J Radiat Oncol Biol Phys 2003;57(5):1297–303.
25. Kollmeier MA, Pei X, Algur E, et al. A comparison of the impact of isotope ((125)I vs. (103)Pd) on toxicity and biochemical outcome after interstitial brachytherapy and external beam radiation therapy for clinically localized prostate cancer. Brachytherapy 2012;11(4):271–6.

26. Peschel RE, Colberg JW, Chen Z, et al. Iodine 125 versus palladium 103 implants for prostate cancer: clinical outcomes and complications. Cancer J 2004;10(3):170–4.
27. Rosenthal SA, Bittner NH, Beyer DC, et al. American Society for Radiation Oncology (ASTRO) and American College of Radiology (ACR) practice guideline for the transperineal permanent brachytherapy of prostate cancer. Int J Radiat Oncol Biol Phys 2011;79(2):335–41.
28. Ash D, Flynn A, Battermann J, et al. ESTRO/EAU/EORTC recommendations on permanent seed implantation for localized prostate cancer. Radiother Oncol 2000;57(3):315–21.
29. Crook J, McLean M, Catton C, et al. Factors influencing risk of acute urinary retention after TRUS-guided permanent prostate seed implantation. Int J Radiat Oncol Biol Phys 2002;52(2):453–60.
30. Terk MD, Stock RG, Stone NN. Identification of patients at increased risk for prolonged urinary retention following radioactive seed implantation of the prostate. J Urol 1998;160(4):1379–82.
31. Martens C, Pond G, Webster D, et al. Relationship of the International Prostate Symptom score with urinary flow studies, and catheterization rates following 125I prostate brachytherapy. Brachytherapy 2006;5(1):9–13.
32. Tanaka N, Asakawa I, Anai S, et al. Periodical assessment of genitourinary and gastrointestinal toxicity in patients who underwent prostate low-dose-rate brachytherapy. Radiat Oncol 2013;8:25.
33. Gutman S, Merrick GS, Butler WM, et al. Severity categories of the International Prostate Symptom Score before, and urinary morbidity after, permanent prostate brachytherapy. BJU Int 2006;97(1):62–8.
34. Wallner K, Lee H, Wasserman S, et al. Low risk of urinary incontinence following prostate brachytherapy in patients with a prior transurethral prostate resection. Int J Radiat Oncol Biol Phys 1997;37(3):565–9.
35. Moran BJ, Stutz MA, Gurel MH. Prostate brachytherapy can be performed in selected patients after transurethral resection of the prostate. Int J Radiat Oncol Biol Phys 2004;59(2):392–6.
36. Mark R, Akins S, Manning M, et al. Previous transurethral resection of the prostate (TURP) is not a contraindication for interstitial high dose rate (HDR) brachytherapy for prostate cancer. Am J Clin Oncol 2011;34(2):205.
37. Ragde H, Blasko JC, Grimm PD, et al. Interstitial iodine-125 radiation without adjuvant therapy in the treatment of clinically localized prostate carcinoma. Cancer 1997;80(3):442–53.
38. Fukada J, Shigematsu N, Nakashima J, et al. Predicting pubic arch interference in prostate brachytherapy on transrectal ultrasonography-computed tomography fusion images. J Radiat Res 2012;53(5):753–9.
39. Solhjem MC, Davis BJ, Pisansky TM, et al. Prostate volume before and after permanent prostate brachytherapy in patients receiving neoadjuvant androgen suppression. Cancer J 2004;10(6):343–8.
40. Kucway R, Vicini F, Huang R, et al. Prostate volume reduction with androgen deprivation therapy before interstitial brachytherapy. J Urol 2002;167(6):2443–7.
41. Petit JH, Gluck C, Kiger WS 3rd, et al. Bicalutamide alone prior to brachytherapy achieves cytoreduction that is similar to luteinizing hormone-releasing hormone analogues with less patient-reported morbidity. Urol Oncol 2008;26(4):372–7.
42. Syed AM, Puthawala A, Austin P, et al. Temporary iridium-192 implant in the management of carcinoma of the prostate. Cancer 1992;69(10):2515–24.

43. Angelopoulos A, Baras P, Sakelliou L, et al. Monte Carlo dosimetry of a new 192Ir high dose rate brachytherapy source. Med Phys 2000;27(11):2521–7.
44. Schwartz DJ, Davis BJ, Vetter RJ, et al. Radiation exposure to operating room personnel during transperineal interstitial permanent prostate brachytherapy. Brachytherapy 2003;2(2):98–102.
45. Nag S, Dobelbower R, Glasgow G, et al. Inter-society standards for the performance of brachytherapy: a joint report from ABS, ACMP and ACRO. Crit Rev Oncol Hematol 2003;48(1):1–17.
46. Yamada Y, Rogers L, Demanes DJ, et al. American Brachytherapy Society consensus guidelines for high-dose-rate prostate brachytherapy. Brachytherapy 2012;11(1):20–32.
47. Hoskin PJ, Colombo A, Henry A, et al. GEC/ESTRO recommendations on high dose rate afterloading brachytherapy for localised prostate cancer: an update. Radiother Oncol 2013;107(3):325–32.
48. Edge SB, Compton CC. The American Joint Committee on Cancer: the 7th edition of the AJCC cancer staging manual and the future of TNM. Ann Surg Oncol 2010;17(6):1471–4.
49. Rodrigues G, Warde P, Pickles T, et al. Pre-treatment risk stratification of prostate cancer patients: a critical review. Can Urol Assoc J 2012;6(2):121–7.
50. Roach M 3rd, Weinberg V, Sandler H, et al. Staging for prostate cancer: time to incorporate pretreatment prostate-specific antigen and Gleason score? Cancer 2007;109(2):213–20.
51. Thompson I, Thrasher JB, Aus G, et al. Guideline for the management of clinically localized prostate cancer: 2007 update. J Urol 2007;177(6):2106–31.
52. Heidenreich A, Aus G, Bolla M, et al. EAU guidelines on prostate cancer. Eur Urol 2008;53(1):68–80.
53. Horwich A, Parker C, Bangma C, et al. Prostate cancer: ESMO clinical practice guidelines for diagnosis, treatment and follow-up. Ann Oncol 2010;21(Suppl 5): v129–33.
54. Eifler JB, Feng Z, Lin BM, et al. An updated prostate cancer staging nomogram (Partin tables) based on cases from 2006 to 2011. BJU Int 2013;111(1):22–9.
55. Pisansky TM, Blute ML, Hillman DW, et al. The relevance of prostatectomy findings for brachytherapy selection in patients with localized prostate carcinoma. Cancer 2002;95(3):513–9.
56. Davis BJ, Pisansky TM, Wilson TM, et al. The radial distance of extraprostatic extension of prostate carcinoma: implications for prostate brachytherapy. Cancer 1999;85(12):2630–7.
57. Butzbach D, Waterman FM, Dicker AP. Can extraprostatic extension be treated by prostate brachytherapy? An analysis based on postimplant dosimetry. Int J Radiat Oncol Biol Phys 2001;51(5):1196–9.
58. Davis BJ, Haddock MG, Wilson TM, et al. Treatment of extraprostatic cancer in clinically organ-confined prostate cancer by permanent interstitial brachytherapy: is extraprostatic seed placement necessary? Tech Urol 2000;6(2):70–7.
59. Schwartz DJ, Sengupta S, Hillman DW, et al. Prediction of radial distance of extraprostatic extension from pretherapy factors. Int J Radiat Oncol Biol Phys 2007;69(2):411–8.
60. Keane FK, Chen MH, Zhang D, et al. Androgen deprivation therapy and the risk of death from prostate cancer among men with favorable or unfavorable intermediate-risk disease. Cancer 2015;121(16):2713–9.

61. Merrick GS, Butler WM, Galbreath RW, et al. Stratification of brachytherapy-treated intermediate-risk prostate cancer patients into favorable and unfavorable cohorts. J Contemp Brachytherapy 2015;7(6):430–6.
62. Grimm P, Billiet I, Bostwick D, et al. Comparative analysis of prostate-specific antigen free survival outcomes for patients with low, intermediate and high risk prostate cancer treatment by radical therapy. Results from the Prostate Cancer Results Study Group. BJU Int 2012;109(Suppl 1):22–9.
63. Kishan AU, Shaikh T, Wang PC, et al. Clinical outcomes for patients with Gleason score 9-10 prostate adenocarcinoma treated with radiotherapy or radical prostatectomy: a multi-institutional comparative analysis. Eur Urol 2016. [Epub ahead of print].
64. Lee WR, Dignam JJ, Amin MB, et al. Randomized phase III noninferiority study comparing two radiotherapy fractionation schedules in patients with low-risk prostate cancer. J Clin Oncol 2016;34(20):2325–32.
65. Pollack A, Walker G, Horwitz EM, et al. Randomized trial of hypofractionated external-beam radiotherapy for prostate cancer. J Clin Oncol 2013;31(31): 3860–8.
66. Morgan TM, Meng MV, Cooperberg MR, et al. A risk-adjusted definition of biochemical recurrence after radical prostatectomy. Prostate Cancer Prostatic Dis 2014;17(2):174–9.
67. Rosenberg JE, Chen MH, Nguyen PL, et al. Hormonal therapy or external-beam radiation with brachytherapy and the risk of death from prostate cancer in men with intermediate risk prostate cancer. Clin Genitourin Cancer 2012;10(1):21–5.
68. Beyer DC, McKeough T, Thomas T. Impact of short course hormonal therapy on overall and cancer specific survival after permanent prostate brachytherapy. Int J Radiat Oncol Biol Phys 2005;61(5):1299–305.
69. Merrick GS, Butler WM, Wallner KE, et al. Long-term urinary quality of life after permanent prostate brachytherapy. Int J Radiat Oncol Biol Phys 2003;56(2): 454–61.
70. Merrick GS, Butler WM, Wallner KE, et al. Late rectal function after prostate brachytherapy. Int J Radiat Oncol Biol Phys 2003;57(1):42–8.
71. Krupski T, Petroni GR, Bissonette EA, et al. Quality-of-life comparison of radical prostatectomy and interstitial brachytherapy in the treatment of clinically localized prostate cancer. Urology 2000;55(5):736–42.
72. Yorozu A, Kuroiwa N, Takahashi A, et al. Permanent prostate brachytherapy with or without supplemental external beam radiotherapy as practiced in Japan: outcomes of 1300 patients. Brachytherapy 2015;14(2):111–7.
73. Serrano N, Moghanaki D, Asher D, et al. Comparative study of late rectal toxicity in prostate cancer patients treated with low-dose-rate brachytherapy: With or without supplemental external beam radiotherapy. Brachytherapy 2016;15(4): 435–41.
74. Michalski JM, Yan Y, Watkins-Bruner D, et al. Preliminary toxicity analysis of 3-dimensional conformal radiation therapy versus intensity modulated radiation therapy on the high-dose arm of the Radiation Therapy Oncology Group 0126 prostate cancer trial. Int J Radiat Oncol Biol Phys 2013;87(5):932–8.
75. Zelefsky MJ, Kollmeier M, Cox B, et al. Improved clinical outcomes with high-dose image guided radiotherapy compared with non-IGRT for the treatment of clinically localized prostate cancer. Int J Radiat Oncol Biol Phys 2012;84(1): 125–9.

76. Taira AV, Merrick GS, Butler WM, et al. Long-term outcome for clinically localized prostate cancer treated with permanent interstitial brachytherapy. Int J Radiat Oncol Biol Phys 2011;79(5):1336–42.
77. Merrick GS, Wallner KE, Galbreath RW, et al. Is supplemental external beam radiation therapy necessary for patients with higher risk prostate cancer treated with 103Pd? Results of two prospective randomized trials. Brachytherapy 2015;14(5):677–85.
78. Merrick GS, Wallner KE, Butler WM, et al. 20 Gy versus 44 Gy of supplemental external beam radiotherapy with palladium-103 for patients with greater risk disease: results of a prospective randomized trial. Int J Radiat Oncol Biol Phys 2012;82(3):e449–455.
79. Prestidge BR, Winter K, Sanda MG, et al. Initial report of NRG Oncology/RTOG 0232: a phase 3 study comparing combined external beam radiation and transperineal interstitial permanent brachytherapy with brachytherapy alone for selected patients with intermediate-risk prostatic carcinoma. Int J Radiat Oncol Biol Phys 2016;96(2S):S4.
80. Coen JJ, Zietman AL, Thakral H, et al. Radical radiation for localized prostate cancer: local persistence of disease results in a late wave of metastases. J Clin Oncol 2002;20(15):3199–205.
81. Spratt DE, Zumsteg ZS, Ghadjar P, et al. Comparison of high-dose (86.4 Gy) IMRT vs combined brachytherapy plus IMRT for intermediate-risk prostate cancer. BJU Int 2014;114(3):360–7.
82. Smith GD, Pickles T, Crook J, et al. Brachytherapy improves biochemical failure-free survival in low- and intermediate-risk prostate cancer compared with conventionally fractionated external beam radiation therapy: a propensity score matched analysis. Int J Radiat Oncol Biol Phys 2015;91(3):505–16.
83. Shilkrut M, Merrick GS, McLaughlin PW, et al. The addition of low-dose-rate brachytherapy and androgen-deprivation therapy decreases biochemical failure and prostate cancer death compared with dose-escalated external-beam radiation therapy for high-risk prostate cancer. Cancer 2013;119(3):681–90.
84. Hoskin PJ, Rojas AM, Bownes PJ, et al. Randomised trial of external beam radiotherapy alone or combined with high-dose-rate brachytherapy boost for localised prostate cancer. Radiother Oncol 2012;103(2):217–22.
85. Morris WJ, Tyldesley S, Pai HH, et al. ASCENDE-RT*: a multicenter, randomized trial of dose-escalated external beam radiation therapy (EBRT-B) versus low-dose-rate brachytherapy (LDR-B) for men with unfavorable-risk localized prostate cancer. J Clin Oncol 2015;33(7):Suppl 7, Abstract 3.
86. Xiang M, Nguyen PL. Significant association of brachytherapy boost with reduced prostate cancer-specific mortality in contemporary patients with localized, unfavorable-risk prostate cancer. Brachytherapy 2015;14(6):773–80.
87. Stone NN, Potters L, Davis BJ, et al. Multicenter analysis of effect of high biologic effective dose on biochemical failure and survival outcomes in patients with Gleason score 7-10 prostate cancer treated with permanent prostate brachytherapy. Int J Radiat Oncol Biol Phys 2009;73(2):341–6.
88. Wallner K, Roy J, Harrison L. Low risk of perioperative infection without prophylactic antibiotics for transperineal prostate brachytherapy. Int J Radiat Oncol Biol Phys 1996;36(3):681–3.
89. Mabjeesh NJ, Chen J, Stenger A, et al. Preimplant predictive factors of urinary retention after iodine 125 prostate brachytherapy. Urology 2007;70(3):548–53.

90. Hauswald H, Kamrava MR, Fallon JM, et al. High-dose-rate monotherapy for localized prostate cancer: 10-year results. Int J Radiat Oncol Biol Phys 2016; 94(4):667–74.
91. Jawad MS, Dilworth JT, Gustafson GS, et al. Outcomes associated with 3 treatment schedules of high-dose-rate brachytherapy monotherapy for favorable-risk prostate cancer. Int J Radiat Oncol Biol Phys 2016;94(4):657–66.
92. Keyes M, Miller S, Moravan V, et al. Predictive factors for acute and late urinary toxicity after permanent prostate brachytherapy: long-term outcome in 712 consecutive patients. Int J Radiat Oncol Biol Phys 2009;73(4):1023–32.
93. Zamboglou N, Tselis N, Baltas D, et al. High-dose-rate interstitial brachytherapy as monotherapy for clinically localized prostate cancer: treatment evolution and mature results. Int J Radiat Oncol Biol Phys 2013;85(3):672–8.
94. Mohammed N, Kestin L, Ghilezan M, et al. Comparison of acute and late toxicities for three modern high-dose radiation treatment techniques for localized prostate cancer. Int J Radiat Oncol Biol Phys 2012;82(1):204–12.
95. Hoskin P, Rojas A, Lowe G, et al. High-dose-rate brachytherapy alone for localized prostate cancer in patients at moderate or high risk of biochemical recurrence. Int J Radiat Oncol Biol Phys 2012;82(4):1376–84.
96. Keyes M, Miller S, Pickles T, et al. Late urinary side effects 10 years after low-dose-rate prostate brachytherapy: population-based results from a multiphysician practice treating with a standardized protocol and uniform dosimetric goals. Int J Radiat Oncol Biol Phys 2014;90(3):570–8.
97. Ohashi T, Yorozu A, Saito S, et al. Urinary and rectal toxicity profiles after permanent iodine-125 implant brachytherapy in Japanese Men: Nationwide J-POPS multi-institutional prospective cohort study. Int J Radiat Oncol Biol Phys 2015; 93(1):141–9.
98. Strom TJ, Cruz AA, Figura NB, et al. Health-related quality-of-life changes due to high-dose-rate brachytherapy, low-dose-rate brachytherapy, or intensity-modulated radiation therapy for prostate cancer. Brachytherapy 2015;14(6): 818–25.
99. Crook J, Fleshner N, Roberts C, et al. Long-term urinary sequelae following 125iodine prostate brachytherapy. J Urol 2008;179(1):141–5 [discussion: 146].
100. Keyes M, Spadinger I, Liu M, et al. Rectal toxicity and rectal dosimetry in low-dose-rate (125)I permanent prostate implants: a long-term study in 1006 patients. Brachytherapy 2012;11(3):199–208.
101. Zelefsky MJ, Yamada Y, Cohen GN, et al. Five-year outcome of intraoperative conformal permanent I-125 interstitial implantation for patients with clinically localized prostate cancer. Int J Radiat Oncol Biol Phys 2007;67(1):65–70.
102. Gelblum DY, Potters L. Rectal complications associated with transperineal interstitial brachytherapy for prostate cancer. Int J Radiat Oncol Biol Phys 2000; 48(1):119–24.
103. Ghilezan M, Martinez A, Gustason G, et al. High-dose-rate brachytherapy as monotherapy delivered in two fractions within one day for favorable/intermediate-risk prostate cancer: preliminary toxicity data. Int J Radiat Oncol Biol Phys 2012;83(3):927–32.
104. Duchesne GM, Williams SG, Das R, et al. Patterns of toxicity following high-dose-rate brachytherapy boost for prostate cancer: mature prospective phase I/II study results. Radiother Oncol 2007;84(2):128–34.
105. Sanda MG, Dunn RL, Michalski J, et al. Quality of life and satisfaction with outcome among prostate-cancer survivors. N Engl J Med 2008;358(12): 1250–61.

106. Zelefsky MJ, Poon BY, Eastham J, et al. Longitudinal assessment of quality of life after surgery, conformal brachytherapy, and intensity-modulated radiation therapy for prostate cancer. Radiother Oncol 2016;118(1):85–91.
107. Crook JM, Gomez-Iturriaga A, Wallace K, et al. Comparison of health-related quality of life 5 years after SPIRIT: surgical prostatectomy versus interstitial radiation intervention trial. J Clin Oncol 2011;29(4):362–8.
108. Wallis CJ, Mahar AL, Choo R, et al. Second malignancies after radiotherapy for prostate cancer: systematic review and meta-analysis. BMJ 2016;352:i851.
109. Murray L, Mason J, Henry AM, et al. Modelling second malignancy risks from low dose rate and high dose rate brachytherapy as monotherapy for localised prostate cancer. Radiother Oncol 2016;120(2):293–9.
110. Hamilton SN, Tyldesley S, Hamm J, et al. Incidence of second malignancies in prostate cancer patients treated with low-dose-rate brachytherapy and radical prostatectomy. Int J Radiat Oncol Biol Phys 2014;90(4):934–41.
111. Hinnen KA, Schaapveld M, van Vulpen M, et al. Prostate brachytherapy and second primary cancer risk: a competitive risk analysis. J Clin Oncol 2011; 29(34):4510–5.
112. Michalski J, Mutic S, Eichling J, et al. Radiation exposure to family and household members after prostate brachytherapy. Int J Radiat Oncol Biol Phys 2003; 56(3):764–8.
113. Hanada T, Yorozu A, Shinya Y, et al. Prospective study of direct radiation exposure measurements for family members living with patients with prostate (125)I seed implantation: evidence of radiation safety. Brachytherapy 2016;15(4): 412–9.
114. Grado GL. Benefits of brachytherapy as salvage treatment for radiorecurrent localized prostate cancer. Urology 1999;54(2):204–7.
115. Aaronson DS, Yamasaki I, Gottschalk A, et al. Salvage permanent perineal radioactive-seed implantation for treating recurrence of localized prostate adenocarcinoma after external beam radiotherapy. BJU Int 2009;104(5):600–4.
116. Moman MR, van der Poel HG, Battermann JJ, et al. Treatment outcome and toxicity after salvage 125-I implantation for prostate cancer recurrences after primary 125-I implantation and external beam radiotherapy. Brachytherapy 2010;9(2):119–25.
117. Rose JN, Crook JM, Pickles T, et al. Salvage low-dose-rate permanent seed brachytherapy for locally recurrent prostate cancer: association between dose and late toxicity. Brachytherapy 2015;14(3):342–9.
118. Chen CP, Weinberg V, Shinohara K, et al. Salvage HDR brachytherapy for recurrent prostate cancer after previous definitive radiation therapy: 5-year outcomes. Int J Radiat Oncol Biol Phys 2013;86(2):324–9.
119. Wojcieszek P, Szlag M, Glowacki G, et al. Salvage high-dose-rate brachytherapy for locally recurrent prostate cancer after primary radiotherapy failure. Radiother Oncol 2016;119(3):405–10.
120. Nguyen PL, Chen MH, D'Amico AV, et al. Magnetic resonance image-guided salvage brachytherapy after radiation in select men who initially presented with favorable-risk prostate cancer: a prospective phase 2 study. Cancer 2007;110(7):1485–92.
121. Hsu CC, Hsu H, Pickett B, et al. Feasibility of MR imaging/MR spectroscopy-planned focal partial salvage permanent prostate implant (PPI) for localized recurrence after initial PPI for prostate cancer. Int J Radiat Oncol Biol Phys 2013;85(2):370–7.

122. Crehange G, Roach M 3rd, Martin E, et al. Salvage reirradiation for locoregional failure after radiation therapy for prostate cancer: who, when, where and how? Cancer Radiother 2014;18(5–6):524–34.
123. Strom TJ, Wilder RB, Fernandez DC, et al. High-dose-rate brachytherapy with or without intensity modulated radiation therapy as salvage treatment for an isolated, gross local recurrence of prostate cancer post-prostatectomy. Brachytherapy 2014;13(2):123–7.
124. Kumar AM, Smith KL, Reddy CA, et al. Safety and efficacy of salvage low-dose-rate brachytherapy for prostate bed recurrences following radical prostatectomy. J Contemp Brachytherapy 2015;7(4):241–6.
125. Traudt K, Ciezki J, Klein EA. Low-dose-rate brachytherapy as salvage treatment of local prostate cancer recurrence after radical prostatectomy. Urology 2011; 77(6):1416–9.
126. Valicenti RK, Thompson I Jr, Albertsen P, et al. Adjuvant and salvage radiation therapy after prostatectomy: American Society for Radiation Oncology/American Urological Association guidelines. Int J Radiat Oncol Biol Phys 2013; 86(5):822–8.
127. Mariados N, Sylvester J, Shah D, et al. Hydrogel spacer prospective multicenter randomized controlled pivotal trial: dosimetric and clinical effects of perirectal spacer application in men undergoing prostate image guided intensity modulated radiation therapy. Int J Radiat Oncol Biol Phys 2015;92(5):971–7.
128. Beydoun N, Bucci JA, Chin YS, et al. First report of transperineal polyethylene glycol hydrogel spacer use to curtail rectal radiation dose after permanent iodine-125 prostate brachytherapy. Brachytherapy 2013;12(4):368–74.
129. Yeh J, Lehrich B, Tran C, et al. Polyethylene glycol hydrogel rectal spacer implantation in patients with prostate cancer undergoing combination high-dose-rate brachytherapy and external beam radiotherapy. Brachytherapy 2016; 15(3):283–7.
130. Oberlin D, Miller F, Casalino D, et al. Increased utilization of multiparametric magnetic resonance imaging for detection and management of prostate cancer. J Urol 2016;195(4):E41.
131. Pugh TJ, Frank SJ, Achim M, et al. Endorectal magnetic resonance imaging for predicting pathologic T3 disease in Gleason score 7 prostate cancer: implications for prostate brachytherapy. Brachytherapy 2013;12(3):204–9.
132. Mason J, Al-Qaisieh B, Bownes P, et al. Multi-parametric MRI-guided focal tumor boost using HDR prostate brachytherapy: a feasibility study. Brachytherapy 2014;13(2):137–45.
133. Al-Qaisieh B, Mason J, Bownes P, et al. Dosimetry modeling for focal low-dose-rate prostate brachytherapy. Int J Radiat Oncol Biol Phys 2015;92(4):787–93.
134. Banerjee R, Park SJ, Anderson E, et al. From whole gland to hemigland to ultra-focal high-dose-rate prostate brachytherapy: A dosimetric analysis. Brachytherapy 2015;14(3):366–72.
135. Nguyen PL, Chen MH, Zhang Y, et al. Updated results of magnetic resonance imaging guided partial prostate brachytherapy for favorable risk prostate cancer: implications for focal therapy. J Urol 2012;188(4):1151–6.
136. Kittel JA, Reddy CA, Smith KL, et al. Long-term efficacy and toxicity of low-dose-rate (1)(2)(5)I prostate brachytherapy as monotherapy in low-, intermediate-, and high-risk prostate cancer. Int J Radiat Oncol Biol Phys 2015;92(4):884–93.
137. Funk RK, Davis BJ, Mynderse LA, et al. Permanent prostate brachytherapy monotherapy with I-125 for low- and intermediate-risk prostate cancer: outcome in 966 patients. Int J Radiat Oncol 2015;93(3):E213–4.

138. Tran AT, Mandall P, Swindell R, et al. Biochemical outcomes for patients with intermediate risk prostate cancer treated with I-125 interstitial brachytherapy monotherapy. Radiother Oncol 2013;109(2):235–40.
139. Sylvester JE, Grimm PD, Wong J, et al. Fifteen-year biochemical relapse-free survival, cause-specific survival, and overall survival following I(125) prostate brachytherapy in clinically localized prostate cancer: Seattle experience. Int J Radiat Oncol Biol Phys 2011;81(2):376–81.
140. Henry AM, Al-Qaisieh B, Gould K, et al. Outcomes following iodine-125 monotherapy for localized prostate cancer: the results of Leeds 10-year single-center brachytherapy experience. Int J Radiat Oncol Biol Phys 2010;76(1):50–6.
141. Zelefsky MJ, Kuban DA, Levy LB, et al. Multi-institutional analysis of long-term outcome for stages T1-T2 prostate cancer treated with permanent seed implantation. Int J Radiat Oncol Biol Phys 2007;67(2):327–33.
142. Guedea F, Aguilo F, Polo A, et al. Early biochemical outcomes following permanent interstitial brachytherapy as monotherapy in 1050 patients with clinical T1-T2 prostate cancer. Radiother Oncol 2006;80(1):57–61.
143. Grimm PD, Blasko JC, Sylvester JE, et al. 10-year biochemical (prostate-specific antigen) control of prostate cancer with (125)I brachytherapy. Int J Radiat Oncol Biol Phys 2001;51(1):31–40.
144. Blasko JC, Grimm PD, Sylvester JE, et al. Palladium-103 brachytherapy for prostate carcinoma. Int J Radiat Oncol Biol Phys 2000;46(4):839–50.
145. Yoshioka Y, Suzuki O, Isohashi F, et al. High-dose-rate brachytherapy as monotherapy for intermediate- and high-risk prostate cancer: clinical results for a median 8-year follow-up. Int J Radiat Oncol Biol Phys 2016;94(4):675–82.
146. Rogers CL, Alder SC, Rogers RL, et al. High dose brachytherapy as monotherapy for intermediate risk prostate cancer. J Urol 2012;187(1):109–16.

Novel Opportunities to Use Radiation Therapy with Immune Checkpoint Inhibitors for Melanoma Management

Kamran A. Ahmed, MD, Sungjune Kim, MD, PhD, Louis B. Harrison, MD*

KEYWORDS

- Abscopal effect • Bystander effect • Immune checkpoint inhibitors
- Radiation therapy

KEY POINTS

- Anti–cytotoxic T lymphocyte antigen 4 and anti–programmed cell death 1 agents are immune checkpoint inhibitors with a proven role in the management of advanced melanoma.
- Preclinical models have revealed radiation therapy to stimulate the immune system.
- Based on preclinical evidence, numerous prospective studies are currently underway to assess radiation therapy in the management of advanced melanoma alongside immune checkpoint inhibitors.

INTRODUCTION

Immunotherapy is shifting the oncologic landscape in the management of malignancies. The immune system plays a critical role in the body's ability to clear neoplastic cells. Tumor evasion of the host immune system is crucial to its survival and proliferation. Through various mechanisms, tumors are able to evade the body's innate and adaptive immune system. Immune checkpoint inhibitors (ICIs) are a new class of targeted agents, which directly target various machineries used by tumor cells to suppress the immune system. These drugs have displayed impressive results in both solid tumors and hematological malignancies. Nowhere have these impressive survival results been more detailed than in melanoma. Melanoma was the first tumor model to study the efficacy of ICIs. As a result, substantial survival benefits have been noted in the use of these agents over conventional chemotherapy.[1]

Disclosures: The authors have nothing to disclose.
Department of Radiation Oncology, H. Lee Moffitt Cancer Center and Research Institute, 12902 Magnolia Drive, Tampa, FL 33612, USA
* Corresponding author.
E-mail address: louis.harrison@moffitt.org

Surg Oncol Clin N Am 26 (2017) 515–529
http://dx.doi.org/10.1016/j.soc.2017.01.007
surgonc.theclinics.com

The role of radiation therapy (RT) in advanced metastatic melanoma has traditionally been part of the larger effort to improve local tumor control either intracranially or extracranially.[2,3] However, over the past decade studies have suggested the potential for RT to work synergistically with ICIs priming the immune system to enhance the efficacy of these systemic agents. Although the exact mechanism behind this synergistic effect is not known, several theories have been proposed.[4–7] These theories include the use of RT microenvironment modification with cytokine and danger signal release resulting in immunogenic cell death.[8] Multiple case reports have reported on the existence of such an effect whereby localized radiation alongside immunomodulating agents may have an effect in treating distant sites of disease.[9–13] In addition, several case series detailing results both systemically and intracranially with combined modality management have been reported. The purpose of this review is to highlight the research, which has been conducted to date with ICIs alone and in combination with RT for the management of advanced melanoma.

ANTI–CYTOTOXIC T LYMPHOCYTE ANTIGEN 4 THERAPY

Numerous receptors on the antigen-presenting cells and T cell are responsible for the immune response to tumor cells[7] (**Fig. 1**). Cytotoxic T lymphocyte antigen 4 (CTLA-4) is a receptor expressed on the surface of T cells that interacts with CD80 and CD86 on antigen-presenting cells to downregulate the T-cell response on tumors.[14] The anti–CTLA-4 monoclonal antibody, ipilimumab, inhibits the effect of the CTLA-4 receptor in inhibiting the immune response. The effect of CTLA-4 blockade is to allow CD28 (T

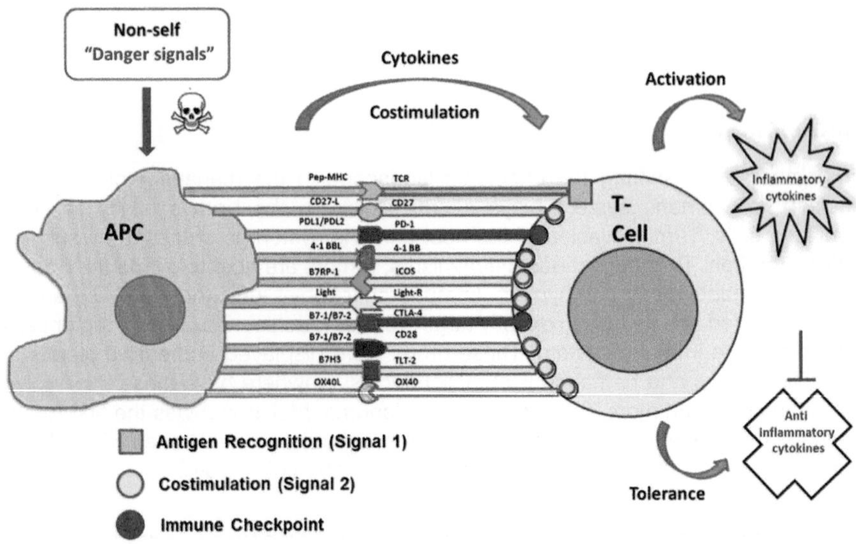

Fig. 1. Immune synapse. A snapshot of an immune synapse between antigen-presenting cell (APC) and effector cell (T cell) during immune priming is depicted. The APC stimulated by the danger signal will present antigen (signal 1) and costimulation (signal 2) via ligand-receptor interaction or cytokines. The immune response is restrained by immune checkpoint receptors and antiinflammatory cytokines. CTLA-4, cytotoxic T lymphocyte antigen 4; MHC, major histocompatibility complex; PD-1, programmed cell death 1. (*From* Grass GD, Krishna N, Kim S. The immune mechanisms of abscopal effect in radiation therapy. Curr Probl Cancer 2016;40:12; with permission.)

cell) to bind to the B7-1 receptor (antigen-presenting cell), thus, allowing for immune stimulation and cytotoxic T-cell activation and proliferation. Following extensive preclinical and pilot studies, a phase II study was undertaken to assess the response to ipilimumab. A double-blind phase II study revealed a dose-dependent response with an overall response rate (ORR) of 11.0% for 10.0 mg/kg and 4.2% for 3.0 mg/kg but 0% for 0.3 mg/kg (P = .0015).[15] However, improved efficacy was also associated with increased adverse events. Phase III data have also revealed improved responses with ipilimumab.[16] Ipilimumab ± glycoprotein100 peptide (gp100) vaccine was compared with gp100 vaccine monotherapy in patients with unresectable stage III or stage IV melanoma. Ipilimumab significantly improved overall survival (OS) compared with gp100 vaccine alone with a median OS of 10 months compared with 6.4 months in patients receiving the vaccine alone. Improved OS of approximately 2 months was also confirmed by a second randomized phase III trial assessing ipilimumab (10 mg/kg) and dacarbazine (850 mg/m^2) compared with dacarbazine (850 mg/m^2) plus placebo.[17] A pooled analysis of data from 1861 patients enrolled in 10 prospective and 2 retrospective trials revealed that survival curves begin to plateau around 3 years after treatment.[18] The rates of OS at 3 years were found to be 22%, 26%, and 20% for all, treatment-naive, and previously treated patients, respectively.

It should be noted that the response to ipilimumab can be preceded by an increase in diameter of tumor lesions owing to the distinct immune response patterns and T-cell recall at the tumor site.[19] This unique response pattern makes clear the need for distinct evaluation criteria of treated lesions. In addition to response evaluation criteria in solid tumors (RECIST) criteria,[20] the immune-related response criteria are often used to evaluate lesions treated with immunotherapy.[19] Separate guidelines have been developed for the evaluation of cranial lesions treated with immunotherapy by the Response Assessment in Neuro-Oncology group.[21]

ANTI–PROGRAMMED CELL DEATH 1 THERAPY

Following chronic T-cell activation, the inhibitory receptor programmed cell death 1 (PD-1) is induced on T cells, which engages with one of its ligands, programmed death-ligand 1 (PD-L1), found on tissue-based macrophages, antigen-presenting cells, and tumor cells. This interaction along the PD-1/PD-L1 axis mediates the immune escape of tumor cells by promoting T-cell exhaustion.[22] PD-L1 is expressed in various tumors, is thought to be one of the main mechanisms of immune escape, and is associated with worse prognosis. The discovery of the PD-1/PD-L1 axis led to the development of specific anti–PD-1 inhibitors. Two anti–PD-1 inhibitors, the monoclonal antibodies nivolumab (a fully human anti–PD-1 immunoglobulin G4 [IgG4]) and pembrolizumab (a humanized anti–PD-1 IgG4) have both gained widespread use in the management of advanced melanoma.[23] Several phase III studies have confirmed improved response rates with anti–PD-1 therapy. A randomized study of nivolumab versus dacarbazine in BRAF wild-type untreated melanoma revealed a superior ORR of 40% versus 14% with an improved OS rate of 73% versus 42%.[24] Improved toxicity profiles were also noted with anti–PD-1 therapy with a 12% treatment-related adverse effect rate versus 18% with dacarbazine. In the CheckMate 037 phase III trial, patients were randomly assigned 1:2 to either the investigator's choice of chemotherapy or to nivolumab 3 mg/kg every 2 weeks.[25] In the first reported interim analysis, objective responses were reported in 32% of the first 120 patients in the nivolumab group and 11% of the 47 patients in the investigator's choice group. The rate of grade 3 to 4 drug-related adverse events was fairly similar between the two groups: 5% and 9% in nivolumab and chemotherapy groups, respectively.

The efficacy of pembrolizumab has also been well studied in the management of advanced-stage melanoma. KEYNOTE-002 was a phase II study assessing 2 different doses of pembrolizumab, including 2 mg/kg and 10 mg/kg, compared with investigator's choice chemotherapy.[1] Results revealed an improvement in progression-free survival (PFS) at 6 months as assessed by independent central review. Grade 3 to 4 treatment-related adverse events were more common in patients receiving chemotherapy than pembrolizumab. Improved rates of PFS were noted with pembrolizumab compared with ipilimumab in a large phase III randomized study of 834 patients.[26] Patients were randomized to 10 mg/kg every 2 weeks, 10 mg/kg every 3 weeks, or to 4 doses of ipilimumab 3 mg/kg every 3 weeks. The 6-month PFS rates were 47%, 46%, and 27%, respectively, with 1-year OS rates of 74%, 68%, and 58%, respectively. Treatment-related adverse events (grades 3–5) were slightly lower in the pembrolizumab groups: 13% and 10% versus 20% with ipilimumab.

COMBINATION THERAPY WITH ANTI–PROGRAMMED CELL DEATH 1 AND ANTI–CYTOTOXIC T LYMPHOCYTE ANTIGEN 4 AGENTS

Combining ICIs in various sequences offers a new treatment option in the management of advanced melanoma. Data have revealed that combined therapy may offer improved results over single-agent therapy alone. In a double blind study of 142 patients who were previously untreated, patients were randomly assigned 2:1 to receive ipilimumab (3 mg/kg) combined with nivolumab (1 mg/kg) or placebo once every 3 weeks for 4 doses followed by nivolumab 3 mg/kg or placebo every 2 weeks until disease progression or severe toxicity.[27] In patients with BRAF wild-type tumors, ORR was 61% in the group that received both ipilimumab and nivolumab versus 11% in the group that received ipilimumab and placebo. Median PFS was not reached with the combination therapy and was 4.4 months with ipilimumab monotherapy groups. These results were similar to those obtained in 3 patients with BRAF mutated tumors. These results are similar to another phase III study involving 945 patients who were randomized 1:1:1 to either ipilimumab or nivolumab alone or to combination therapy in stage III or IV melanoma.[28] Patients treated with the combination therapy had a PFS of 11.5 months, compared with 2.9 months for those treated with ipilimumab alone and 6 months for those treated with nivolumab alone. However, combination therapy was associated with a higher incidence of grade 3 to 4 immune-related adverse events commonly involving more than one organ. Combination therapy was also compared with ipilimumab alone in treatment-naive patients in the phase II CheckMate 064 study. In this trial, 2 sequences of combination therapy were tested. These regimens included ipilimumab followed by nivolumab versus nivolumab followed by ipilimumab.[29] The response rate was higher for the latter sequence: 41% versus 20% with a higher 12-month OS rate of 76% versus 54%. This study suggests that the sequence of treatment with combined immune checkpoint inhibition effects outcomes with improved response and survival noted with nivolumab followed by ipilimumab.

RADIATION THERAPY AND IMMUNE CHECKPOINT INHIBITORS: PRECLINICAL DATA

RT has long been a standard component of the treatment paradigm for many solid malignancies with curative or palliative intent, including melanoma. The effect of radiation on DNA damage has been thought to be from the generation of double-strand breaks leading to mitotic and apoptotic cell death.[30] However, evidence also suggests the immune system plays a larger influence on the response of malignant cells to radiation. A robust immune system has been shown to play an important role in RT's effect, with studies revealing that in T-cell–deficient mice, tumor control by RT is reduced compared with those mice that are immunocompetent. The study by Lugade and colleagues[31] revealed immune responses in mice after treatment of B16 melanoma with single 15-Gy or fractionated 5 $\times$ 3-Gy doses of RT (**Table 1**). Irradiated mice were more capable of presenting tumor antigens and specific T cells secreting interferon (IFN)-C on peptide stimulation within tumor draining lymph nodes than nonirradiated mice. Activation of the immune system in lymph nodes correlated with an increase in the CD45+ cells infiltrating single dose irradiated tumors compared with nonirradiated mice. Other studies have also revealed the influence of RT enhancing major histocompatibility complex class I (MHC-I) expression and inducing antitumor immunity and the radiation-induced IFN-gamma production within the microenvironment of the tumor.[32] In addition, the absence of toll-like receptor signaling has been shown to impair the effect of RT-mediated tumor control. RT has been shown to prime the immune system augmenting T-cell activation.[5,33,34]

The immunomodulatory effects of RT have also been associated with cross presentation of tumor-derived antigens by dendritic cells. The activation of T-cell response requires the cross presentation of these antigens with type I IFN. Through upregulation of the MHC-I, adhesion molecules, death receptors, and NKG2D ligands, which enable identification and elimination of damaged cancer cells, RT is also able to initiate the effector phase by recruiting effector T cells at the tumor site.[35,36] However, radiation may also have immunosuppressive effects. It has been noted that regulatory

Table 1
Preclinical data supporting role of radiotherapy with immune checkpoint inhibitors

Author, Year of Publication	Key Points
Lugade et al,[31] 2005	Irradiated mice are more capable of presenting tumor antigens and T cells secreting IFN-C on peptide stimulation within tumor draining lymph nodes than nonirradiated mice.
Reits et al,[32] 2006	Cell surface expression of MHC class I molecules was increased for many days in a radiation dose-dependent manner. Immunotherapy was successful in eradicating a murine colon adenocarcinoma only when preceded by radiotherapy of tumor tissue.
Dewan et al,[42] 2009	Fractionated rather than single-dose radiation found to produce immune mediated abscopal effect alongside anti–CTLA-4 therapy with the same effect locally.
Apetoh et al,[34] 2008	Patients with breast cancer who carry a toll-like receptor 4 (TLR4) loss-of-function allele relapse quicker after radiotherapy and chemotherapy than those carrying the normal TLR4 allele.
Matsumura et al,[36] 2008	Radiation enhances recruitment of CD8 T cells in mouse and human breast cancer cell lines through the chemokine CXCL16.
Deng et al,[40] 2014	PD-L1 is upregulated in the tumor microenvironment following RT with a reduction in the local accumulation of tumor-infiltration myeloid-derived suppressor cells.
Twyman-Saint Victor et al,[41] 2015	Differing roles of RT and ICIs were noted with anti–CTLA-4 inhibiting Treg cells, RT enhanced diversity of T-cell repertoire of intratumoral T cells, and PD-L1 blockade reversed T-cell exhaustion.

T cells (Tregs) are more radioresistant than conventional T-cells and are upregulated following RT.[37] Tregs play an important immunosuppressive role in antitumor immunity. In addition, RT can enhance tumor infiltration by myeloid-derived suppressor cells, which are responsible for sustaining chronic immunosuppression. It has also been shown that RT can induce Langerhans cells to migrate to the lymph nodes from the skin where they upregulate Tregs.[38,39] Given both these immunosuppressive and immunostimulatory effects, it is no surprise that the use of RT is a unique interplay between both the upregulation and downregulation of effects on the immune system and their effects on ICIs. The balance between these signals determines the direct effect RT will have alongside ICIs in tumor management. Therefore, understanding how RT can be optimized in terms of total dose, fractions, and timing to enhance the immunogenicity of ICIs is key.

Preclinical models have revealed the potential of RT to enhance the efficacy of anti–PD-1 therapy. Deng and colleagues[40] demonstrated PD-L1 to be upregulated in the tumor microenvironment following RT. Concomitant with RT-mediated tumor regression, combined therapy reduced the local accumulation of tumor-infiltrating myeloid-derived suppressor cells, which suppress T-cell action against tumors. Twyman-Saint Victor and colleagues[41] have suggested further preclinical support for combined modality management and ICIs. The group reported optimal response to management with combined therapy with ICIs and RT, noting anti–CTLA-4 predominantly inhibits Treg cells and RT enhances the diversity of the T-cell receptor repertoire of intratumoral T cells. Together, anti–CTLA-4 promotes expansion of T cells, whereas radiation shapes the T-cell receptor repertoire of the expanded peripheral clones. The addition of PD-L1 blockade reverses T-cell exhaustion. These results paralleled findings in patients on a melanoma clinical trial at the institution. These findings support the distinct but complementary roles ICIs and RT have in tumor regression.

The optimal radiation dose to enhance immunogenicity remains an open question. The use of fractionated radiation has been shown to be more immunogenic than single-dose radiation with a dose of 24 Gy in 3 fractions or 30 Gy in 5 fractions inducing an immune-mediated abscopal effect alongside anti–CTLA-4 therapy with the same effect locally.[42] However, the benefits of fractionated radiation were not observed in another study by Lugade and colleagues,[31] which revealed 15 Gy in 5 fractions to be inferior to 15 Gy in 1 fraction in primary tumor control with equivocal T-cell activation. Moving forward, it will be important for us to better understand the underlying relationship of radiation fractionation and immunogenicity in order to take advantage of the priming effect of radiation to induce the greatest immunogenicity from ICIs.

RADIATION THERAPY AND IMMUNE CHECKPOINT INHIBITORS: SYSTEMIC CLINICAL DATA

Case Reports

One of the prime areas in which involvement of the immune system with RT has been observed is the bystander effect or the abscopal effect whereby local radiation can prompt a response in tumor cells outside the radiation field. Several cases have been reported since that time on complete responses to disease outside the irradiated field using combined modality treatment[10–13,43] and are summarized in **Table 2**. The abscopal effect was first reported by Mole[44] in 1953 and has subsequently been reported in numerous tumor types. Although the exact mechanism by which the abscopal effect takes place remains to be elucidated, there is a suggestion that the immune system plays a critical role. Local radiation elicits a large, immune-mediated systemic response implicated by local inflammatory reactions that can unmask tumor antigens.

Table 2
Case reports of the abscopal effect

Citation	Age (y) and Sex	Dose and Fractionation	Site Treated
Kingsley,[9] 1975	28/M	14.4 Gy in 35 fractions with fast neutrons	Right inguinal lymph nodes
Abood et al,[10] 2009	63/M	50 Gy in 25 fractions	Neck
Postow et al,[11] 2012	33/F	28.5 Gy in 3 fractions with maintenance ipilimumab	Pleural-based paraspinal mass
Hiniker et al,[12] 2012	57/M	54 Gy in 3 fractions with ipilimumab	2 of 7 melanoma liver metastases
Stamell et al,[13] 2013	67/M	24 Gy in 3 fractions with electrons	Primary melanoma lesion on skin of scalp
Thallinger et al,[43] 2015	44/M	30 Gy in 10 fractions with concurrent temozolomide alongside ipilimumab	Melanoma brain metastases

Abbreviations: F, female; M, male.

A sudden reappearance of these antigens by tumor can stimulate the immune system to identify previously unrecognized tumor antigens. Studies have now revealed that in addition to the classic radiation-mediated generation of free radicals leading to DNA double-strand breaks, in vivo radiation may also induce immunologic cell death.[5,45,46] Radiation damage may lead to an increased release of damage-associated molecular patterns, which, when engulfed by antigen-presenting cells, present these to T cells, thereby initiating an immune response.[47–49]

Several additional case reports of the abscopal effect have been reported in the management of advanced melanoma since the report by Mole[44]. In 1975, Kingsley[9] published a report of a 28-year-old man who experienced a complete response to lymphadenopathy in the right inguinal region 9 months following 14.4 Gy in 35 fractions of neutrons. Demaria and colleagues[8] detailed the case of irradiation to an implanted mammary carcinoma leading to tumor shrinkage of not only the irradiated flank but also the nonirradiated flank in the same host. This effect did not take place when the patient had severe combined immunodeficiency. One of the primary explanations is that tumor-specific epitopes were generated and presented to T cells leading to immune activation and cell death of tumors outside the irradiated field. Stamell and colleagues[13] reported further clinical evidence of the abscopal effect in a patient with a scalp melanoma. After RT to the area, the patient experienced a complete remission including resolution of nodal metastases with an increase of melanoma-specific antigens. In addition, Park and colleagues[50] found that in preclinical renal cell carcinoma and melanoma models, the combination of stereotactic RT and anti–PD-1 therapy was able to induce complete regression of the tumor to not only the irradiated lesion but also to lesions outside the irradiated field. Although reports of the abscopal effect are rare, the effects may be dramatic and a better understanding of the molecular mechanisms behind such responses is vital.

Case Series

Several institutions have reported larger case series detailing the response of ICIs alongside RT (**Table 3**). A retrospective review from Grimaldi and colleagues[51]

Table 3
Case series assessing both the systemic and intracranial response of radiotherapy with immune checkpoint inhibitors

Author, Publication Year	Therapeutic Agent	Comments
Systemic Disease		
Grimaldi et al,[51] 2014	Ipilimumab	13 patients receiving RT to the brain and 8 to extracranial sites; abscopal response in 11 patients (52%), OS 22.4 mo vs 8.3 mo with and without abscopal response
Chandra et al,[52] 2015	Ipilimumab	47 patients with metastatic melanoma with 65 courses of radiation; 28-mo median survival with 20% estimated 5-y survival
Qin et al,[53] 2016	Ipilimumab	88 patients treated with or without RT, no significant differences in OS, PFS, and immune-related and non–immune-related toxicity despite RT group with worse baseline characteristics
Barker et al,[54] 2013	Ipilimumab	29 patients treated with 33 courses of nonbrain RT; 9-mo and 39-mo median OS in patients receiving RT during induction and maintenance with ipilimumab, respectively
Theurich et al,[55] 2016	Ipilimumab	127 patients either ipilimumab alone or ipilimumab alongside electro-chemotherapy or radiotherapy; local therapy produced longer OS (median OS 93 vs 42 wk)
Intracranial Disease		
Silk et al,[58] 2013	Ipilimumab	33 patients treated with ipilimumab and 37 without, ipilimumab with improved OS 18.3 vs 5.3 mo
Knisely et al,[60] 2012	Ipilimumab	77 patients, 35% received ipilimumab with 21.3 mo vs 4.9 mo in those that did not
Mathew et al,[59] 2013	Ipilimumab	58 patients treated with SRS and ipilimumab with median LC, freedom from new brain metastases, and OS of 8.7, 4.3, and 5.9 mo, respectively
Kiess et al,[61] 2015	Ipilimumab	46 patients treated to 113 brain metastases with single fraction SRS with improved OS and distant brain metastases control with SRS administered before or during ipilimumab administration
Ahmed et al,[63] 2015	Nivolumab	26 patients treated to 73 brain metastases; improved OS and distant brain metastases control noted over historical controls

reported on 21 patients with advanced melanoma followed by RT. Thirteen of these patients received RT to treat metastases in the brain and 8 received RT to extracranial sites. The investigators reported an abscopal response in 11 patients (52%). The authors reported a median time to an abscopal response of 1 month with a median OS of 13 months and a median OS in patients exhibiting an abscopal response of 22.4 months versus 8.3 months without. Similarly, Chandra and colleagues[52] reported on 47 patients with metastatic melanoma treated with ipilimumab and a total of 65 courses of radiation. The median survival was 28 months with an estimated 20% 5-year survival. In 68% of cases, the investigators reported radiotherapy was associated with a favorable index lesion response (*P* = .014).

A recent report from Duke University reported on 88 patients treated with ipilimumab with or without RT.[53] Although the ipilimumab plus RT groups had more unfavorable characteristics, OS, PFS, and immune-related and non–immune-related toxicity between the groups was not statistically significant. The investigators reported that patients who received RT before ipilimumab had an increased duration of irradiated tumor response compared with patients receiving ipilimumab after RT (75% vs 45% at 12 months; *P* = .01). Nonstatistically significant improvements in OS were noted in patients treated with ablative hypofractionated radiation over conventionally fractionated RT.

Memorial Sloan Kettering reported their experience of 29 patients treated with 33 courses of nonbrain radiotherapy between their first and last dose of ipilimumab.[54] The median OS was 9 and 39 months in patients receiving radiotherapy during induction and maintenance with ipilimumab, respectively. Higher rates of adverse events with RT were not associated with combined treatment.

Theurich and colleagues[55] recently reported on data from 127 consecutively treated patients with melanoma in 4 centers in Germany and Switzerland. Patients received either ipilimumab (n = 82) or ipilimumab and additional local treatment including electro-chemotherapy or radiotherapy if indicated for local control. The addition of local therapy to ipilimumab significantly prolonged OS (median OS 93 vs 42 weeks). The investigators reported that combined treatment did not increase immune-related adverse events. The investigators stated that antitumor immune responses were most likely the underlying mechanism leading to improved outcomes.

Initial results from Hiniker and colleagues[56] have been reported in abstract form from a phase II trial of 20 patients with stage IV melanoma treated with palliative doses of RT and ipilimumab (3 mg/kg) for a total of 4 doses. Patients underwent radiation to 1 to 2 sites, and at least 1 measurable nonirradiated site was assessed for the abscopal response. A grade 3 to 4 combined toxicity rate was noted in 15% of patients. Of 20 evaluable patients, 11 (55%) had an initial response to therapy with a median follow-up of 38 weeks, whereas 9 patients (45%) had progressive disease at the first posttreatment scan. Initial results from this prospective study reveal combination therapy to be safe with the suggestion of improved outcomes supporting future prospective analyses.

Several clinical trials are currently underway to assess anti–PD-1 therapy and RT in the prospective setting. These trials include a phase II trial assessing stereotactic body radiotherapy (SBRT) with concurrent anti–PD-1 treatment in metastatic melanoma (NCT02821182). In the trial, a dose of 24 Gy in 3 fractions will be administered before the second cycle of anti–PD-1 treatment. Another phase I/II trial open at Yale University will assess combination pembrolizumab and SBRT in metastatic melanoma (NCT02407171). Patients who progress on pembrolizumab will be treated to a single target lesion with SBRT and then pembrolizumab will be restarted. The radiation dose will be escalated in the phase I portion with a dose of 30 Gy in 5 fractions escalated to 30 Gy in 3 fractions with de-escalation to 10 Gy in 1 fraction if necessary. A phase I trial (NCT02303990) opened by the University of Pennsylvania is testing hypofractionated radiotherapy to an isolated index lesion in combination with pembrolizumab in patients with metastatic melanoma or non–small cell lung cancer (NSCLC) who have failed anti–PD-1 therapy. Combined ipilimumab and nivolumab alongside radiation is being tested in NCT02659540. This is a multicenter phase I study in which RT will be initiated after the first dose and before the second dose of immunotherapy. Following 4 doses of ipilimumab and nivolumab at 3-week intervals, nivolumab at 2-week intervals will be administered. Two radiation regimens will be tested including 30 Gy in 10 fractions and 27 Gy in 3 fractions. Results from these trials among others are awaited to determine how ICIs can be combined with RT to enhance the efficacy of either agent alone.

RADIATION THERAPY AND IMMUNE CHECKPOINT INHIBITORS: INTRACRANIAL CLINICAL DATA

Similar improvements in survival and disease response to those reported in systemic disease have been revealed with intracranial disease in melanoma (**Table 3**). Historically, patients with melanoma brain metastases have been known to have a very poor prognosis with a median OS of 6 months.[57] These reports have focused on the safety as well as the optimal timing of RT to maximize the immunogenicity of ICIs.[58–61] Silk and colleagues[58] reported on 70 patients with melanoma with brain metastases treated between 2005 and 2012; 33 patients received ipilimumab and 37 did not. Patients who received ipilimumab had a median survival of 18.3 months compared with 5.3 months for patients who did not receive ipilimumab. Patients were treated with either stereotactic radiosurgery (SRS) or whole-brain radiation treatment. The possibility for improved rates of OS was further reported by Knisely and colleagues[60] in 77 patients treated between 2002 and 2010 with SRS for melanoma brain metastases. Thirty-five percent of patients received ipilimumab. The median survival in this group was 21.3 months as compared with 4.9 months in those that did not receive ipilimumab.

Kiess and colleagues[61] also confirmed improved response rates with combination therapy. From 2005 to 2011, a total of 46 patients were treated to a total of 113 brain metastases with single fraction SRS. Timing between SRS and administration of ipilimumab was assessed as SRS before, SRS during, or SRS after ipilimumab administration. The group found patients treated with SRS either before or during ipilimumab administration had improved outcomes over those patients treated with SRS after ipilimumab, with 1-year OS of 65% and 56% versus 40%, respectively. In addition, regional recurrences in the brain statistically differed with the timing of SRS and ipilimumab administration, with 1-year regional recurrence rates of 69% and 64% versus 92%. Interestingly, the investigators noted an increase in brain metastases diameter to greater than 150% in 50% of patients treated before or during ipilimumab but only in 13% of patients treated after ipilimumab.

A report from Berghoff and colleagues[62] revealed that more than half of melanoma brain metastases stain positive for PD-L1 by immunohistochemistry accompanied by lymphocytic infiltrates, which supports the potential for anti–PD-1 therapies in melanoma brain metastases. With this understanding, the authors undertook an analysis of patients enrolled in 2 prospective trials at their institution.[63] The protocol for unresectable disease, NCT01176461, was a phase I study of nivolumab with or without a multi-peptide vaccine (MART-1, NY-ESO, gp100 peptides emulsified in Montanide ISA 51VG) in patients with unresectable stage III or IV melanoma.[64] The protocol in the resected (adjuvant) setting, NCT01176474, was a phase I study of nivolumab plus the same multi-peptide vaccine in patients with resected stage IIIC or IV melanoma.[65] Patients were included in the analysis if they were treated with SRS within 6 months of receiving anti–PD-1 therapy. A total of 26 patients treated to a total of 73 brain metastases treated over 30 sessions were identified. Radiation was administered before, during, and after nivolumab in 33 lesions (45%), 5 lesions (7%), and 35 lesions (48%), respectively. The treatment was well tolerated. Kaplan-Meier estimates for local brain metastases control following radiation at 6 and 12 months were 91% and 85%, respectively. The median OS from the date of stereotactic radiation and nivolumab initiation was 11.8 and 12.0 months, respectively, in patients receiving nivolumab for unresected disease (median OS was not reached in patients treated in the resected setting). Rates of 6- and 12-month distant brain control for all treatment sessions were 66% and 53%, respectively. Both the rates of OS and distant brain metastases seemed improved over the historical control.

This finding led the authors' group to further assess responses with SRS alongside other systemic regimens. The authors recently published results of a comparative analysis of 96 patients treated with SRS to 314 brain metastases within 3 months of receipt of anti–PD-1 therapy, anti–CTLA-4 therapy, BRAF/MEK inhibitors (i), BRAFi, or conventional chemotherapy.[66] Twelve-month distant brain control rates were 38%, 21%, 20%, 8%, and 5% ($P = .008$) for SRS with anti–PD-1 therapies, anti–CTLA-4 therapy, BRAF/MEKi, BRAFi, and conventional chemotherapy, respectively. On multivariate analysis, the authors noted anti–PD-1 therapy as well as BRAF/MEKi regimens to significantly improve distant brain control over conventional chemotherapy.

Prospective evaluations assessing the use of stereotactic radiation with anti–PD-1 therapy in the management of melanoma brain metastases are currently underway. These evaluations include NCT02716948, a phase I trial assessing the side effects of SRS and nivolumab in treating patients with newly diagnosed melanoma that has spread to the brain or spine. In addition, NCT02858869 is a pilot study assessing the side effects of pembrolizumab together with SRS to treat patients with melanoma or NSCLC that has spread to the brain.

SUMMARY

Immunotherapy has revolutionized and will continue to shape the way in which we treat a cancer. Melanoma is at the forefront of this paradigm shift. A paradigm shift in the potential synergistic effect of combining RT and ICIs is emerging as well. Preclinical models have long suggested the synergy of RT to enhance the immune response. Retrospective clinical data reveal the potential for RT to enhance the immune response, improving outcomes over treatment with ICIs alone both systemically and intracranially. Numerous questions remain regarding the optimal dose fractionation schedule and timing of therapy to generate the optimal response, which may also be affected by the tumor microenvironment and its unique radiosensitivity. Ultimately, these answers will be found in prospective clinical trials, which are actively underway and accruing patients.

REFERENCES

1. Ribas A, Puzanov I, Dummer R, et al. Pembrolizumab versus investigator-choice chemotherapy for ipilimumab-refractory melanoma (KEYNOTE-002): a randomised, controlled, phase 2 trial. Lancet Oncol 2015;16(8):908–18.
2. Shaw E, Scott C, Souhami L, et al. Single dose radiosurgical treatment of recurrent previously irradiated primary brain tumors and brain metastases: final report of RTOG protocol 90-05. Int J Radiat Oncol Biol Phys 2000;47(2):291–8.
3. Burmeister BH, Henderson MA, Ainslie J, et al. Adjuvant radiotherapy versus observation alone for patients at risk of lymph-node field relapse after therapeutic lymphadenectomy for melanoma: a randomised trial. Lancet Oncol 2012;13(6): 589–97.
4. Golden EB, Pellicciotta I, Demaria S, et al. The convergence of radiation and immunogenic cell death signaling pathways. Front Oncol 2012;2:88.

5. Apetoh L, Ghiringhelli F, Tesniere A, et al. Toll-like receptor 4-dependent contribution of the immune system to anticancer chemotherapy and radiotherapy. Nat Med 2007;13(9):1050–9.
6. Demaria S, Pilones KA, Vanpouille-Box C, et al. The optimal partnership of radiation and immunotherapy: from preclinical studies to clinical translation. Radiat Res 2014;182(2):170–81.
7. Grass GD, Krishna N, Kim S. The immune mechanisms of abscopal effect in radiation therapy. Curr Probl Cancer 2016;40(1):10–24.
8. Demaria S, Ng B, Devitt ML, et al. Ionizing radiation inhibition of distant untreated tumors (abscopal effect) is immune mediated. Int J Radiat Oncol Biol Phys 2004; 58(3):862–70.
9. Kingsley DP. An interesting case of possible abscopal effect in malignant melanoma. Br J Radiol 1975;48(574):863–6.
10. Abood A, Saleh DB, Watt DA. Malignant melanoma and vitiligo: can radiotherapy shed light on the subject? J Plast Reconstr Aesthet Surg 2009;62(5):e119–20.
11. Postow MA, Callahan MK, Barker CA, et al. Immunologic correlates of the abscopal effect in a patient with melanoma. N Engl J Med 2012;366(10):925–31.
12. Hiniker SM, Chen DS, Knox SJ. Abscopal effect in a patient with melanoma. N Engl J Med 2012;366(21):2035 [author reply: 2035–6].
13. Stamell EF, Wolchok JD, Gnjatic S, et al. The abscopal effect associated with a systemic anti-melanoma immune response. Int J Radiat Oncol Biol Phys 2013; 85(2):293–5.
14. Korman AJ, Peggs KS, Allison JP. Checkpoint blockade in cancer immunotherapy. Adv Immunol 2006;90:297–339.
15. Wolchok JD, Neyns B, Linette G, et al. Ipilimumab monotherapy in patients with pretreated advanced melanoma: a randomised, double-blind, multicentre, phase 2, dose-ranging study. Lancet Oncol 2010;11(2):155–64.
16. Hodi FS, O'Day SJ, McDermott DF, et al. Improved survival with ipilimumab in patients with metastatic melanoma. N Engl J Med 2010;363(8):711–23.
17. Robert C, Thomas L, Bondarenko I, et al. Ipilimumab plus dacarbazine for previously untreated metastatic melanoma. N Engl J Med 2011;364(26):2517–26.
18. Schadendorf D, Hodi FS, Robert C, et al. Pooled analysis of long-term survival data from phase II and phase III trials of Ipilimumab in unresectable or metastatic melanoma. J Clin Oncol 2015;33(17):1889–94.
19. Wolchok JD, Hoos A, O'Day S, et al. Guidelines for the evaluation of immune therapy activity in solid tumors: immune-related response criteria. Clin Cancer Res 2009;15(23):7412–20.
20. Eisenhauer EA, Therasse P, Bogaerts J, et al. New response evaluation criteria in solid tumours: revised RECIST guideline (version 1.1). Eur J Cancer 2009;45(2): 228–47.
21. Okada H, Weller M, Huang R, et al. Immunotherapy response assessment in neuro-oncology: a report of the RANO working group. Lancet Oncol 2015; 16(15):e534–42.
22. McDermott DF, Atkins MB. PD-1 as a potential target in cancer therapy. Cancer Med 2013;2(5):662–73.
23. Metcalfe W, Anderson J, Trinh VA, et al. Anti-programmed cell death-1 (PD-1) monoclonal antibodies in treating advanced melanoma. Discov Med 2015; 19(106):393–401.
24. Robert C, Long GV, Brady B, et al. Nivolumab in previously untreated melanoma without BRAF mutation. N Engl J Med 2015;372(4):320–30.

25. Weber JS, D'Angelo SP, Minor D, et al. Nivolumab versus chemotherapy in patients with advanced melanoma who progressed after anti-CTLA-4 treatment (CheckMate 037): a randomised, controlled, open-label, phase 3 trial. Lancet Oncol 2015;16(4):375–84.
26. Robert C, Schachter J, Long GV, et al. Pembrolizumab versus ipilimumab in advanced melanoma. N Engl J Med 2015;372(26):2521–32.
27. Postow MA, Chesney J, Pavlick AC, et al. Nivolumab and ipilimumab versus ipilimumab in untreated melanoma. N Engl J Med 2015;372(21):2006–17.
28. Larkin J, Chiarion-Sileni V, Gonzalez R, et al. Combined nivolumab and ipilimumab or monotherapy in untreated melanoma. N Engl J Med 2015;373(1):23–34.
29. Weber JS, Gibney G, Sullivan RJ, et al. Sequential administration of nivolumab and ipilimumab with a planned switch in patients with advanced melanoma (CheckMate 064): an open-label, randomised, phase 2 trial. Lancet Oncol 2016;17(7):943–55.
30. Khanna KK, Jackson SP. DNA double-strand breaks: signaling, repair and the cancer connection. Nat Genet 2001;27(3):247–54.
31. Lugade AA, Moran JP, Gerber SA, et al. Local radiation therapy of B16 melanoma tumors increases the generation of tumor antigen-specific effector cells that traffic to the tumor. J Immunol 2005;174(12):7516–23.
32. Reits EA, Hodge JW, Herberts CA, et al. Radiation modulates the peptide repertoire, enhances MHC class I expression, and induces successful antitumor immunotherapy. J Exp Med 2006;203(5):1259–71.
33. Zitvogel L, Apetoh L, Ghiringhelli F, et al. Immunological aspects of cancer chemotherapy. Nat Rev Immunol 2008;8(1):59–73.
34. Apetoh L, Tesniere A, Ghiringhelli F, et al. Molecular interactions between dying tumor cells and the innate immune system determine the efficacy of conventional anticancer therapies. Cancer Res 2008;68(11):4026–30.
35. Demaria S, Golden EB, Formenti SC. Role of local radiation therapy in cancer immunotherapy. JAMA Oncol 2015;1(9):1325–32.
36. Matsumura S, Wang B, Kawashima N, et al. Radiation-induced CXCL16 release by breast cancer cells attracts effector T cells. J Immunol 2008;181(5):3099–107.
37. Soto-Pantoja DR, Terabe M, Ghosh A, et al. CD47 in the tumor microenvironment limits cooperation between antitumor T-cell immunity and radiotherapy. Cancer Res 2014;74(23):6771–83.
38. Zitvogel L, Kroemer G. Subversion of anticancer immunosurveillance by radiotherapy. Nat Immunol 2015;16(10):1005–7.
39. Price JG, Idoyaga J, Salmon H, et al. CDKN1A regulates Langerhans cell survival and promotes Treg cell generation upon exposure to ionizing irradiation. Nat Immunol 2015;16(10):1060–8.
40. Deng L, Liang H, Burnette B, et al. Irradiation and anti-PD-L1 treatment synergistically promote antitumor immunity in mice. J Clin Invest 2014;124(2):687–95.
41. Twyman-Saint Victor C, Rech AJ, Maity A, et al. Radiation and dual checkpoint blockade activate non-redundant immune mechanisms in cancer. Nature 2015; 520(7547):373–7.
42. Dewan MZ, Galloway AE, Kawashima N, et al. Fractionated but not single-dose radiotherapy induces an immune-mediated abscopal effect when combined with anti-CTLA-4 antibody. Clin Cancer Res 2009;15(17):5379–88.
43. Thallinger C, Prager G, Ringl H, et al. Abscopal effect in the treatment of malignant melanoma. Hautarzt 2015;66(7):545–8 [in German].
44. Mole RH. Whole body irradiation; radiobiology or medicine? Br J Radiol 1953; 26(305):234–41.

45. Obeid M, Panaretakis T, Joza N, et al. Calreticulin exposure is required for the immunogenicity of gamma-irradiation and UVC light-induced apoptosis. Cell Death Differ 2007;14(10):1848–50.
46. Perez CA, Fu A, Onishko H, et al. Radiation induces an antitumour immune response to mouse melanoma. Int J Radiat Biol 2009;85(12):1126–36.
47. Kroemer G, Galluzzi L, Kepp O, et al. Immunogenic cell death in cancer therapy. Annu Rev Immunol 2013;31:51–72.
48. Krysko DV, Garg AD, Kaczmarek A, et al. Immunogenic cell death and DAMPs in cancer therapy. Nat Rev Cancer 2012;12(12):860–75.
49. Kim S, Ramakrishnan R, Lavilla-Alonso S, et al. Radiation-induced autophagy potentiates immunotherapy of cancer via up-regulation of mannose 6-phosphate receptor on tumor cells in mice. Cancer Immunol Immunother 2014;63(10): 1009–21.
50. Park SS, Dong H, Liu X, et al. PD-1 restrains radiotherapy-induced abscopal effect. Cancer Immunol Res 2015;3(6):610–9.
51. Grimaldi AM, Simeone E, Giannarelli D, et al. Abscopal effects of radiotherapy on advanced melanoma patients who progressed after ipilimumab immunotherapy. Oncoimmunology 2014;3:e28780.
52. Chandra RA, Wilhite TJ, Balboni TA, et al. A systematic evaluation of abscopal responses following radiotherapy in patients with metastatic melanoma treated with ipilimumab. Oncoimmunology 2015;4(11):e1046028.
53. Qin R, Olson A, Singh B, et al. Safety and efficacy of radiation therapy in advanced melanoma patients treated with ipilimumab. Int J Radiat Oncol Biol Phys 2016;96(1):72–7.
54. Barker CA, Postow MA, Khan SA, et al. Concurrent radiotherapy and ipilimumab immunotherapy for patients with melanoma. Cancer Immunol Res 2013;1(2): 92–8.
55. Theurich S, Rothschild SI, Hoffmann M, et al. Local tumor treatment in combination with systemic ipilimumab immunotherapy prolongs overall survival in patients with advanced malignant melanoma. Cancer Immunol Res 2016;4(9):744–54.
56. Hiniker SM, Maecker HT, Swetter SM, et al. A prospective clinical trial combining radiation therapy with systemic immunotherapy in metastatic melanoma. Int J Radiat Biol Phys 2015;93(Suppl 3):S95.
57. Sperduto PW, Kased N, Roberge D, et al. Summary report on the graded prognostic assessment: an accurate and facile diagnosis-specific tool to estimate survival for patients with brain metastases. J Clin Oncol 2012;30(4):419–25.
58. Silk AW, Bassetti MF, West BT, et al. Ipilimumab and radiation therapy for melanoma brain metastases. Cancer Med 2013;2(6):899–906.
59. Mathew M, Tam M, Ott PA, et al. Ipilimumab in melanoma with limited brain metastases treated with stereotactic radiosurgery. Melanoma Res 2013;23(3):191–5.
60. Knisely JP, Yu JB, Flanigan J, et al. Radiosurgery for melanoma brain metastases in the ipilimumab era and the possibility of longer survival. J Neurosurg 2012; 117(2):227–33.
61. Kiess AP, Wolchok JD, Barker CA, et al. Stereotactic radiosurgery for melanoma brain metastases in patients receiving ipilimumab: safety profile and efficacy of combined treatment. Int J Radiat Oncol Biol Phys 2015;92(2):368–75.
62. Berghoff AS, Ricken G, Widhalm G, et al. Tumour-infiltrating lymphocytes and expression of programmed death ligand 1 (PD-L1) in melanoma brain metastases. Histopathology 2015;66(2):289–99.

63. Ahmed KA, Stallworth DG, Kim Y, et al. Clinical outcomes of melanoma brain metastases treated with stereotactic radiation and anti-PD-1 therapy. Ann Oncol 2016;27(3):434–41.
64. Weber JS, Kudchadkar RR, Yu B, et al. Safety, efficacy, and biomarkers of nivolumab with vaccine in ipilimumab-refractory or -naive melanoma. J Clin Oncol 2013;31(34):4311–8.
65. Gibney GT, Kudchadkar RR, DeConti RC, et al. Safety, correlative markers, and clinical results of adjuvant nivolumab in combination with vaccine in resected high-risk metastatic melanoma. Clin Cancer Res 2015;21(4):712–20.
66. Ahmed KA, Abuodeh YA, Echevarria MI, et al. Clinical outcomes of melanoma brain metastases treated with stereotactic radiosurgery and anti-PD-1 therapy, anti-CTLA-4 therapy, BRAF/MEK inhibitors, BRAF inhibitor, or conventional chemotherapy. Ann Oncol 2016;27(12):2288–94.

93. [illegible] patients treated with [illegible] radiation [illegible]
94. [illegible] safety, efficacy, and [illegible]
95. [illegible] SR, et al. [illegible]
96. [illegible] 2017;[illegible]

Printed and bound by CPI Group (UK) Ltd, Croydon, CR0 4YY
07/10/2024
01040505-0016